Flexible Parametric Survival Analysis Using Stata: Beyond the Cox Model

Flexible Parametric Survival Analysis Using Stata: Beyond the Cox Model

PATRICK ROYSTON
MRC Clinical Trials Unit, United Kingdom

PAUL C. LAMBERT
Department of Health Sciences, University of Leicester, United Kingdom and Medical Epidemiology and Biostatistics, Karolinska Institute, Stockholm, Sweden

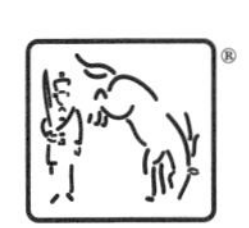

A Stata Press Publication
StataCorp LP
College Station, Texas

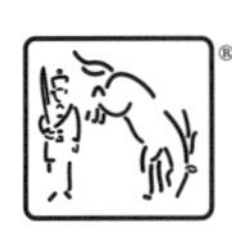

Published by Stata Press, 4905 Lakeway Drive, College Station, Texas 77845
Typeset in $\LaTeX\,2_\varepsilon$
Printed in the United States of America
10 9 8 7 6 5 4 3 2 1

ISBN-10: 1-59718-079-3
ISBN-13: 978-1-59718-079-5

Library of Congress Control Number: 2011921921

Contents

Tables

Figures

Preface

We would first like to quote from the preface of a well-known and respected Stata Press book on survival analysis in Stata (Cleves et al. 2010):

> This is a book about survival analysis for the professional data analyst, whether a health scientist, an economist, a political scientist, or any of a wide range of scientists who have found that survival analysis is applicable to their problems. This is a book for researchers who want to understand what they are doing and to understand the underpinnings and assumptions of the tools they use; in other words, this is a book for all researchers.

In a way, the aims of our book are similar to those of Cleves et al. (2010). We extend their book in particular directions: flexible, parametric, going beyond the standard models, particularly the Cox model. We include, for example, detailed treatments of time-dependent effects and relative survival. Our starting point is a basic understanding of survival analysis and how it is done in Stata. We would be surprised, for example, if a reader had not created and plotted Kaplan–Meier curves and fitted a Cox model in Stata. Our aim is that researchers can build on our examples to apply the methodology to their own investigations of survival data. To that end, we have provided the basic tools (ado-files) but also, in the examples, we present Stata code to do many of the analyses and produce many of the graphs. Indeed, presentation of the results of flexible parametric modeling is often best achieved by well-chosen graphs, and we regard that as an important message of our book.

Royston–Parmar models are a key tool in our approach; they are currently available only in Stata. (See section 1.10 for more information.) We would like to see their implementation in other software, such as R or SAS. However, we are very unlikely to implement this ourselves! If anyone has attempted such an implementation (or plans to do so) and would value our input, we would encourage them to contact us.

This book uses Stata version 12 throughout, but is fully compatible with Stata 11.1 or later, with only minor cosmetic differences across versions.

Finally, we would like to thank the folk who have contributed to our understanding of survival analysis and those who have undertaken the seemingly thankless task of commenting on our draft text. We are particularly grateful to

Therese Andersson, Karolinska Institute
Carol Coupland, University of Nottingham

Paul Dickman, Karolinska Institute
Sandra Eloranta, Karolinska Institute
Bobby Gutierrez, StataCorp
Hans van Houwelingen, University of Leiden
Bernard Rachet, London School of Hygiene and Tropical Medicine
Bill Rising, StataCorp
Mark Rutherford, University of Leicester
Willi Sauerbrei, University of Freiburg Medical Center
Michael Schemper, University of Vienna

London and Leicester
July 2011

Patrick Royston
Paul C. Lambert

1 Introduction

1.1 Goals

Most books on survival analysis devote a substantial section of their material to the Cox proportional hazards (PH) model (Cox 1972). The Cox model has played a vital role in applied survival analysis during the last three decades. The model and its software implementations have popularized survival analysis and made it accessible to researchers in varied disciplines who are not necessarily statisticians. It has been so successful that it is probably used in most practical analyses of the effects of covariates on survival.

Some years ago, Sir David Cox, in a revealing interview with Nancy Reid (Reid 1994), was asked what he thought of the cottage industry that had grown up around "his" model. He responded by saying that he would normally wish to attack a problem parametrically, because operations such as prediction were so much easier. Prediction (really estimation) of relevant features of survival data is a key theme in the present book.

Our main goals are to describe and to illustrate the use and applications of flexible parametric survival models, programmed in Stata, which in some important respects go beyond the Cox model and beyond the standard parametric survival models (such as the Weibull). These flexible models overcome the problems of potentially poor fit of standard parametric models and of the "noisy" estimates of the hazard and survival functions associated with the Cox model and with nonparametric estimators such as the Kaplan–Meier.

Flexible parametric survival models can help us in a number of ways. For example, they allow us to obtain an estimate of the baseline survival function and its uncertainty which vary smoothly over time. Prediction of survival probabilities and differences, hazard functions, hazard differences and ratios, time-dependent effects of covariates, and excess mortality rates in the context of relative survival are just some of the possible outputs from the models. Furthermore, the Stata commands are easy to use and to apply to real problems in a variety of settings.

Other than in chapter 1, we give extensive code showing how to implement the methods we describe in Stata. We present results graphically in many cases, but do not present code for all graphs because many are similar in style. More details of the structure and content of our book are outlined briefly in section 1.11.

1.2 A brief review of the Cox proportional hazards model

The Cox PH model is by far the most common model used in survival analysis. Many texts, some excellent, have been published on the model; we recommend, for example, Hosmer, Lemeshow, and May (2008) for a good, practical introduction and Grambsch and Therneau (2000) for extensions of the model. The quantities estimated from a Cox model are *hazard ratios* (HRs), which measure how much a covariate increases or decreases the rate of a particular event, assuming that it acts multiplicatively. For example, if the event were mortality and we applied a Cox model that estimated an HR of two for males compared with females, the mortality rate would be twice as high in males as in females.

A basic assumption of the Cox model is that the estimated parameters are not associated with time. In other words, we assume that any two hazard rates predicted by the model are proportional over time. In the above example, we assume that the doubling of the rate for males holds at 1 week, 1 month, 1 year, etc.

We can write the Cox model algebraically, as follows:

$$h_i(t|\mathbf{x}_i) = h_0(t)\exp(\mathbf{x}_i\beta)$$

The hazard function for the ith individual, $h_i(t|\mathbf{x}_i)$, is conditional on covariates $\mathbf{x}_i$, where $\beta = \beta_1, \dots, \beta_k$ is the vector of regression coefficients. The baseline hazard function $h_0(t)$ is $h_i(t|\mathbf{x} = 0)$. One of the most recognized features of the Cox model is that we do not need to assume that the baseline hazard function has a specific shape. For this reason, the Cox model is often called *semiparametric*: we make parametric assumptions about the effects of covariates on the hazard function, but not about the shape of the hazard function itself. This is an important and appealing feature of the Cox model. If we were interested only in the HR, we could disregard distributional assumptions about the event times.

1.3 Beyond the Cox model

1.3.1 Estimating the baseline hazard

Consider arguably the simplest possible situation in survival modeling: a randomized, controlled clinical trial (say, in cancer) with right-censored time-to-event outcomes and a single covariate, `trt` (treatment), coded 0 for control or standard therapy and 1 for the experimental treatment arm. The data in the following example are taken from a Medical Research Council trial in 347 patients with advanced kidney cancer (Medical Research Council Renal Cancer Collaborators 1999). The primary outcome measure in the trial was all-cause mortality. The control and experimental treatments are the drugs medroxyprogesterone acetate (MPA) and interferon-α (IFN), respectively. To compare IFN with MPA, we fit a Cox model (`stcox trt`) with the following results:

```
. use kidney_ca
(kidney cancer data)

. stcox trt, nolog

         failure _d:  cens
   analysis time _t:  survtime/365.25

Cox regression -- Breslow method for ties

No. of subjects =          347                  Number of obs   =        347
No. of failures =          322
Time at risk    =  375.6769336
                                                LR chi2(1)      =       6.81
Log likelihood  =   -1610.1366                  Prob > chi2     =     0.0091

------------------------------------------------------------------------------
          _t | Haz. Ratio   Std. Err.      z    P>|z|     [95% Conf. Interval]
-------------+----------------------------------------------------------------
         trt |   .7464934   .0836699    -2.61   0.009     .5992665    .9298907
------------------------------------------------------------------------------
```

What do we get directly from the analysis? Principally, two things: an estimate (with confidence interval [CI]) of the HR comparing MPA with IFN, and a test of significance of the treatment effect. We can infer from the Stata output that IFN has reduced the mortality (hazard) rate by 25% with a 95% CI of $(7\%, 40\%)$. The treatment effect is significant at the 1% level.

If (in Stata 11 or Stata 12) the `predict` command is used, or (in Stata 10 and earlier) we include certain options of the `stcox` command, we can obtain several additional outputs, including an estimate of the baseline survival function (in this case, $S(t)$ for the control arm), Schoenfeld residuals (which can be used to test the PH assumption), martingale residuals (which are useful for assessing the functional form for continuous predictors), and several other quantities. However, we find no option to get a useful estimate of the baseline hazard function when using `predict`.

Why is the hazard function useful? Because

- in medicine, it is a clinically meaningful measure of disease course, and
- it is the "ground" against which relative hazard effects are estimated.

The thicker pair of lines in figure 1.1 show an estimate of the hazard function in the control and experimental arms of the kidney cancer dataset. We estimated them under the PH assumption by fitting a Royston–Parmar (RP) model, a major theme of this book. RP models are implemented in the `stpm2` command (Lambert and Royston 2009). We outline the `stpm2` command in section 1.6 and describe the models in detail in chapter 5.

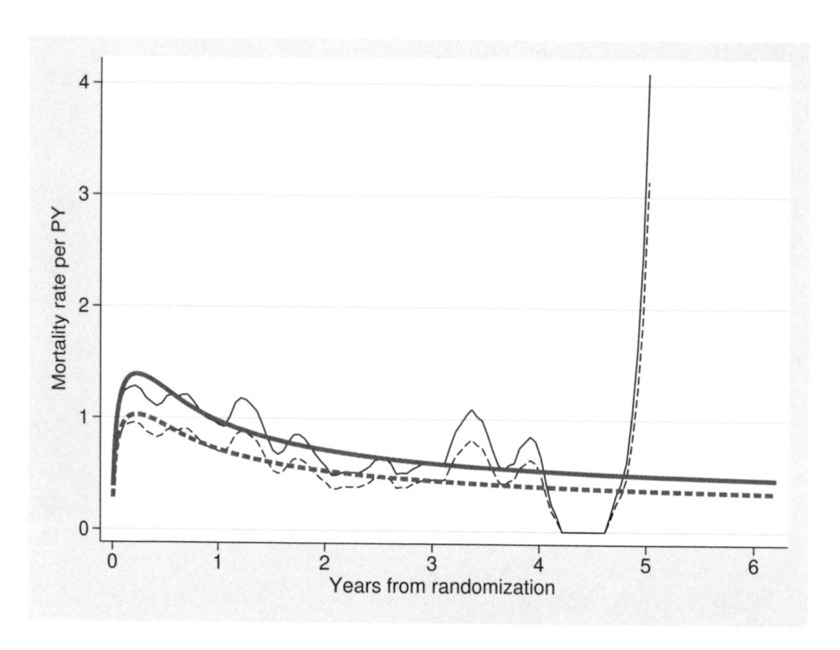

Figure 1.1. Kidney cancer data. Hazard functions in two treatment groups estimated under the PH assumption. Thick lines are from `stpm2` with two degrees of freedom for the baseline log cumulative-hazard function. Thin lines are from `stcurve` following `stcox`. Solid lines show the control group; dashed lines, the experimental group. PY stands for person-year.

The figure tells us the following:

- The death rate from advanced kidney cancer seems to be highest about 3 months after randomization, and it decreases after that time.
- The hazard is substantially reduced by the experimental treatment at all time points. (Under the PH assumption, the curves are forced to be proportional to each other.)
- Even after 4 years, the hazard is still substantial. The fact that it does not approach zero suggests that the disease is fatal, which is nearly always the case.

We have harvested quite a lot of useful information. Even if we relax the PH assumption, the plot of the ensuing hazard functions (not shown) is very similar to the thick lines in figure 1.1, so our conclusion about the treatment effect seems to be robust.

The thin lines in figure 1.1 are a nonparametric estimate of the hazard (mortality) rate. We estimated them with the `stcurve` command, which uses a technique known as kernel smoothing. The code that produced figure 1.1 is as follows:

```
. use kidney_ca
(kidney cancer data)
. stpm2 trt, df(2) scale(hazard)
Iteration 0:   log likelihood =  -564.1407
Iteration 1:   log likelihood = -564.09236
Iteration 2:   log likelihood = -564.09235
Log likelihood = -564.09235                     Number of obs   =        347

------------------------------------------------------------------------------
             |      Coef.   Std. Err.      z    P>|z|     [95% Conf. Interval]
-------------+----------------------------------------------------------------
xb           |
         trt |  -.3005732   .1118951    -2.69   0.007    -.5198836   -.0812628
       _rcs1 |   1.224624   .0629679    19.45   0.000     1.101209    1.348039
       _rcs2 |   .1814725   .0426715     4.25   0.000     .0978379     .265107
       _cons |  -.4535717   .0863545    -5.25   0.000    -.6228235   -.2843199
------------------------------------------------------------------------------
. predict h0, at(trt 0) hazard
. predict h1, at(trt 1) hazard
. stcox trt, noshow nolog nohead
Cox regression -- Breslow method for ties
No. of subjects =          347                  Number of obs   =        347
No. of failures =          322
Time at risk    =  375.6769336
                                                LR chi2(1)      =       6.81
Log likelihood  =   -1610.1366                  Prob > chi2     =     0.0091

------------------------------------------------------------------------------
          _t | Haz. Ratio   Std. Err.      z    P>|z|     [95% Conf. Interval]
-------------+----------------------------------------------------------------
         trt |   .7464934   .0836699    -2.61   0.009     .5992665    .9298907
------------------------------------------------------------------------------
. stcurve, hazard at1(trt=0) at2(trt=1) kernel(epan2)
> legend(off) lpattern(l -) title("") ylabel(0(1)4, angle(h))
> xscale(range(0 6.2)) xlabel(0(1)6) lwidth(medthin ..)
> addplot(line h0 h1 _t, sort lpattern(l -) lwidth(thick ..)
> lcolor(gs6 ..) xtitle("Years from randomization")
> ytitle("Mortality rate per person year"))
```

We obtained the curves after fitting the Cox model to the `trt` variable, assuming PH. Notice how wiggly and hard to interpret they are compared with those from `stpm2`. We think that the apparent sharp increase in mortality rate after four years is an artifact; the data there are sparse, the feature is not biologically plausible, and it is not seen in the curves from `stpm2`.

Finally, the HRs were 0.746 (standard error [SE] 0.084) and 0.740 (SE 0.083) according to the Cox and RP models, respectively—for practical purposes, they are identical.

1.3.2 The baseline hazard contains useful information

One of the consequences of a method that only estimates relative risk and not absolute risk is that users may ignore the importance of absolute risk. If we are told that the mortality rate is double for individuals with a particular exposure, then we want to know what reference value this doubling refers to. In a survival model, the reference is usually the baseline hazard rate, which usually changes as a function of time. Thus even if the PH assumption is reasonable, the impact of a particular exposure in absolute terms depends on how long has passed since the time origin (diagnosis, randomization, start of treatment, etc.) and the magnitude of the underlying hazard rate.

An example to illustrate the importance of the baseline hazard is in survival from colon cancer. Figure 1.2(a) shows data from England and Wales where the time from diagnosis to death from colon cancer in those ages < 50 years has been modeled and smooth estimates of the hazard function derived for two time periods, 1981–1985 and 1986–1990. The event is death from any cause and thus the hazard rate can be considered as a mortality rate. The model assumes that the two hazard rates are proportional. The figure shows that the mortality rate is high in the first few months after diagnosis, but then decreases. By about 8 years, the mortality rate is very close to zero. We can infer that very few colon cancer patients who have survived to this time will actually die between 8 and 10 years. When the mortality rate associated with a diagnosis of a particular disease approaches zero, we have what is know as "statistical" or "population" cure (Lambert et al. 2007). The HR between the two time periods is 0.92, implying that the mortality rate is 8% lower in the more recent period. As the model assumes PH, the estimated relative effect is forced to be the same over the whole time period.

Figure 1.2(b) shows the difference in the hazard (mortality) rates. The absolute difference decreases with increasing follow-up time. Thus the 8% reduction in the mortality rate has little impact beyond about 6 years.

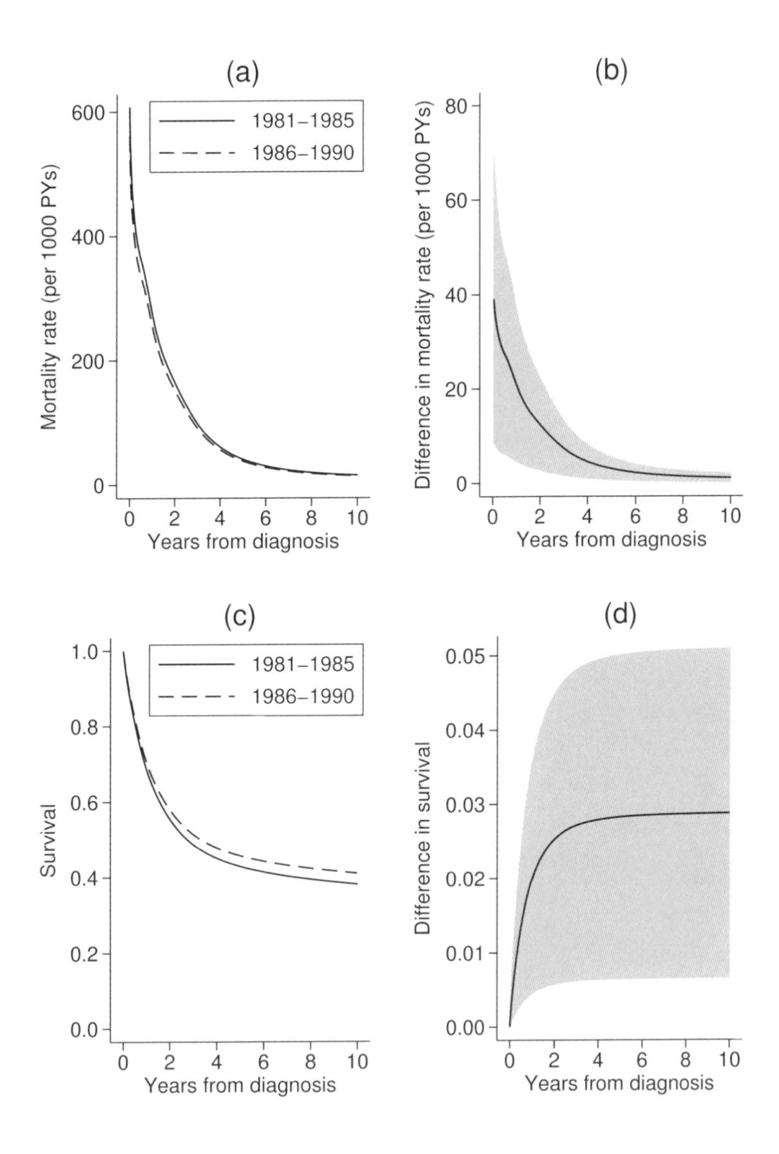

Figure 1.2. Cancer of the colon in England and Wales 1981–1985 and 1986–1990 for subjects aged < 50 years: (a) hazard rates, (b) difference in hazard rates, (c) survival functions, and (d) difference in survival functions. PYs stands for person-years.

Figure 1.2(c) shows the estimated survival functions and figure 1.2(d) shows the difference in the two survival curves. Figure 1.2(d) shows an improvement of just under 3% in absolute terms in survival in the more recent period. This should be expected given that the more recent period has a lower mortality rate. When we look at the difference in the survival curves, we see that most of the improvement has been in the first 2–3 years.

We feel that the graphs shown in figure 1.2 give a better understanding of the disease and of the improvement in the more recent period than just quoting a hazard ratio of 0.92.

1.3.3 Advantages of smooth survival functions

A Kaplan–Meier plot of the survival function, $S(t)$, is an important feature of most survival analyses and is widely presented in publications of applied work. For the Cox model, Stata's `predict` command after `stcox` with the `basesurv()` option provides an estimate of the baseline survival function, $S_0(t) = S(t|\mathbf{x} = 0)$. From the baseline survival and the HR, we can predict the survival function for any combination of covariate values. However, all such survival functions are step functions and typically are not particularly smooth. However, it is reasonable to suppose that the underlying function is smooth. Also, the least precise parts of the curve get the most visual weight, a general criticism of Kaplan–Meier survival curves.

Kaplan–Meier-type estimates of $S(t)$ are composed of a sequence of point estimates of the survival function that are highly serially correlated. Accordingly, Kaplan–Meier plots tend to display "runs" of values that move away from and back toward the general trend, giving an undulating appearance. This may make the curve difficult to interpret and may lead to overemphasis of local features.

An example of these aspects, which is particularly a problem in smaller samples, appears in the kidney cancer data (see figure 1.3).

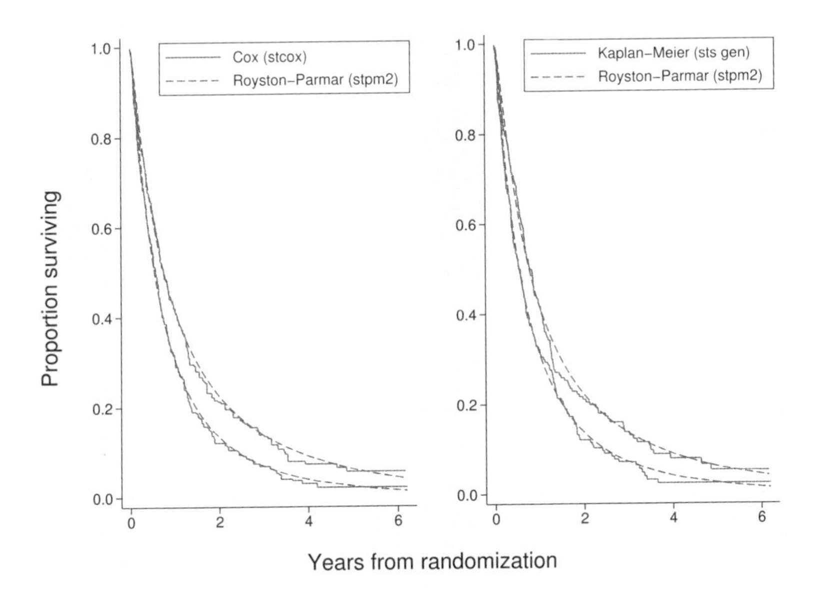

Figure 1.3. Kidney cancer data. Survival curves. Left panel: estimates of $S_0(t)$ and $S_1(t)$ assuming PH. Right panel: estimates of $S_0(t)$ and $S_1(t)$ not assuming PH. Solid lines are for `stcox` (left panel) or `sts generate` (right panel); dashed lines are for `stpm2`.

The left-hand panel shows that the survival curves estimated by `stpm2` are smoother than the Kaplan–Meier-like survival curves predicted from a Cox model. The right-hand panel compares Kaplan–Meier curves calculated separately in each treatment group with `stpm2` estimates in which we do not assume PH. The Kaplan–Meier curves seem to converge temporarily (they do not actually cross) at about $t = 18$ months. This feature, which does not appear in the left-hand graph nor in the `stpm2` estimates, is almost certainly due to chance.

1.3.4 Some requirements of a practical survival analysis

The main purpose of the Cox model in its simplest form is to estimate HRs assuming PH. Because of its embedding in counting-process theory (see, for example, Andersen et al. [1997]), it can be extended in many different ways to answer scientific questions across a remarkable range of contexts. In our book, we are dealing with the more basic types of survival analysis, where the researcher needs to obtain satisfactory estimates of quantities that include hazard rates and their differences and ratios, survival curves and their differences, HRs (both fixed and time varying), and survival at given time points. By "satisfactory" we mean smooth (for functions) and unbiased. Easy availability of the curves and estimates with Stata software is also of practical importance.

As an example, figure 1.4 shows the estimated differences in hazard (mortality) rate and survival probability for the kidney cancer data.

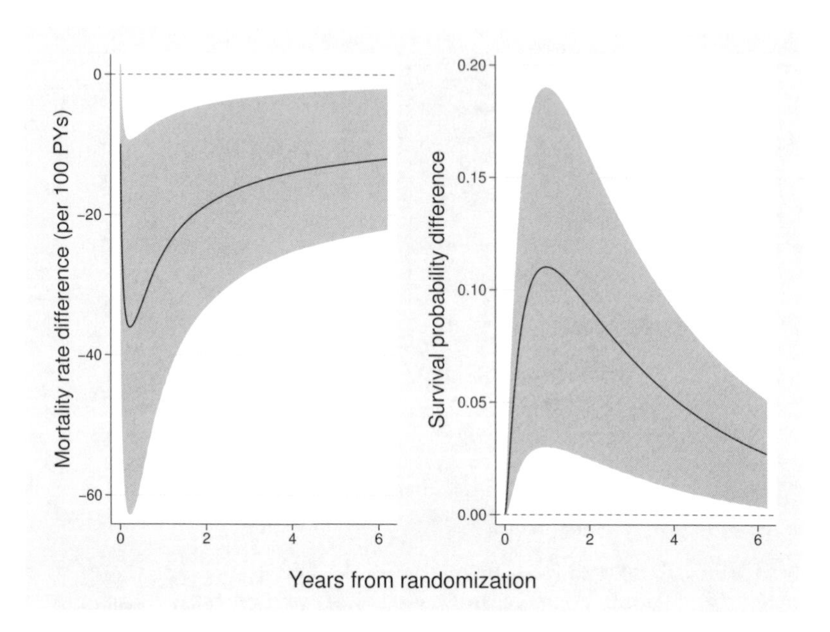

Figure 1.4. Kidney cancer data. Differences in hazard rates and survival probabilities, with pointwise 95% CIs, estimated by a flexible parametric survival model. PYs stands for person-years.

The curves were derived from a RP PH model, using simple `predict` commands following use of `stpm2` to fit the model. The treatment reduces the mortality rate in absolute terms immediately after randomization, whereas the biggest differences in survival probabilities between the treatment arms come rather later, after about 1 year. Note, however, the large uncertainty in the curves, despite the respectable sample size of 347 patients, of whom 322 died.

1.3.5 When the proportional-hazards assumption is breached

Stata provides tools to assess possible nonproportional hazards of covariate effects. For example, `stphplot` gives a graphical assessment of the PH assumption for a categorical covariate. We illustrate this in the kidney cancer data for the covariate `who` (World Health Organization performance status), which in the present dataset takes the values 0, 1, and 2. Patients with `who` status 0 are able to carry out normal everyday duties, whereas those with `who` status 2 are quite unwell (see
http://www.cancerhelp.org.uk/about-cancer/cancer-questions/performance-status
for the definition of World Health Organization performance status). Figure 1.5 shows the result of running `stphplot, by(who)`.

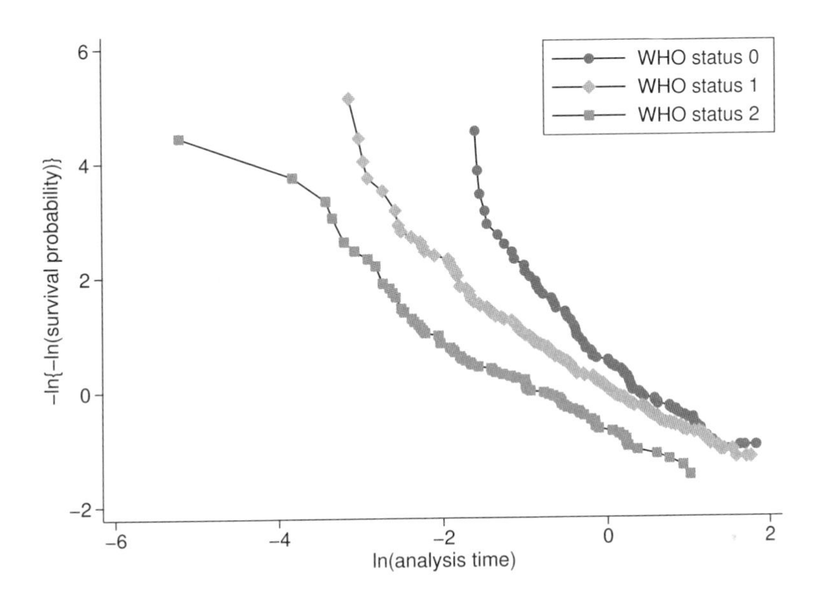

Figure 1.5. Kidney cancer data. Results of applying `stphplot` to the covariate `who`. Nonproportional hazards are evidenced by the nonparallel lines. The vertical axis is an estimate of minus the log cumulative-hazard function for each `who` group, and the horizontal axis is log survival-time.

If PH holds, the 3 lines should be approximately parallel. Certainly, they do not look parallel; rather, the lines for `who` 1 and `who` 2 are roughly parallel, but not to the line for `who` 0. We can check our suspicion of nonproportional hazards by applying a Grambsch–Therneau test (Grambsch and Therneau 1994) of the scaled Schoenfeld residuals from a Cox model on the two dummy variables for `who`:

```
. use kidney_ca, clear
(kidney cancer data)

. stcox i.who, nolog

         failure _d:  cens
   analysis time _t:  survtime/365.25

Cox regression -- Breslow method for ties

No. of subjects =          347                  Number of obs   =        347
No. of failures =          322
Time at risk    =  375.6769336
                                                LR chi2(2)      =      49.53
Log likelihood  =   -1588.7762                  Prob > chi2     =     0.0000

------------------------------------------------------------------------------
          _t | Haz. Ratio   Std. Err.      z    P>|z|     [95% Conf. Interval]
-------------+----------------------------------------------------------------
         who |
          1  |   1.378984   .1886655     2.35   0.019     1.054635    1.803085
          2  |   3.070376   .4835384     7.12   0.000     2.254966    4.180643
------------------------------------------------------------------------------

. stphtest, rank detail

      Test of proportional-hazards assumption

      Time:  Rank(t)
      ----------------------------------------------------------------
                  |       rho            chi2       df       Prob>chi2
      ------------+---------------------------------------------------
      0b.who      |          .              .        1             .
      1.who       |   -0.16007           8.13        1         0.0043
      2.who       |   -0.22602          14.89        1         0.0001
      ------------+---------------------------------------------------
      global test |                     15.51        2         0.0004
      ----------------------------------------------------------------
```

The tests of nonproportional hazards for each dummy variable (comparing `who` 1 and `who` 2 with `who` 0) overall are highly significant.

The question is, having detected nonproportional hazards in a Cox model, what do we do next? In section 7.3 we show that we can split the time scale into a number of intervals and estimate a separate HR within each interval, or we can make the log HR a linear function of $\ln(t)$. Further extensions of the Cox model to cope with nonproportional hazards effects are available (for example, Sauerbrei, Royston, and Look [2007b]), but they can be complex. For moderate or large sample sizes, those extensions demand considerable computer memory and processing power. We need methods of modeling that are simple, efficient, tractable, and informative in such situations. The extensions to RP models described in chapter 7 provide one useful approach.

Under nonproportional hazards, how is a single HR that is estimated by a Cox model, for example, to be interpreted? Is it indeed useful at all? The question is very relevant when analyzing data with a nonproportional treatment effect in a clinical trial with a time-to-event endpoint. Researchers sometimes report a single HR even when survival curves cross (for example, Mok et al. [2009]). We sometimes see it described as an "average" HR (Schemper, Wakounig, and Heinze 2009), the intuitive idea being that the Cox model somehow smooths or averages the HR over time. While it is mathematically possible to define such an average HR, we doubt its usefulness, because the issue of noninterpretability remains. The HR is by definition a ratio of hazard functions. For example, a HR function that starts > 1 for small t and becomes < 1 for large t is not meaningfully summarized by a single value near 1. We therefore regard the single HR as a meaningless summary under nonproportional hazards unless the departures from proportionality are so small as to be unimportant. We prefer to allow the HR to be a function of time, as described for some of the models in chapters 5 and 7.

1.4 Why parametric models?

1.4.1 Smooth baseline hazard and survival functions

Parametric survival models generally provide smooth estimates of the hazard and survival functions for any combination of covariate values. Exceptions are piecewise models—for example, the piecewise exponential (see section 4.3.1), for which the hazard function is a step function and the survival function has discontinuities in the first derivative.

1.4.2 Time-dependent HRs

With parametric models, we can obtain essentially any type of output—for example, a time-dependent HR (see section 7.6)—as a function of the estimated model parameters (the covariates and time). Furthermore, we can use Stata's powerful `predictnl` command, which implements the delta method using numeric derivatives, to get SEs and CIs quite easily (see section 1.9).

1.4.3 Modeling on different scales

Sometimes, a covariate whose effect is nonproportional on the hazards scale may be (much closer to) proportional on another scale, such as the odds or probit (inverse normal probability) scales (see chapter 5). We may be able to take advantage of the different possible scales to build a parsimonious and efficient alternative to a PH model.

1.4.4 Relative survival

In cancer survival, we often want to know the impact of covariates on the mortality rate for a particular cancer. However, because cancer is usually a disease of old age, many people may die of diseases other than the cancer they were originally diagnosed with. In relative survival models, we deal with this issue by incorporating expected mortality, which we can usually obtain from routine data sources. Traditionally, simple piecewise models have been used for relative survival, but all the advantages of standard parametric survival models also apply to relative survival models. See chapter 8 for details.

1.4.5 Prediction out of sample

The baseline survival function in a Cox model (estimated by `predict` *varname*, `basesurv()` following use of `stcox`) is available only in the estimation sample. To predict survival outside the estimation sample, we need special measures, such as interpolation or even extrapolation. Using special measures limits the applications of the Cox model in some situations. An important case arises when we wish to validate a survival model in an independent sample, a task that necessitates out-of-sample prediction (see section 6.8).

1.4.6 Multiple time scales

In a Cox model, we can consider only one time scale—for example, time from diagnosis of disease or time from randomization in a clinical trial. Sometimes, for example, in age–period–cohort models (Clayton and Schifflers 1987), we might want to consider more than one time scale. See section 7.9 for an example of using multiple time scales.

1.5 Why not standard parametric models?

We have outlined some advantages of working with parametric models. In chapter 13 of Cleves et al. (2010)—an excellent introduction to survival analysis in Stata—the authors describe six standard parametric survival models—exponential, Weibull, Gompertz, lognormal, loglogistic, and generalized gamma. The models, together with a rich set of extensions, are implemented in the portmanteau command `streg`. Cleves et al. (2010) give formulas for the hazard and survival functions for these models, together with detailed examples and their implementation in Stata. We do not repeat the material here.

With such riches available, why do we need to go beyond `streg`? There are two main reasons. First, the simpler parametric models in `streg` may not be flexible enough to adequately represent, say, the hazard function—in other words, they may not fit the data well enough. (Concern about possible lack of fit of parametric models is one of the main reasons for the popularity of the Cox model; the shape of the baseline distribution does not influence estimates of HRs.) For example, the main parametric PH model, the Weibull, has a hazard function that always goes in the same direction with time—up, down, or constant. Many real-life datasets have hazards that peak after some period of time and then decline, so the Weibull model can never fit such data well. Second, in our book, we present new classes of parametric models that include flexible PH models, but also flexible proportional odds (PO) and probit-scale models. These alternative models greatly extend the range of survival distributions that can be estimated.

As an example, consider figure 1.6.

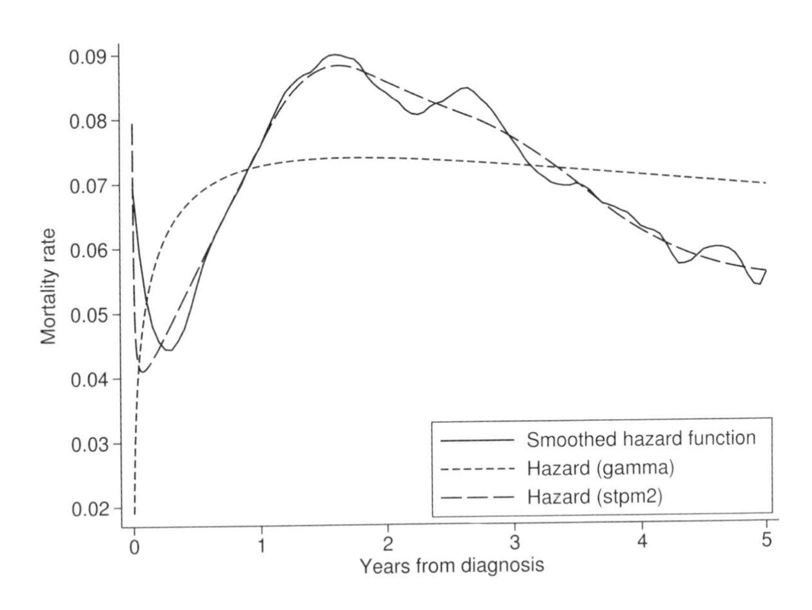

Figure 1.6. England and Wales breast cancer data. Three estimates of the hazard function (mortality rate).

The dataset relates to survival for 24,889 patients with breast cancer in England and Wales (see section 3.3). We have estimated the hazard function (here, the mortality rate) by a nonparametric smoothing technique (as in figure 1.1) and by two parametric survival models. The first model, the generalized gamma distribution, is the most complex parametric survival distribution supported by `streg`. Most of the other distributions are special cases of the gamma. The second is an RP model, which is implemented in `stpm2`. Notice how the shape of the gamma hazard function bears little resemblance to that derived from the other approaches, whereas the estimates from the nonparametric method and the RP model broadly agree (apart from the unconvincing "wiggles" in the nonparametric estimate).

One further issue with standard parametric models is that if a PH model is to be fit using `streg`, then the only choices are the exponential, Weibull, or Gompertz distributions. All of these have monotonic hazard functions in that they either increase or decrease over time (or stay constant, in the case of the exponential distribution). Thus if the underlying hazard function has a turning point it is not possible to find a well-fitting parametric PH survival model. The lognormal, loglogistic, and generalized gamma distributions do have hazard functions with turning points. However, it is not possible using these distributions in `streg` to have PH models because they can only be expressed in the accelerated failure-time metric. Although coefficients from accelerated failure-time models are used in other disciplines, they are not used much in medical research, our main area of application.

We conclude that although there may be some theoretical advantages to using standard parametric survival models, they are generally not sufficiently flexible to represent real data adequately.

1.6 A brief introduction to stpm2

We have implemented RP models in the `stpm2` command, as we describe in chapter 5. For a detailed account of the `stpm2` command with examples of its use, we refer the reader to Lambert and Royston (2009). Here we give a taste of the power of `stpm2` and its essential simplicity.

Like most Stata estimation commands, `stpm2` has two parts: parameter estimation (that is, model fitting) and postestimation facilities (prediction). The former is accomplished by `stpm2`, the latter by `predict`.

1.6.1 Estimation (model fitting)

The syntax of `stpm2` is basically simple:

`stpm2` [*varlist*] [*if*] [*in*], `scale(hazard|odds|normal) df(#)` [`tvc(`*varlist*`)` `dftvc(`*df-list*`)` *other_options*]

The covariates are included in *varlist*. There are two key options: `df()` and `scale()`. The first controls the complexity (degrees of freedom) of the baseline distribution function. The second determines whether the model is to be fit on the `hazard`, `odds`, or `normal` scale. With the `df(1)` option, Weibull, loglogistic, and lognormal models, respectively, can be fit, albeit with a parametrization that differs from the standard one used by Stata's `streg` command—see sections 5.2.3, 5.4.4, and 5.5.3 for details. With `df(#)` and $\# > 1$, `stpm2` fits what we call PH, PO, and probit flavors of RP models.

Models with time-dependent effects require the `tvc()` and `dftvc()` options. See section 7.6 for more details of these models.

Some examples are

```
stpm2, scale(hazard) df(3)
stpm2 trt, scale(hazard) df(2) eform
stpm2 trt, scale(odds) df(2)
stpm2 trt, scale(hazard) df(2) tvc(trt) dftvc(1)
```

1.6.2 Postestimation facilities (prediction)

The `predict` command, used after fitting a model with `stpm2`, has many options that provide considerable richness in what we can estimate. The most important options are probably `survival`, `hazard`, `ci`, and `zeros`, followed by `hrnumerator()`, `hrdenominator()`, `hdiff1()`, `hdiff2()`, `sdiff1()`, `sdiff2()`, `at()`, and `timevar()`. The `hrnumerator()` and `hrdenominator()` options give HRs (which may vary with time `_t`), irrespective of the `scale()` that we have assumed for covariate effects. The `ci` option generally provides a CI for whatever is being predicted. The `zeros` option predicts with all covariates set to zero, thus giving baseline values.

Some examples:

```
stpm2 trt, scale(hazard) df(2)
predict basesurv, survival zeros
predict surv1, at(trt 1)
predict hazarddiff, hdiff1(trt 1) ci
predict survdiff, sdiff1(trt 1) ci
stpm2 trt, scale(hazard) df(2) tvc(trt) dftvc(1)
predict hr, hrnumerator(trt 1) hrdenominator(trt 0) ci
```

1.7 Basic relationships in survival analysis

Our book is meant to be practical. Apart from sections marked with an asterisk, we assume only a fairly low mathematical level. However, readers should understand the three key mathematical functions in survival analysis—the *survival function*, $S(t)$; the *hazard function*, $h(t)$; and the *cumulative hazard function*, $H(t)$. The three functions are essentially just transformations of one another. Let the random variable T be the survival time (that is, time to event) since the origin of the study ($t = 0$). The functions' definitions are as follows:

$$\begin{aligned} S(t) &= \Pr(T > t) \\ h(t) &= \lim_{\delta t \to 0} \frac{\Pr(t \le T < t + \delta t | T \ge t)}{\delta t} \\ &= -\frac{d \log S(t)}{dt} \\ H(t) &= \int_0^t h(u)\, du \end{aligned}$$

The survival function describes the proportion of the population who have not experienced an event by time t. In studies of mortality, the hazard function is known as the "force of mortality", the mortality rate, or the death rate; it may be expressed per 100; 1,000; 10,000; or even 100,000 head of population, depending on the rarity of the condition in question. Also important are the identities that relate $S(t)$ and $H(t)$:

$$S(t) = \exp\{-H(t)\}$$
$$H(t) = -\ln\{S(t)\}$$

Additionally, the cumulative distribution function, $F(t)$, equals $1 - S(t)$.

A survival dataset of n individuals includes the time to event or censoring (t_i), the censoring indicator (δ_i, taking the value 1 for an event and 0 for a censored observation), and a vector of covariates $\mathbf{x}_i$ that may influence survival. In our book, we often use the term survival in a generic sense to mean nonoccurrence of the event of interest. Survival does not necessarily signify "not dying", and its meaning is apparent from the context.

The contribution of the ith individual to the log likelihood function for a parametric survival model is given by

$$\ln L_i = \delta_i \ln h(t_i) + \ln S(t_i) \tag{1.1}$$

In the above equation, we assume that each individual becomes at risk at time 0. While this is a sensible assumption for many applications—for example time from diagnosis or time from randomization—in some situations we want individuals to become at risk after time 0. This is known as *late entry* or *delayed entry*. One application of this would be used under the following conditions: when age is used as the time scale, when time 0 is an individual's date of birth, and that the individual would not become at risk until the age of diagnosis with a disease. We describe an analysis using age as the time scale in section 7.8. We need a simple modification of (1.1) to accommodate delayed entry at t_{0i}:

$$\ln L_i = \delta_i \ln h(t_i) + \ln S(t_i) - \ln S(t_{0i})$$

Further examples of the use of delayed entry include splitting the time scale to incorporate time-dependent effects (section 7.3) and period analysis (section 9.8).

1.8 Comparing models

A useful criterion of model fit is the Akaike information criterion (AIC) (Akaike 1973), defined as the deviance (minus twice the maximized log likelihood) plus $2k$, where k is the dimension of the model (that is, the number of fitted parameters). We first use the AIC in section 4.8.4 for comparing models with a different number of knots when using splines. The candidate model with the lowest AIC may be preferred. The models we are comparing do not have to be nested.

An alternative to AIC is the Bayes information criterion (BIC) (Schwarz 1978), which is the deviance penalized by adding $k \log n$, where k is the model dimension and n is the sample size. In survival analysis, n is interpreted as the number of events rather than the number of individuals. The model that minimizes the BIC among a set of candidates is said to be "best" in the sense that BIC asymptotically selects the true model, provided that model is one of the candidate models.

Because parametric models are fit by maximum likelihood, we always get an AIC value and a BIC value. We can therefore compare parametric models quite easily. The parameters of a Cox model, however, are estimated by maximum partial likelihood, and we do not get AIC or BIC values comparable with those from parametric models. We can compare different Cox models on the same dataset using partial-likelihood versions of AIC or BIC, but we cannot compare a Cox model with a parametric model.

We interpret AIC and BIC in a rather informal way in our book. We view information criteria as guides to selecting a model rather than as hard-and-fast rules for doing so. We frequently find that with large sample sizes, minimizing the AIC (and sometimes even the BIC) seems to cause overfitting. Consequently, we often have to choose a suitable model subjectively.

See Burnham and Anderson (2004) for many details of the use of information criteria in model comparisons.

1.9 The delta method

The delta method is a useful general procedure in statistics; it can compute variances (and hence CIs) of nonlinear transformations of one or more random variables. After fitting a model, we have a vector of estimated parameters, $\boldsymbol{\beta}$, and its associated variance–covariance matrix, $V(\boldsymbol{\beta})$. We may be interested in a nonlinear transformation of the parameters or in a nonlinear transformation of the parameters and the data. In Stata, the `nlcom` command can be used for the former and the `predictnl` command can be used for the latter. Variances obtained using the delta method are based on a Taylor series expansion of the nonlinear transformation $g(\boldsymbol{\beta}|\mathbf{x})$ of the parameters $\boldsymbol{\beta}$ and data $\mathbf{x}$, and involve calculation of the derivatives of $g(\boldsymbol{\beta}|\mathbf{x})$ with respect to $\boldsymbol{\beta}$. The use of `predictnl` in Stata is particularly useful because the derivatives are obtained numerically.

The postestimation `predict` command for `stpm2` makes extensive use of `predictnl`, for example, to obtain CIs for hazard rates, time-dependent HRs, and differences in survival functions. An important question is "how well does the delta method perform when compared with a computationally intensive method such as the bootstrap?" In our experience, the delta method performs exceptionally well. Figure 1.7 shows the baseline hazard rate, the time-dependent HR, the difference in the hazard rates, and the difference in the survival functions from the Rotterdam breast cancer data, which are described in more detail in section 3.2. The model fit is a PO model with a single binary covariate, `recent`, that describes whether each individual was recruited in a more recent time period. CIs obtained from the delta method (shaded area) and from 10,000 bootstrap samples (dashed lines) are shown. There is excellent agreement between the delta method and the computationally much more intensive bootstrap. Except in datasets with tiny sample sizes, we usually see very good agreement between the two methods.

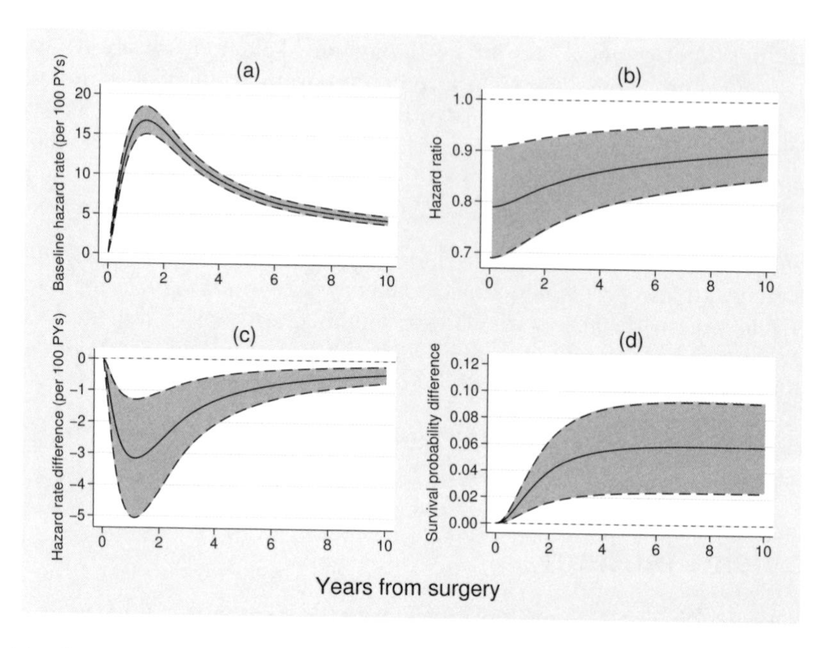

Figure 1.7. Rotterdam breast cancer data. Comparison of delta method versus bootstrap estimation of CIs. (a) Baseline hazard rate, (b) HR, (c) hazard difference, and (d) survival difference. The shaded area corresponds to the delta method, and the dashed lines are obtained from the bootstrap. PYs stands for person-years.

1.10 Ado-file resources

Some of the analyses we demonstrate, particularly in chapter 6, require ado-files that are not part of official Stata. For convenience, all of these ado-files may be installed from the Statistical Software Components (SSC) archive (often called the Boston College Archive) at http://www.repec.org. For further details of managing SSC components, see [R] **ssc**. Table 1.1 gives a list of these routines with a brief indication of their functions.

Table 1.1. Ado-files used in our book and available from the SSC archive.

Routine	Description
`fracdydx`	evaluate derivatives of fractional polynomials
`rcsgen`	generate restricted cubic spline variables
`running`	symmetric nearest-neighbor smoothing
`stcstat2`	Harrell's concordance index for flexible parametric models
`stpm2`	fit flexible parametric survival models
`stpm2cm`	calculation of crude mortality
`str2d`	explained variation in survival analysis
`stsurvdiff`	difference between two Kaplan–Meier survival curves
`stsurvimpute`	impute censored survival times
`xriml`	reference interval estimation by maximum likelihood

Any problems encountered with any of these programs should be reported to Patrick Royston or Paul Lambert. Their email addresses are given in the help files.

1.11 How our book is organized

In the first three chapters, we set the scene for the main body of the material in chapters 4 through 9. Readers familiar with Stata's `stset` command can skip chapter 2. Chapter 3 introduces datasets that are used more than once in the book. In chapter 4, we show how the Poisson distribution provides a rich family of flexible parametric survival models, initially under the PH assumption but extensible to accommodate time-dependent effects. Because the Poisson is a generalized linear model and is fit using Stata's `glm` command, we can use the rich set of tools and techniques available with generalized linear models. In chapter 5, we provide a gentle introduction to RP parametric survival models, which are at the heart of our book. In chapter 6, we describe how to use RP models to derive prognostic survival models, and in chapter 7 we extend both Poisson and RP models to allow for time-dependent effects of covariates. In chapter 8, we talk about how to broaden the models to accommodate relative survival, an important concept in population cancer statistics. Finally, in chapter 9 we discuss several additional applications of the models.

We give passages of Stata code throughout our book so that users can repeat the analyses if they wish to or adapt the code for their own analyses. Instructions for downloading Stata materials (do-files and datasets) are available at
http://www.stata-press.com/data/fpsaus.html.

2 Using stset and stsplit

2.1 What is the stset command?

The stset command tells Stata about the format of the survival data. Stata only needs to be informed once of the format. All subsequent survival analysis commands (the st commands) use this information. For example, a Cox proportional hazards model with age and sex as covariates can be fit after using stset by typing the following command:

```
. stcox age sex
```

At the minimum, stset needs to inform Stata of the survival time (for example, years from diagnosis), but should nearly always include the failure variable (for example, whether the patient died). However, the stset command is flexible and powerful for setting up survival data with a more complicated format. In this chapter, the use of the stset command is explained through several examples.

2.2 Some key concepts

Before we explain some details of using stset, it is important to explain some key concepts about what we mean by time.

Time origin This defines time 0—that is, when the clock starts and we start recording time. Examples of time 0 include date of diagnosis, date of randomization, and date of birth.

Exit time This defines the time (or date) when a subject stops being at risk, either by experiencing the event or being censored.

Failure indicator This defines whether a subject experiences the event or is censored.

Entry time This defines when the subject starts being at risk. In many cases, this is the same as the time origin—that is, time 0.

Analysis time This is the amount of time the person was at risk—that is, the difference between the exit and the entry times.

See Cleves et al. (2010) and Stata manual [ST] **stset** for more explanation.

2.3 Syntax of the stset command

`stset` *timevar* [*if*] [*weight*] [, `failure(`*failvar*[== *numlist*]`)` *other_options*]

- The *timevar* variable is compulsory. It is the survival time (or a date) of the event or the censoring time.
- The `failure(`*failvar*[==*numlist*]`)` option is optional, but it is good practice to always use it. If this option is omitted, it is assumed that all subjects experience the event. It is a number list giving the values of *failvar* that indicate a failure; all other values indicate a censoring. In many cases, *failvar* is a single number, but a number list is useful if, for example, different codes are used for different causes of death.
- The `exit()` option gives the latest time at which the subject is at risk. The default is `exit(failure)`; that is, the subject is removed from the risk set after the first event, even if there are subsequent records indicating additional failures for the subject. This command is useful if follow-up time is to be restricted. For example, you may be using dates to define survival times but may wish to restrict the follow-up time to 12/31/2007; this restriction can be done by specifying `exit(time mdy(12,31,2007))`. Multiple failures need to be specified as `exit(time .)`, because the default behavior is to remove the subject from the risk set after the first failure.
- The `origin()` option gives the time origin of the time scale. The default is zero. This option is particularly useful when dates or age define the time scale. For example, the origin may be the date of diagnosis or the date of birth.
- The `enter()` option gives the time at which the subject becomes at risk of experiencing the event. This option is useful if age is to be taken as the time scale. For example, if there were a date of diagnosis (`datediag`), you would use `enter(datediag)`. It is also useful if patients are only considered to be at risk after a certain date. It is useful in period analysis when the survival time is artificially left-truncated. For example, if information on subjects at risk after 1/1/2001 were to be included, one would use `enter(time mdy(1,1,2001))`.
- The `scale(`*#*`)` option transforms the survival time. For example, to transform the time scale from days to years, use `scale(365.24)`.
- The `id(`*varname*`)` option specifies an identification (ID) number for each subject. This option is not compulsory, but it is good practice to specify it because the `stsplit` command requires an ID variable. If there are multiple observations per subject, the `id()` option is mandatory.

The options above are the most common. See the Stata manual [ST] **stset** for other options.

2.4 Variables created by the stset command

The `stset` command usually creates four new variables. It creates five new variables if the `origin()` option is used. These variables contain all the necessary information about the structure of the survival data for the `st` survival analysis commands. The created variables are

`_t`	analysis time when record ends
`_d`	1 if failure, 0 if censored
`_t0`	analysis time when record begins
`_st`	1 if the record is included, 0 if excluded
`_origin`	the time origin if the `origin()` option of `stset` is used.

2.5 Examples of using stset

We use an example dataset to illustrate the `stset` command. A small, fictitious dataset includes three subjects whose dates of birth, diagnosis, event (death) and treatment change are known. The data are listed below:

```
. list, noobs ab(9)
```

id	event	tx	datebirth	datediag	dateexit	datetreat	sdays	syears
1	0	1	27mar1969	18jun2000	31dec2006	05jul2002	2387	6.535
2	1	1	05sep1975	16apr1999	03jun2004	06sep2000	1875	5.134
3	1	0	13feb1974	02nov2001	19jan2005	.	1174	3.214

The variables are as follows:

`id`	identification number
`event`	event indicator (0 = censored, 1 = dead)
`tx`	treatment indicator (0 = standard, 1 = new)
`datebirth`	date of birth
`datediag`	date of diagnosis
`dateexit`	date of death or censoring
`datetreat`	date of change in treatment
`sdays`	survival time in days
`syears`	survival time in years

One subject (`id` = 3) did not change treatment, and `datetreat` is recorded as missing for that subject. The variables `sdays` and `syears` were calculated using

```
. generate sdays = dateexit - datediag
. generate syears = (dateexit - datediag)/365.24
```

The variable `datetreat` is used to demonstrate how to incorporate time-varying covariates in an analysis.

2.5.1 Standard survival data

If the survival time and censoring indicator have already been created, then stset can be used as follows:

```
. stset syears, failure(event == 1) id(id)

                id:  id
     failure event:  event == 1
obs. time interval:  (syears[_n-1], syears]
 exit on or before:  failure

------------------------------------------------------------------------------
        3  total obs.
        0  exclusions
------------------------------------------------------------------------------
        3  obs. remaining, representing
        3  subjects
        2  failures in single failure-per-subject data
 14.88336  total analysis time at risk, at risk from t =         0
                             earliest observed entry t =         0
                                  last observed exit t =  6.535429

. list id _t0 _t _d _st event sdays syears, noobs ab(7)
```

id	_t0	_t	_d	_st	event	sdays	syears
1	0	6.5354285	0	1	0	2387	6.535
2	0	5.1336107	1	1	1	1875	5.134
3	0	3.2143247	1	1	1	1174	3.214

The id() option is not compulsory here because there should be only one row of data per subject. However, it is good practice to include it, because when the time scale is later split using stsplit, the data must previously have been stset with the id() option.

The output gives some summary information. This output should be checked for exclusions (for example, for zero or negative survival times), that the number of events corresponds to what is expected, and so on.

The stset command has created four new variables. For this example, _t0 is 0 for all subjects because all subjects become at risk at time 0—that is, when they are diagnosed. The variable _t gives the survival or censoring time (that is, when the subject stops being at risk due to death or censoring), which in this case is the same as syears. The _d variable is the event indicator (0 if censored, and 1 if an event), and it is the same as the event variable here. The _st variable specifies whether the observation should be included in the analysis (1 = include, 0 = exclude). _st is zero if survival times are recorded as zero (or are negative) or if a case was excluded by use of an if or in filter specified in the stset command.

2.5.2 Using the scale( ) option

Suppose that survival time is measured in days but that the analysis time is to be in years. The `scale()` option can be used, for example, as follows:

```
. stset sdays, failure(event == 1) id(id) scale(365.24)

                id:  id
     failure event:  event == 1
obs. time interval:  (sdays[_n-1], sdays]
 exit on or before:  failure
    t for analysis:  time/365.24

------------------------------------------------------------------------------
        3  total obs.
        0  exclusions
------------------------------------------------------------------------------
        3  obs. remaining, representing
        3  subjects
        2  failures in single failure-per-subject data
 14.88336  total analysis time at risk, at risk from t =         0
                             earliest observed entry t =         0
                                  last observed exit t =  6.535429

. list id _t0 _t _d _st event sdays syears, noobs ab(7)
```

id	_t0	_t	_d	_st	event	sdays	syears
1	0	6.5354288	0	1	0	2387	6.535
2	0	5.1336108	1	1	1	1875	5.134
3	0	3.2143248	1	1	1	1174	3.214

The survival time (in days) is divided by 365.24 to give survival time in years. This is noted in the output from the `stset` command.

The variables created by `stset` (`_t0`, `_t`, `_d`, and `_st`) are exactly the same as those in the previous example. This is to be expected because the `syears` variable was calculated in the same way `stset` did. It is usually safer to let `stset` do the rescaling. There are other advantages; for example, with the `stsplit` command, you can specify options that account for the fact that the data have been rescaled.

2.5.3 Date of diagnosis and date of exit

It is common to have data consisting of various dates. Examples include the date of diagnosis of a particular disease, the date of death, the end of follow-up, the date of birth, or the date patients were given particular treatments. Given these dates, it is easy to calculate the various relevant times, but the `stset` command can do most of this work for you.

Stata records dates as the number of days from 1 January 1960. It is necessary to ensure that dates have either been read in or converted to this format. We recommend either reading in the date as a string (for example, "3/27/1969") and then using the `date()` function, such as

```
. generate datediag = date(sdatediag, "MDY")
```

or reading in the day, month, and year separately and using the `mdy()` function:

```
. generate datediag = mdy(monthdiag, daydiag, yeardiag)
```

When working with dates, the `origin()` option should be used. If this is not done, the time origin is 1/1/1960. The `stset` command is as follows:

```
. stset dateexit, failure(event == 1) id(id) origin(datediag)

                id:  id
     failure event:  event == 1
obs. time interval:  (dateexit[_n-1], dateexit]
 exit on or before:  failure
    t for analysis:  (time-origin)
            origin:  time datediag

------------------------------------------------------------------------------
        3  total obs.
        0  exclusions
------------------------------------------------------------------------------
        3  obs. remaining, representing
        3  subjects
        2  failures in single failure-per-subject data
     5436  total analysis time at risk, at risk from t =         0
                                 earliest observed entry t =         0
                                      last observed exit t =      2387
. list id _t0 _t _d _st _origin event sdays syears, noobs ab(7)
```

id	_t0	_t	_d	_st	_origin	event	sdays	syears
1	0	2387	0	1	14779	0	2387	6.535
2	0	1875	1	1	14350	1	1875	5.134
3	0	1174	1	1	15281	1	1174	3.214

In the output from `stset`, it is reported that `t for analysis: (time - origin)`, which is what is wanted. Just as the dates are stored in units of days, the analysis time is also in units of days. A new Stata variable, `_origin`, has been created that stores the time origin (in days from 1/1/1960). To have analysis time in units of years, the `scale()` option should be used.

2.5.4 Date of diagnosis and date of exit with the scale( ) option

By adding the `scale()` option, the analysis time can be transformed to units of years, which is usually easier for interpretation.

```
. stset dateexit, failure(event == 1) id(id) origin(datediag) scale(365.24)

                id:  id
     failure event:  event == 1
obs. time interval:  (dateexit[_n-1], dateexit]
 exit on or before:  failure
    t for analysis:  (time-origin)/365.24
            origin:  time datediag

------------------------------------------------------------------------------
        3  total obs.
        0  exclusions
------------------------------------------------------------------------------
        3  obs. remaining, representing
        3  subjects
        2  failures in single failure-per-subject data
 14.88336  total analysis time at risk, at risk from t =         0
                             earliest observed entry t =         0
                                  last observed exit t =  6.535429

. list id _t0 _t _d _st _origin event sdays syears, noobs ab(7)
```

id	_t0	_t	_d	_st	_origin	event	sdays	syears
1	0	6.5354288	0	1	14779	0	2387	6.535
2	0	5.1336108	1	1	14350	1	1875	5.134
3	0	3.2143248	1	1	15281	1	1174	3.214

The variables created by `stset` (`_t0`, `_t`, `_d`, and `_st`) are exactly the same as in sections 2.5.1 and 2.5.2.

2.5.5 Restricting the follow-up time

In some instances, it may be necessary to define the maximum follow-up time. This may be because follow-up information after a certain date may be unreliable. Alternatively, you may be interested only in follow-up to a certain time after diagnosis. For example, if only a few individuals survive after five years, you may want to restrict follow-up to 5 years.

In the following example, the censoring date is 12/31/2005 and anyone still alive at this date is censored at this time. The `mdy()` function is combined with the `exit()` option:

```
. stset dateexit, failure(event == 1) id(id) origin(datediag) scale(365.24)
> exit(time mdy(12,31,2005))

                id:  id
     failure event:  event == 1
obs. time interval:  (dateexit[_n-1], dateexit]
 exit on or before:  time mdy(12,31,2005)
    t for analysis:  (time-origin)/365.24
            origin:  time datediag

------------------------------------------------------------------------------
        3  total obs.
        0  exclusions
------------------------------------------------------------------------------
        3  obs. remaining, representing
        3  subjects
        2  failures in single failure-per-subject data
 13.88402  total analysis time at risk, at risk from t =         0
                             earliest observed entry t =         0
                                  last observed exit t =  5.536086

. list id _t0 _t _d _st _origin event sdays syears, noobs ab(7)
```

id	_t0	_t	_d	_st	_origin	event	sdays	syears
1	0	5.5360859	0	1	14779	0	2387	6.535
2	0	5.1336108	1	1	14350	1	1875	5.134
3	0	3.2143248	1	1	15281	1	1174	3.214

The option `exit(time mdy(12,31,2005))` truncates the time scale at this date. This truncation affects subject 1, who had a censoring date of 12/31/2006, so the survival time has been reduced by one year. The other two individuals are unaffected because they were not at risk at this date as they had already experienced an event.

If the interest lies in restricting the follow-up time to five years, then you can use

```
. stset dateexit, failure(event == 1) id(id) origin(datediag) scale(365.24)
> exit(time datediag + 365.24*5)

                id:  id
     failure event:  event == 1
obs. time interval:  (dateexit[_n-1], dateexit]
 exit on or before:  time datediag + 365.24*5
    t for analysis:  (time-origin)/365.24
            origin:  time datediag

------------------------------------------------------------------------------
        3  total obs.
        0  exclusions
------------------------------------------------------------------------------
        3  obs. remaining, representing
        3  subjects
        1  failure in single failure-per-subject data
 13.21432  total analysis time at risk, at risk from t =         0
                             earliest observed entry t =         0
                                  last observed exit t =         5
```

```
. list id _t0 _t _d _st _origin event sdays syears, noobs ab(7)
```

id	_t0	_t	_d	_st	_origin	event	sdays	syears
1	0	5	0	1	14779	0	2387	6.535
2	0	5	0	1	14350	1	1875	5.134
3	0	3.2143248	1	1	15281	1	1174	3.214

Note the use of `exit(time datediag + 365.24*5)`. This is on the original time scale in days, so the number of days per year (365.24) has been multiplied by the desired follow-up time. The analysis time (`_t`) is now 5 years for subject 1. Subject 2 also has an analysis time of 5 years, but the event indicator (`_d`) has changed from 1 to 0 because the event occurred after 5 years of follow-up.

2.5.6 Left-truncation

We can left-truncate the time scale using the `enter()` option. This command is also used when age is the time scale in section 2.5.7. An example of left-truncation is in *period analysis*, in which only the survival experience of subjects who are at risk in a recent time period are included in the analysis (see section 9.8). For example, if we only want to include the survival times after 1/1/2001, we can use `enter(time mdy(1,1,2001))`.

```
. stset dateexit, failure(event == 1) id(id) origin(datediag) scale(365.24)
> enter(time mdy(1,1,2001))

                id:  id
     failure event:  event == 1
obs. time interval:  (dateexit[_n-1], dateexit]
 enter on or after:  time mdy(1,1,2001)
 exit on or before:  failure
    t for analysis:  (time-origin)/365.24
            origin:  time datediag

------------------------------------------------------------------------------
        3  total obs.
        0  exclusions
------------------------------------------------------------------------------
        3  obs. remaining, representing
        3  subjects
        2  failures in single failure-per-subject data
 12.63005  total analysis time at risk, at risk from t =         0
                             earliest observed entry t =         0
                                  last observed exit t =  6.535429

. list id _t0 _t _d _st _origin event sdays syears, noobs ab(7)
```

id	_t0	_t	_d	_st	_origin	event	sdays	syears
1	.53937137	6.5354288	0	1	14779	0	2387	6.535
2	1.7139415	5.1336108	1	1	14350	1	1875	5.134
3	0	3.2143248	1	1	15281	1	1174	3.214

This is the first time we have observed that _t0 is not 0. This is because the first two subjects were diagnosed before 1/1/2001 and we have specified that we are only interested in analyzing the survival times after this date. The variable _t0 is still 0 for subject 3 because that subject was diagnosed after 1/1/2001. Left-truncation is also known as delayed entry.

2.5.7 Age as the time scale

It has become increasingly popular to use age as the time scale in epidemiological cohort studies. This is an alternative (and often better) way of adjusting for age. See section 7.8 for more details of this approach.

With age as the time scale, we need the enter() and origin() options. Because we are interested in age, the time origin must be the date of birth, and the entry time in the study is the date of diagnosis.

```
. stset dateexit, failure(event == 1) id(id) origin(datebirth)
> enter(datediag) scale(365.24)

                id:  id
     failure event:  event == 1
obs. time interval:  (dateexit[_n-1], dateexit]
 enter on or after:  time datediag
 exit on or before:  failure
    t for analysis:  (time-origin)/365.24
            origin:  time datebirth

------------------------------------------------------------------------------
        3  total obs.
        0  exclusions
------------------------------------------------------------------------------
        3  obs. remaining, representing
        3  subjects
        2  failures in single failure-per-subject data
 14.88336  total analysis time at risk, at risk from t =         0
                             earliest observed entry t =  23.61187
                                  last observed exit t =  37.76421

. list id _t0 _t _d _st _origin event sdays syears, noobs ab(9)
```

id	_t0	_t	_d	_st	_origin	event	sdays	syears
1	31.228781	37.76421	0	1	3373	0	2387	6.535
2	23.611872	28.745482	1	1	5726	1	1875	5.134
3	27.71876	30.933085	1	1	5157	1	1174	3.214

In the above results, the variable _t0 denotes the age at which the subject was diagnosed with the disease. The variable _t denotes the age at which the subject died or ceased to be at risk due to censoring.

2.6 The stsplit command

The stsplit command splits the time scale into two or more episodes. It is useful for dealing with multiple events, time-varying covariates, and time-dependent effects. It is described in more detail in section 4.3. Here we briefly explain how it can be used to set up data with time-dependent effects and for time-varying covariates.

2.6.1 Time-dependent effects

When the effect of a covariate depends on the time since follow-up, it is a time-dependent effect. As explained in section 7.3, one way of dealing with the situation is to split the time-scale into a number of intervals and estimate a separate parameter for a covariate of interest for each interval. The stsplit command makes the process simple. For example, suppose that we want the effect of the treatment variable to be different for the first year of follow-up than in subsequent years. The following code splits the time scale at one year and calculates two dummy variables, tx1 and tx2.

```
. stset dateexit, failure(event == 1) id(id) origin(datediag) scale(365.24)

                id:  id
     failure event:  event == 1
obs. time interval:  (dateexit[_n-1], dateexit]
 exit on or before:  failure
    t for analysis:  (time-origin)/365.24
            origin:  time datediag

------------------------------------------------------------------------------
        3  total obs.
        0  exclusions
------------------------------------------------------------------------------
        3  obs. remaining, representing
        3  subjects
        2  failures in single failure-per-subject data
 14.88336  total analysis time at risk, at risk from t =         0
                             earliest observed entry t =         0
                                  last observed exit t =  6.535429

. stsplit sp_time, at(1)
(3 observations (episodes) created)

. generate tx1 = tx*(sp_time==0)

. generate tx2 = tx*(sp_time==1)

. list id _t0 _t _d _st sp_time tx tx1 tx2, noobs sepby(id)
```

id	_t0	_t	_d	_st	sp_time	tx	tx1	tx2
1	0	1	0	1	0	1	1	0
1	1	6.5354288	0	1	1	1	0	1
2	0	1	0	1	0	1	1	0
2	1	5.1336108	1	1	1	1	0	1
3	0	1	0	1	0	0	0	0
3	1	3.2143248	1	1	1	0	0	0

If a survival model is now fit including covariates (`tx1` and `tx2`), then a separate treatment effect would be estimated for the first year after diagnosis and for subsequent years.

2.6.2 Time-varying covariates

When incorporating time-varying covariates in survival analysis, we must split the follow-up at the time where the covariate changes value. This time usually differs between subjects. We can use `stsplit`, but we need to invoke a new facility, splitting along *another* time scale.

The origin of another time scale can be specified by the option `after()`. In this case, we use the variable `datetreat` as the origin of the new time scale. Then we ask to have the data split at only one point on this time scale, `0`, which by definition equals the date the new treatment started.

The variable created, `changetx`, has values corresponding to the left endpoint of the intervals. Stata codes the left endpoint as `-1` for intervals prior to `datetreat`.

```
. stset dateexit, failure(event == 1) id(id) origin(datediag) scale(365.24)

                id:  id
     failure event:  event == 1
obs. time interval:  (dateexit[_n-1], dateexit]
 exit on or before:  failure
    t for analysis:  (time-origin)/365.24
            origin:  time datediag

------------------------------------------------------------------------------
        3  total obs.
        0  exclusions
------------------------------------------------------------------------------
        3  obs. remaining, representing
        3  subjects
        2  failures in single failure-per-subject data
 14.88336  total analysis time at risk, at risk from t =         0
                             earliest observed entry t =         0
                                  last observed exit t =  6.535429

. replace datetreat = dateexit + 1 if datetreat == .
(1 real change made)

. stsplit changetx, after(datetreat) at(0)
(2 observations (episodes) created)

. replace changetx = changetx + 1
(5 real changes made)
```

```
. list id _t0 _t _d _st changetx event sdays syears, noobs sepby(id) ab(9)
```

id	_t0	_t	_d	_st	changetx	event	sdays	syears
1	0	2.0452305	0	1	0	.	2387	6.535
1	2.0452305	6.5354288	0	1	1	0	2387	6.535
2	0	1.3936042	0	1	0	.	1875	5.134
2	1.3936042	5.1336108	1	1	1	1	1875	5.134
3	0	3.2143248	1	1	0	1	1174	3.214

Following the `stsplit` command, the variable `changetx` has the value `-1` before the treatment change and `0` for the time after the treatment change. Thus the `replace` command changes these to `0` and `1`, respectively. The subject who does not change treatment has only one record.

If there are more treatment changes at other dates or there are other time-varying covariates, then must be declared in another variable and the process repeated.

2.7 Conclusion

The `stset` command is extremely powerful for setting up survival data and is a feature of Stata that we are particularly fond of compared to the implementation of survival analysis in other packages.

3 Graphical introduction to the principal datasets

3.1 Introduction

In this chapter, we introduce the datasets that are most frequently used in our book. We describe their survival distributions and hazard functions using nonparametric techniques (Kaplan–Meier and smoothed hazard functions, respectively) and a flexible parametric technique (Royston–Parmar models, implemented in `stpm2`). At this stage, we give only a flavor of what `stpm2` can do, leaving all the details until later.

3.2 Rotterdam breast cancer data

Sauerbrei, Royston, and Look (2007b) analyzed data from 2,982 patients with primary breast cancer whose records were included in the tumor bank at Rotterdam, The Netherlands. Follow-up time ranged from 1 to 231 months (median, 107 months). We analyze relapse-free survival, defined as the time from primary surgery to disease recurrence or death from breast cancer. Times to death from other causes were treated as censored. For our analyses, we censored the event and censoring times at 120 months (10 years). With the relapse-free survival outcome, 1,477 events were observed in the interval up to 120 months. By using the `exit()` option of `stset` (see section 2.3), the follow-up time was restricted to 10 years, as follows:

```
. use rott2
(Rotterdam breast cancer data, truncated at 10 years)
. stset rf, id(pid) failure(rfi == 1) exit(time 10 * 12) scale(12)
                id:  pid
     failure event:  rfi == 1
obs. time interval:  (rf[_n-1], rf]
 exit on or before:  time 10 * 12
    t for analysis:  time/12
------------------------------------------------------------------------------
     2982  total obs.
        0  exclusions
------------------------------------------------------------------------------
     2982  obs. remaining, representing
     2982  subjects
     1477  failures in single failure-per-subject data
 16262.06  total analysis time at risk, at risk from t =         0
                             earliest observed entry t =         0
                                  last observed exit t =        10
```

In addition to pid (patient identification), year (year of breast surgery, 1978–1993) and the time-to-event variables (rf, rfi), seven prognostic and two treatment variables were recorded. These were age (age at surgery), meno (menopausal status: 0 = pre, 1 = post), size (tumor size in 3 classes), grade (tumor grade 2 or 3), nodes (number of positive lymph nodes), pr (progesterone receptors, fmol/l), er (estrogen receptors, fmol/l), hormon (hormonal therapy: 0 = no, 1 = yes), chemo (chemotherapy: 0 = no, 1 = yes), and recent (dichotomized year: 0 = 1978–87, 1 = 1988–93).

To work with complete data, a single, multivariate, stochastic imputation of missing values of size (1.1% missing), grade (26.6%), nodes (2.2%), pr (5.4%), and er (3.6%) was made. We do not in general recommend working with only a single imputation. For present purposes, however, it is not necessary to complicate matters by fully accommodating the missing data in the analyses we demonstrate.

Figure 3.1 shows the estimated survival and hazard functions for the data.

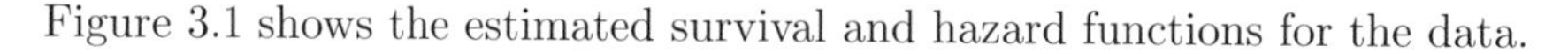

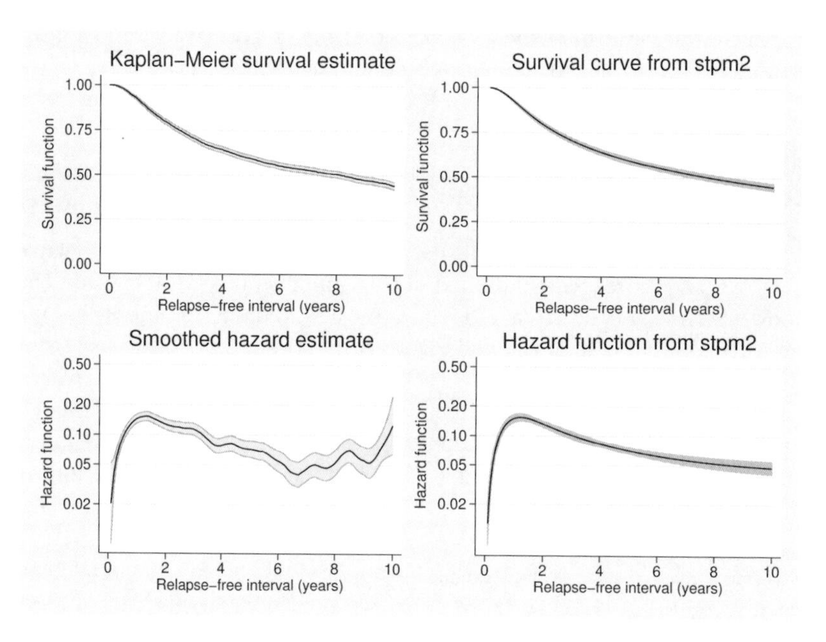

Figure 3.1. Rotterdam breast cancer data. Survival curves and hazard functions are estimated by the Kaplan–Meier method (sts graph), nonparametric kernel smoothing (sts graph, hazard), and stpm2.

The survival curves indicate a median time to event of about eight years. The Kaplan–Meier curve shows a slight downturn after about nine years, which is not reflected in the survival curve from stpm2. The smoothed nonparametric hazard estimate shows a corresponding upturn. Whether the feature is "real" or not is questionable—it seems surprising that the event rate would start to increase after such a long time.

The pointwise confidence intervals (CIs) from the smoothed hazard estimate are wider than that from stpm2. Conditional on a parsimonious parametric model (for example from stpm2), CIs are generally too narrow because they do not take model uncertainty into account. Nonparametric CIs make fewer assumptions and tend to be wider. Also they are implicitly high-dimensional and "noisy".

The commands we used to create the individual graphs in figure 3.1 are as follows:

```
. use rott2
// Survival - Kaplan-Meier
. sts graph, xtitle("Relapse-free interval (years)")                    ///
    ytitle("Survival function") ci xla(0(2)10) legend(off)             ///
    name(g1, replace) ylabel(,angle(h) format(%3.2f))
. // Survival - stpm2 with 2 knots
. stpm2, df(3) scale(hazard) nolog
. predict sstpm, survival ci
. graph twoway (rarea sstpm_lci sstpm_uci _t, pstyle(ci) sort)          ///
    (line sstpm _t, sort clpattern(1)),                                ///
    yscale(r(0 1)) ylabel(0(.25)1, angle(h) format(%3.2f))             ///
    xtitle("Relapse-free interval (years)") ytitle("Survival function") ///
    title("Survival curve from stpm2")                                 ///
    legend(off) name(g2, replace)
. // Hazard - kernel smoothing with Epanechnikov kernel
. sts graph, hazard kernel(epan2) ci                                    ///
    yscale(log) ylabel(0.02 0.05 0.1 0.2 0.5, angle(h) format(%3.2f))  ///
    xtitle("Relapse-free interval (years)") ytitle("Hazard function")  ///
    legend(off) name(g3, replace)
. // Hazard - stpm2 with 2 knots
. stpm2, df(3) scale(hazard) nolog
. predict hstpm, hazard ci
. graph twoway (rarea hstpm_lci hstpm_uci _t, pstyle(ci) sort)          ///
    (line hstpm _t, sort clpattern(1)),                                ///
    yscale(log) ylabel(0.02 0.05 0.1 0.2 0.5, angle(h) format(%3.2f))  ///
    xtitle("Relapse-free interval (years)") ytitle("Hazard function")  ///
    title("Hazard function from stpm2")                                ///
    legend(off) name(g4, replace)
. graph combine g1 g2 g3 g4
```

Note the use of the kernel(epan2) option with sts graph, hazard—the epan2 type of Epanechnikov kernel seems to give better results than the default. However, the resulting curve is still wiggly, with uninterpretable artifacts typical of such an approach.

3.3 England and Wales breast cancer data

We use a second dataset in breast cancer, comprising 115,331 women diagnosed with breast cancer in England and Wales between 1986 and the end of 1990, with follow-up to the end of 1995. The event of interest is death from any cause, with follow-up restricted to 5 years after diagnosis. In chapter 7, where we model time-dependent effects, we analyze a subset of 24,889 women less than 50 years of age. In chapter 8, when describing relative survival models, we analyze the complete dataset. The data include three covariates: dep (quantile group based on the Carstairs deprivation index (Coleman et al. 1999), with 1 = least deprived, ..., 5 = most deprived), region (National Health Service region in 1998, coded 1–9), and `agediag` (age at diagnosis in exact years). Five dummy variables (`dep1`, ..., `dep5`) corresponding to the different `dep` groups have been added.

Figure 3.2 shows the estimated survival and hazard functions for the reduced data of 24,889 women aged 50 or younger.

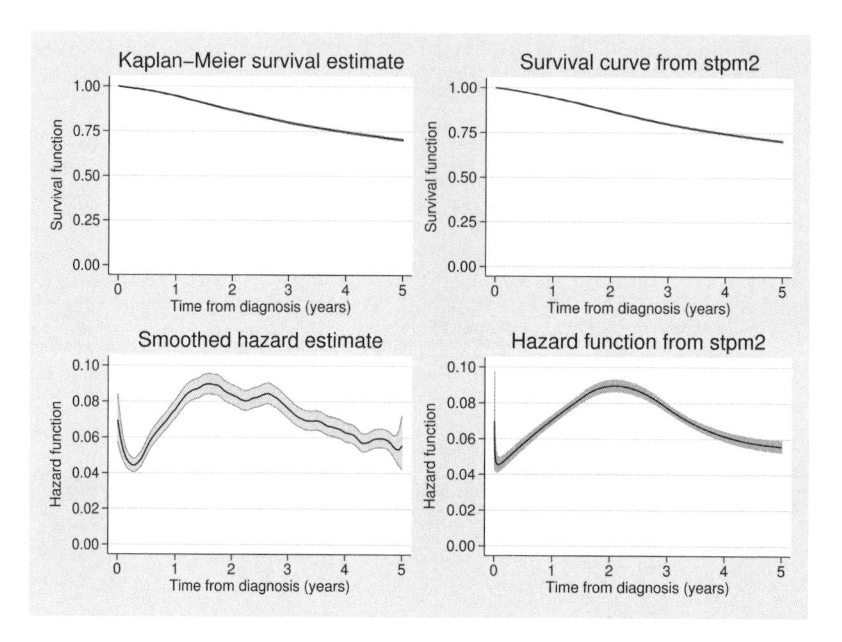

Figure 3.2. England and Wales breast cancer data subset, aged $\leq$ 50 years. Survival curves and hazard functions estimated by the Kaplan–Meier method (`sts graph`), nonparametric kernel smoothing (`sts graph, hazard`), and `stpm2`.

Commands similar to those that created figure 3.1 were used:

```
. use EW_breast2, clear
(England & Wales breast cancer survival: Aged<=50)
. stset survtime, failure(dead = 1) exit(time 5) id(ident)
                id:  ident
     failure event:  dead == 1
obs. time interval:  (survtime[_n-1], survtime]
 exit on or before:  time 5
------------------------------------------------------------------------------
    24889  total obs.
        0  exclusions
------------------------------------------------------------------------------
    24889  obs. remaining, representing
    24889  subjects
     7366  failures in single failure-per-subject data
   104639  total analysis time at risk, at risk from t =         0
                             earliest observed entry t =         0
                                  last observed exit t =         5
```

```
. // Survival - KM
. sts graph, xtitle("Time from diagnosis (years)") ytitle("Survival function")
> ci legend(off) name(g1, replace)

         failure _d:  dead == 1
   analysis time _t:  survtime
  exit on or before:  time 5
                 id:  ident

.
. // Survival - stpm2 with 2 knots
. stpm2, df(3) scale(hazard) nolog

Log likelihood = -22542.381                     Number of obs   =      24889

------------------------------------------------------------------------------
             |      Coef.   Std. Err.      z    P>|z|     [95% Conf. Interval]
-------------+----------------------------------------------------------------
xb           |
       _rcs1 |   .7526083   .0096452    78.03   0.000     .7337041    .7715125
       _rcs2 |  -.0132857   .0080348    -1.65   0.098    -.0290336    .0024623
       _rcs3 |   .0464962     .00312    14.90   0.000     .0403811    .0526113
       _cons |  -1.370018   .0119516  -114.63   0.000    -1.393443   -1.346593
------------------------------------------------------------------------------

. predict sstpm, survival ci

. preserve

. qui bysort _t: drop if _n > 1

. graph twoway (rarea sstpm_lci sstpm_uci _t, pstyle(ci) sort)
> (line sstpm _t, sort lpattern(l)), yscale(r(0 1)) ylabel(0(.25)1)
> xtitle("Time from diagnosis (years)") ytitle("Survival function")
> title("Survival curve from stpm2")
> legend(off) name(g2, replace)

. restore

.
. // Hazard - kernel smoothing with Epanichnikov kernel
. sts graph, hazard kernel(epan2) ci yscale(r(0 .1)) ylabel(0(.02).1)
> xtitle("Time from diagnosis (years)") ytitle("Hazard function")
> legend(off) name(g3, replace)

         failure _d:  dead == 1
   analysis time _t:  survtime
  exit on or before:  time 5
                 id:  ident

.
. // Hazard - stpm2 with 2 knots
. stpm2, df(3) scale(hazard) nolog

Log likelihood = -22542.381                     Number of obs   =      24889

------------------------------------------------------------------------------
             |      Coef.   Std. Err.      z    P>|z|     [95% Conf. Interval]
-------------+----------------------------------------------------------------
xb           |
       _rcs1 |   .7526083   .0096452    78.03   0.000     .7337041    .7715125
       _rcs2 |  -.0132857   .0080348    -1.65   0.098    -.0290336    .0024623
       _rcs3 |   .0464962     .00312    14.90   0.000     .0403811    .0526113
       _cons |  -1.370018   .0119516  -114.63   0.000    -1.393443   -1.346593
------------------------------------------------------------------------------

. predict hstpm, hazard ci

. preserve

. qui bysort _t: drop if _n > 1
```

```
. graph twoway (rarea hstpm_lci hstpm_uci _t, pstyle(ci) sort)
> (line hstpm _t, sort lpattern(l)), yscale(r(0 .1)) ylabel(0(.02).1)
> xtitle("Time from diagnosis (years)") ytitle("Hazard function")
> title("Hazard function from stpm2")
> legend(off) name(g4, replace)
. restore
. graph combine g1 g2 g3 g4, imargin(small)
```

Note the initial high mortality rate of patients who die shortly after diagnosis of breast cancer. It is believed that this is a small group comprises some patients with late-stage breast cancer and some who are diagnosed as a result of investigation of an unrelated fatal condition. Note also the larger peak about two years after diagnosis. Plausibly, the latter is preceded by the peak in breast cancer recurrence rate seen in figure 3.1. The shapes of the estimated hazard functions are broadly similar between the two estimation techniques, although the details differ.

3.4 Orchiectomy data

The dataset we use to illustrate the use of age as the time scale is from a large study of men diagnosed with prostate cancer in Sweden. The orchiectomy study (Dickman et al. 2004a) compares the incidence of hip fracture in three groups: 17,731 prostate cancer patients treated with bilateral orchiectomy (removal of the testicles), 43,230 prostate cancer patients not treated with bilateral orchiectomy, and 362,354 male controls randomly selected from the general population. Five controls not having had a diagnosis of prostate cancer were randomly selected from the general population for each cancer case; they were matched by age and county of residence. The outcome was fracture of the femoral neck of the hip. It is suspected that orchiectomy may lead to increased risk of hip fracture because it is associated with reduced bone mineral density due to androgen deprivation.

Because the risk of hip fracture increases with age, it is appropriate to take age as the main time scale.

Here, to give a feel for the data, we summarize the fracture results with age as the time scale in the control group. Details of modeling the two exposure groups and the control group are given in section 7.8. First, to incorporate attained age as the time scale, we must `stset` the data using variables stored in date format. The following variables are recorded

`enddate`	date of hip fracture or censoring
`startdate`	date of recruitment (6 months postdiagnosis)
`datebirth`	date of birth
`id`	identification number
`fracture`	event indicator

With this information, we stset the data as follows:

```
. use orchiectomy, clear
. stset enddate, failure(fracture = 1) enter(startdate) origin(birthdate)
> id(id) scale(365.24) exit(time birthdate + 100 * 365.24)

                id:  id
     failure event:  fracture == 1
obs. time interval:  (enddate[_n-1], enddate]
 enter on or after:  time startdate
 exit on or before:  time birthdate + 100 * 365.24
    t for analysis:  (time-origin)/365.24
            origin:  time birthdate
------------------------------------------------------------------------------
   423312  total obs.
       14  obs. begin on or after exit
------------------------------------------------------------------------------
   423298  obs. remaining, representing
   423298  subjects
    11002  failures in single failure-per-subject data
  2120262  total analysis time at risk, at risk from t =         0
                             earliest observed entry t =  38.53357
                                  last observed exit t =       100
```

Stata dates are recorded in days, therefore the scale(365.24) option converts the times to years. The age at entry is determined by enter() minus origin()—that is, startdate minus birthdate. The age at the event or censoring is determined by enddate minus startdate. Through use of the exit() option, the maximum age is 100—we chose to exclude the very small number of individuals older than 100. As reported by stset, this had the effect of removing 14 observations from the analysis because the subjects were diagnosed at over 100 years of age. Two dummy variables, exp2 and exp3, denote the prostate cancer patients with and without a bilateral orchiectomy, respectively. The population controls form the reference group.

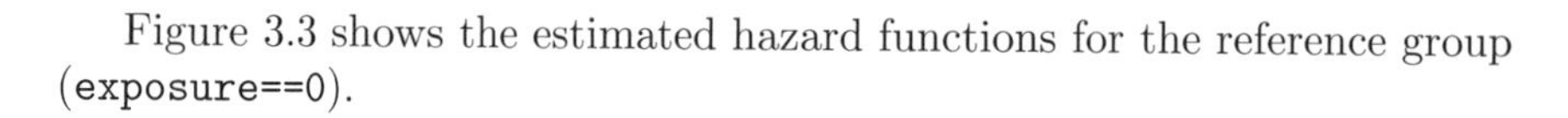

Figure 3.3 shows the estimated hazard functions for the reference group (`exposure==0`).

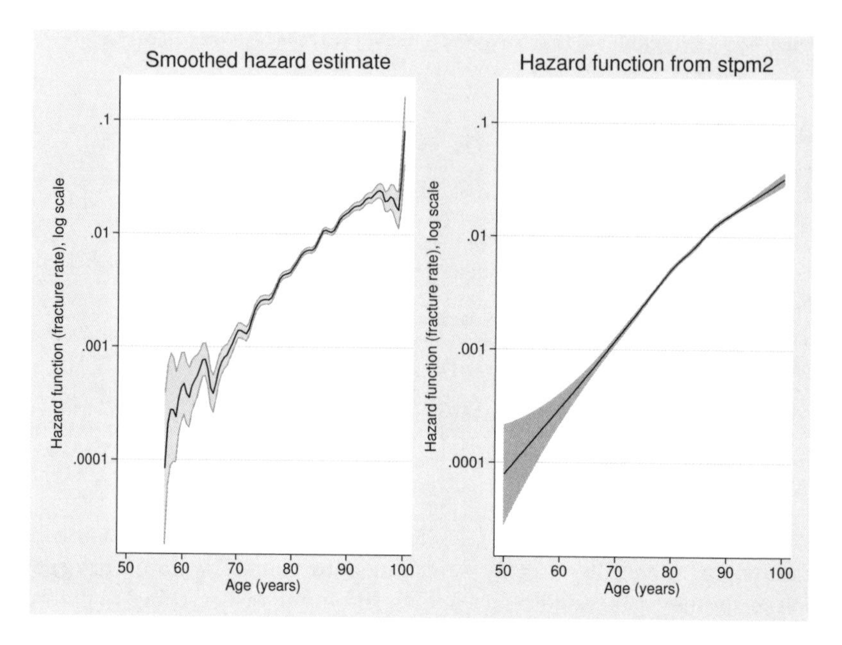

Figure 3.3. Orchiectomy data. Incidence rate for hip fracture in men diagnosed with prostate cancer in Sweden. Left panel, nonparametric estimate; right panel, `stpm2` estimate

Because of the delayed-entry nature of the data caused by using age as the time scale, we have deliberately avoided calculating the survival function, because it is hard to interpret. The hazard function remains interpretable in terms of the risk experienced by people of a given age who have previously been diagnosed with prostate cancer.

There are differences between the two estimates of the hazard function for men older than 95 years. The kernel smoothing method presents a “blip” (a slight drop then a sharp rise) in the fracture rate among the extremely old, whereas `stpm2` presents a smoothly rising trend. Judging by the rather simple behavior of the survival function estimates and the consideration that the “blip” makes little biological sense, the “blip” may be an artifact. For example, it could result from some feature of how the data were recorded.

Unfortunately, the orchiectomy data are not available to be downloaded.

3.5 Conclusion

We have introduced the main datasets graphically to give a feel for their survival and hazard functions. We explore their features further in subsequent chapters.

4 Poisson models

Summary

1. Exponential survival models can be fit as generalized linear models using Poisson regression.
2. Piecewise exponential models can be fit by splitting the time scale into a number of intervals. In such models, the baseline hazard rate is assumed to be constant within intervals, but can vary between intervals.
3. If the number of intervals is defined by the unique event times, then using Poisson regression is mathematically equivalent to fitting a Cox model. Having a smaller number of intervals still gives a good approximation to the Cox model with parameter estimates that are fairly insensitive to the number of intervals under the proportional-hazards (PH) assumption.
4. With large datasets, it can be computationally efficient to collapse the data over covariate patterns of interest.
5. If the time scale is split into a large number of narrow time intervals, then smooth estimates of the baseline hazard function can be obtained using splines or fractional polynomials (FPs).
6. The smoothness of spline functions can be controlled by selection of the number of knots. The Akaike information criterion (AIC) and Bayes information criterion (BIC) are useful tools in this process.

4.1 Introduction

In this chapter, we show how survival data can be modeled within the generalized linear modeling (GLM) framework using Poisson models. We demonstrate how the time scale can be split into several intervals to allow some flexibility in the shape of the baseline hazard function. We show that the Cox model is a special case of these models. We also argue that modeling the baseline hazard function smoothly (using splines or FPs) has several advantages, and we demonstrate how the modeling is implemented in the Poisson approach. This chapter concentrates on PH models, but in chapter 7 we show how the methods can be easily extended to situations where the effect of a covariate on the hazard rate varies over follow-up time—that is, when the hazard rates are not proportional.

4.2 Modeling rates with the Poisson distribution

Suppose that we assume that the hazard rate, $h(t)$, is constant over some time interval—that is, $h(t) = \lambda$. This means that the rate at which people die of a particular disease (or have a recurrence, etc.) does not change over follow-up time. A constant hazard rate implies that the survival times have an exponential distribution, and thus the survival function is

$$S(t) = \exp(-\lambda t)$$

It is possible to fit exponential survival models using `streg`, but we show first that the same parameter estimates, likelihood, etc. are obtained using `glm` with the option `family(poisson)`. We use the Rotterdam breast cancer data described in section 3.2 to demonstrate this practice. The data have been `stset` in the same way as in section 3.2.

We are interested to see if there has been an improvement in relapse-free survival over calendar time. We model the variable `recent`, which (as we have already mentioned) takes the value 0 and 1 for patients registered between 1978–1987 and 1988–1993, respectively.

The code below fits an exponential survival model first using `streg` and then `glm`. We shall explain the `glm` code shortly.

```
. use rott2
(Rotterdam breast cancer data, truncated at 10 years)

. streg recent, dist(exp) nolog nohr noshow

Exponential regression -- log relative-hazard form

No. of subjects =         2982                   Number of obs   =       2982
No. of failures =         1477
Time at risk    =  16262.06298
                                                 LR chi2(1)      =       6.02
Log likelihood  =   -3803.0523                   Prob > chi2     =     0.0141

------------------------------------------------------------------------------
          _t |      Coef.   Std. Err.      z    P>|z|     [95% Conf. Interval]
-------------+----------------------------------------------------------------
      recent |   -.128911   .0523843    -2.46   0.014    -.2315824   -.0262396
       _cons |  -2.324953   .0391031   -59.46   0.000    -2.401593   -2.248312
------------------------------------------------------------------------------
```

```
. glm _d recent, family(poisson) lnoffset(_t) nolog
Generalized linear models                          No. of obs      =      2982
Optimization     : ML                              Residual df     =      2980
                                                   Scale parameter =         1
Deviance         =   4652.10458                    (1/df) Deviance =  1.561109
Pearson          =  9243.149131                    (1/df) Pearson  =  3.101728

Variance function: V(u) = u                        [Poisson]
Link function    : g(u) = ln(u)                    [Log]

                                                   AIC             =  2.552014
Log likelihood   =  -3803.05229                    BIC             = -19188.94

------------------------------------------------------------------------------
             |                 OIM
          _d |      Coef.   Std. Err.      z    P>|z|     [95% Conf. Interval]
-------------+----------------------------------------------------------------
      recent |   -.128911   .0523843    -2.46   0.014    -.2315824   -.0262396
       _cons |  -2.324953   .0391031   -59.46   0.000    -2.401593   -2.248312
       ln(_t) |          1  (exposure)
------------------------------------------------------------------------------
```

The log likelihood, the parameter estimates, their standard errors (SEs) and their confidence intervals (CIs) are identical between `streg` and `glm`. We can interpret the parameters as follows: The hazard rate in 1978–1987 (when `recent` = 0) was exp(`_cons`) = 0.098 or a rate of recurrence or death due to breast cancer of 98 per 1,000 person-years. The hazard ratio is $\exp(-0.129) = 0.88$ in 1988–1993 compared with 1978–1987; that is, the rate of recurrence or death due to breast cancer was 12% lower in the more recent period. For the `glm` model, we include an offset using the `lnoffset()` option because we need to tell Stata how long each subject was at risk for. We now briefly explain why we can use both approaches.

As we have seen in section 1.7, the contribution of the ith subject to the log likelihood of a sample of survival data can be written as

$$\ln L_i = d_i \ln h(t_i) + \ln S(t_i)$$

where d_i is an event indicator (0 for a censored observation, 1 for an event) and t_i is the observed event or censoring time. If we substitute the hazard and survival functions for the exponential distribution into the above formula, we get

$$\ln L_i = d_i \ln \lambda - \lambda t_i$$

After dropping terms that do not depend on the model parameters, the expression is identical to the likelihood for a Poisson distribution with outcome d_i and mean λt_i. The time at risk is a constant and can be incorporated into a linear predictor via an offset. We therefore obtain the same parameter estimates from a GLM with outcome d_i, a Poisson error structure, a log link, and an offset of $\ln(t_i)$. In Stata, we use the event indicator `_d` for the outcome variable and `_t` for the time at risk. There is nothing new here. The Poisson distribution has been used for many years, particularly in epidemiology, to model rates (Breslow and Day 1987).

In fitting exponential survival models, we have assumed that the hazard rate is constant over time. This assumption is unrealistic in most applications. For example, after a diagnosis of cancer, there is usually a high initial mortality rate that decreases over time. Although Poisson modeling of rates is common in epidemiology, the models are usually extended by splitting the time scale into intervals and assuming that the hazard rate is constant within an interval but varies between intervals. These models are known as *piecewise exponential* models. Splitting the time scale is discussed further in the following section.

4.3 Splitting the time scale

Most implementations of survival analysis in Stata have a single row of data (observations) per subject. When we split the time scale into a number of intervals, we obtain more than one row per subject. We initially use time-splitting to fit PH models using Poisson modeling, but time-splitting is also useful with standard Cox or parametric survival models for time-dependent effects (see section 7.3), with time-varying covariates, and in cases when we are interested in multiple time scales (see section 7.9).

In epidemiology, the time scale is often split into a small number of intervals, each of length 1 year. The use of a small number of intervals is mainly for historical reasons in that these models were used when computers were much slower than they are today. Figure 4.1 shows a schematic description in which the time scale has been split into five intervals and the hazard rate is estimated separately within each interval. The hazard rate is assumed to be constant within each interval, which means that we are assuming exponential survival times within each interval. If this is an unreasonable assumption, we can increase the number of intervals.

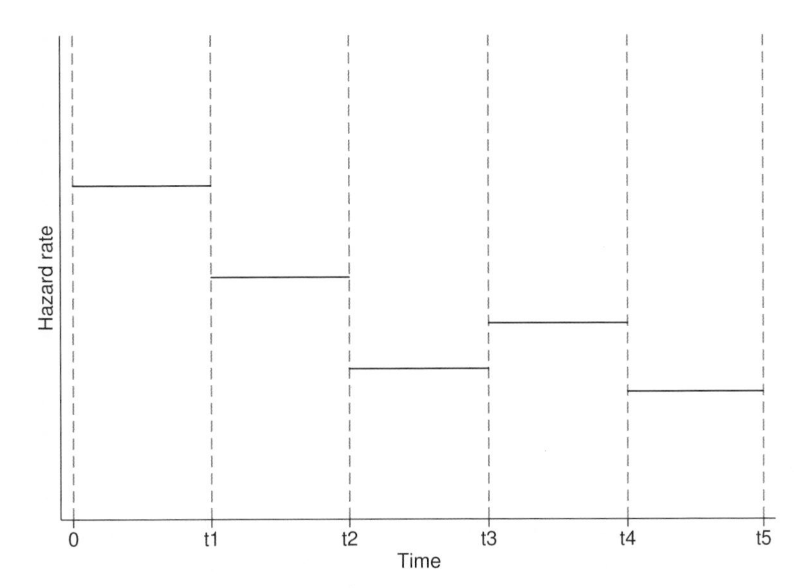

Figure 4.1. Schematic plot to illustrate piecewise constant hazard rates.

As an illustration of the approach, we model the Rotterdam breast cancer data using intervals of one year. To do this, we first split the time scale into yearly intervals. To demonstrate how the structure of the data changes, we have selected three subjects whose details are listed below:

```
. list pid _t0 _t _d if inlist(pid,2553,784,1167), noobs
```

pid	_t0	_t	_d
2553	0	1.6208076	1
1167	0	10	0
784	0	6.5160847	0

By looking at the values of _t, we can see that patient 2553 experienced the event cancer recurrence or death (failed) after 1.62 years (_d = 1 and _t = 1.62), patient 1167 was censored at 10 years (the maximum follow-up time), and patient 784 was censored after 6.52 years. Note that _t0 is 0 for all subjects, indicating that all subjects became at risk at time zero, which has been defined as the time of surgery for primary breast cancer.

We now use stsplit to split the time scale into yearly intervals:

```
. stsplit split_time, every(1)
(14529 observations (episodes) created)
. generate risktime = _t - _t0
. list pid _t0 _t _d split_time risktime if inlist(pid,2553,784,1167),
> sepby(pid) ab(10) noobs
```

pid	_t0	_t	_d	split_time	risktime
2553	0	1	0	0	1
2553	1	1.6208076	1	1	.6208076
1167	0	1	0	0	1
1167	1	2	0	1	1
1167	2	3	0	2	1
1167	3	4	0	3	1
1167	4	5	0	4	1
1167	5	6	0	5	1
1167	6	7	0	6	1
1167	7	8	0	7	1
1167	8	9	0	8	1
1167	9	10	0	9	1
784	0	1	0	0	1
784	1	2	0	1	1
784	2	3	0	2	1
784	3	4	0	3	1
784	4	5	0	4	1
784	5	6	0	5	1
784	6	6.5160847	0	6	.5160847

We have also calculated the time at risk (risktime) within each interval, which is simply _t minus _t0. The time at risk within each interval is needed for the Poisson modeling. stsplit has created a variable split_time, which is the same as _t0 in this case. We see that after using stsplit, there are an extra 14,529 observations in our dataset, making a total of 17,511. The listing for the three example individuals indicates that the increase is due to multiple rows of data per individual. In the split dataset, _t0 represents the start time of each interval, and _t represents either the end time of the interval or the time of an event or censoring within a particular interval. For example, subject 2553 now has two rows of data. The first row indicates that in the first interval (that is, the first year of follow-up) she became at risk at time zero (_t0 = 0) and was censored at the end of the interval (_t = 1 and _d = 0). For the second interval, she became at risk at time _t0 = 1 and failed at time _t = 1.62 years. The risktime variable shows that this subject contributed 1 person-year to the first interval and 0.62 person-years to the second interval. Subject 1167 was censored after 10 years and thus has 10 rows of data after splitting the time scale, with _t0 denoting the start time of each interval and _t denoting the end time of each interval. Finally, subject 784 was censored after 6.52 years and thus has 7 rows of data after splitting. Although there are multiple rows of data per subject, we do not need to be concerned with correlation between observations on the same subject. This is essentially because the time intervals are nonoverlapping.

Now that we have split the time scale using `stsplit`, we are ready to fit a piecewise exponential model.

4.3.1 The piecewise exponential model

We have seen that with an exponential survival model it is unrealistically assumed that the hazard rate is constant over the whole of the follow-up period. With the piecewise exponential model, the time scale is split into several intervals. We assume that the hazard rate is constant within each interval but can vary arbitrarily between the intervals. There is, of course, some subjectivity in choosing the number of intervals and where to place the cutpoints. This is discussed in more detail in section 4.6. For the moment, we assume that splitting into yearly intervals is sufficient.

An exponential survival model can be written as

$$h_i(t|\mathbf{x}_i) = \lambda \exp(\mathbf{x}_i\boldsymbol{\beta})$$

where $h_i(t|\mathbf{x}_i)$ is the hazard rate for the ith subject, λ is the baseline hazard rate that does not vary over time, $\mathbf{x}_i$ is a vector of covariates for the ith subject, and $\boldsymbol{\beta}$ are the regression parameters (log hazard-ratios). We extend this to a piecewise exponential model by adding a subscript, j, to the baseline hazard rate, and thus the model becomes

$$h_{ij}(t|\mathbf{x}_i) = \lambda_j \exp(\mathbf{x}_i\boldsymbol{\beta})$$

The hazard rate for the ith subject now varies over follow-up interval j because of the added subscript for λ_j.

We can fit this model using a Poisson regression as follows

$$\begin{aligned} d_{ij} &\sim \text{Poisson}(\mu_{ij}) \\ \ln(\mu_{ij}) &= \ln(y_{ij}) + \alpha_j + \mathbf{x}_i\boldsymbol{\beta} \end{aligned}$$

where μ_{ij} is the mean of the Poisson distribution. The time at risk, y_{ij}, for the ith subject in the jth interval is incorporated through the offset $\ln(y_{ij})$. We are now modeling on the log-hazard scale, and thus $\alpha_j = \ln(\lambda_j)$. We are not actually assuming that the d_{ij} have independent Poisson distributions. However, when we express the model in this way, it is the likelihood function that is equivalent to that from a piecewise exponential model. We just use the GLM framework as a convenient tool to fit the model.

We can use glm to fit a Poisson model in Stata:

```
. glm _d ibn.split_time recent, family(poisson) lnoffset(risktime) nocons nolog
> eform noheader
```

_d	IRR	OIM Std. Err.	z	P>|z|	[95% Conf.	Interval]
split_time						
0	.0967016	.0067456	-33.49	0.000	.0843445	.1108692
1	.1604905	.0097414	-30.14	0.000	.1424896	.1807654
2	.132105	.0091526	-29.22	0.000	.1153308	.1513189
3	.1014962	.0082949	-27.99	0.000	.0864738	.1191283
4	.088327	.0080601	-26.59	0.000	.0738616	.1056254
5	.076737	.0079604	-24.75	0.000	.0626188	.0940383
6	.0470707	.0065406	-21.99	0.000	.0358488	.0618055
7	.050304	.0073742	-20.39	0.000	.0377417	.0670475
8	.0753501	.0102016	-19.10	0.000	.0577883	.0982488
9	.0678678	.0112165	-16.28	0.000	.0490891	.0938301
recent	.843453	.0444216	-3.23	0.001	.7607311	.9351701
ln(risktime)	1	(exposure)				

We have used the factor-variable notation introduced in Stata 11. The ibn.split_time term indicates that split_time has been treated as a factor variable with no reference group. Using this term in conjunction with nocons estimates the baseline hazard in each interval directly in the model. The baseline hazard rate is a step function when recent = 0, and it represents the hazard rate in the 1978–1987 period. Thus in the first year of follow-up, the rate of recurrence or death due to breast cancer was $0.0967 \times 1000 = 96.7$ per 1,000 person-years, while in the second year it increased to 160 per 1,000 person-years. We can also calculate conditional event probabilities from these estimates (see also section 6.5.1). The probability of not having a recurrence or dying of breast cancer in the first year is $\exp(-0.0967 \times 1) = 0.91$, and the probability of not having a recurrence or dying of breast cancer in the second year *conditional* on not having had one in the first year is $\exp(-0.1605 \times 1) = 0.85$. The multiplication by 1 (the length of the time interval) when calculating these probabilities is important. Although it is not mathematically necessary in this case, it demonstrates that the estimated probability depends on the length of the time interval. Stata has labeled the column of parameter estimates IRR, which stands for incidence-rate ratio. The parameter estimates for the dummy covariates are not incidence-rate ratios, but just incidence (or hazard) rates. The only actual ratio for the parameter estimates is for recent, which is the hazard ratio comparing those registered between 1988–1993 with those registered 1978–1987. The value of 0.843 indicates that the rate of recurrence or death due to breast cancer in 1988–1993 is estimated to be 15.7% lower than in 1978–1987. This is a PH model; the effect of recent does not depend on the time interval. Thus the model assumes that the 15.7% reduction in the rate of recurrence or death due to breast cancer is the same at all time points. We will see in chapter 7 that a nonproportional hazards model can be estimated by including an interaction between the covariate of interest and the dummy variables for the baseline hazard rate.

As already noted, assuming a constant hazard within each time interval is equivalent to assuming an exponential survival distribution within each time interval. We can thus use streg with dist(exp) to fit exactly the same model. This is shown below:

```
. streg ibn.split_time recent, dist(exp) nolog noshow nocons noheader

          _t   Haz. Ratio   Std. Err.      z    P>|z|     [95% Conf. Interval]

  split_time
           0     .0967016    .0067456   -33.49   0.000     .0843445    .1108692
           1     .1604905    .0097414   -30.14   0.000     .1424896    .1807654
           2      .132105    .0091526   -29.22   0.000     .1153308    .1513189
           3     .1014962    .0082949   -27.99   0.000     .0864738    .1191283
           4      .088327    .0080601   -26.59   0.000     .0738616    .1056254
           5      .076737    .0079604   -24.75   0.000     .0626188    .0940383
           6     .0470707    .0065406   -21.99   0.000     .0358488    .0618055
           7      .050304    .0073742   -20.39   0.000     .0377417    .0670475
           8     .0753501    .0102016   -19.10   0.000     .0577883    .0982488
           9     .0678678    .0112165   -16.28   0.000     .0490891    .0938301

      recent      .843453    .0444216    -3.23   0.001     .7607311    .9351701

note: no constant term was estimated in the main equation
```

The estimates are the same (as expected). An advantage of using streg is that it is easy to obtain an estimate of the survival function using the predict command.

```
. predict surv, csurv
. twoway (line surv _t if recent == 0, sort) (line surv _t if recent == 1, sort),
> scheme(sj) legend(order(1 "1978-1987" 2 "1988-1993") ring(0) pos(5) cols(1))
> yscale(range(0 1)) ylabel(0(0.2)1, angle(horizontal) format(%3.1f))
> ytitle("S(t)") xtitle("Time from surgery (years)")
```

We need to use the csurv option rather than the surv option, otherwise we obtain an estimate of the conditional survival function—that is, the probability of the event in each time interval. The csurv option estimates the conditional probabilities and then multiplies them together. The graph is shown in figure 4.2, which clearly shows the difference in survival between the two time periods.

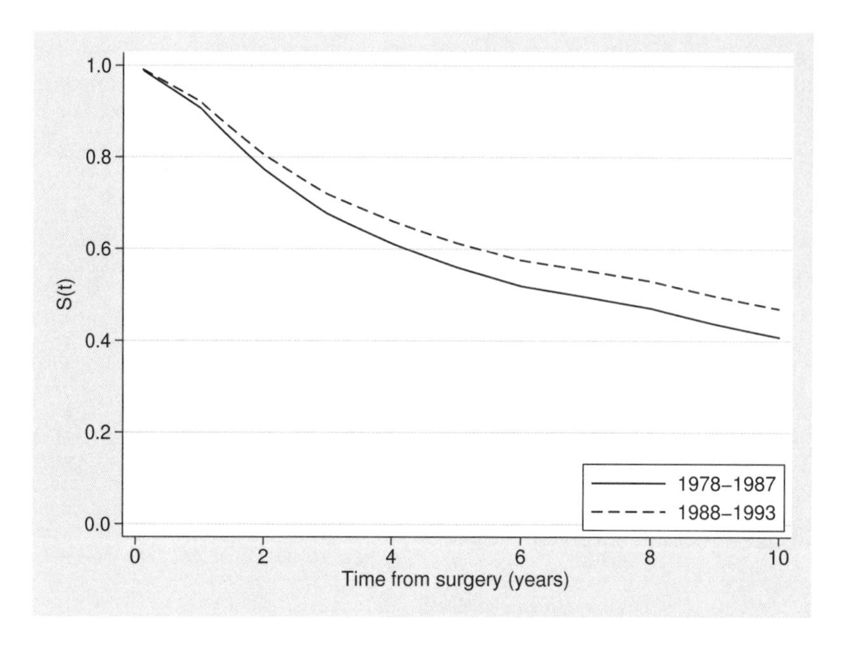

Figure 4.2. Rotterdam breast cancer data. Survival functions from piecewise exponential model.

Unfortunately, it is not possible to calculate the SE of the estimated survival function using the `predict` command to derive CIs. For an explanation of how to calculate a CI for the survival function, see section 4.8.6.

If there are many individuals in the dataset and many intervals are used, the dataset can become very large and it can take a long time to fit these models. Fortunately, it is possible to reduce the size of the data and thus speed up computational time by collapsing the data over the different covariate patterns (where time interval is considered a covariate). However, after collapsing the data it is not possible to use `streg`.

4.3.2 Time as just another covariate

Modeling the data with the Poisson approach allows us to think about survival time in a different way from that in standard survival analysis. Usually, survival time is considered to be the outcome variable and we have to use special methods to account for the censoring process. With the Poisson approach, it perhaps becomes clearer that we are modeling rates. We have a binary variable as an outcome, and our models investigate variation in the corresponding rates. There are many factors that cause systematic variation in rates—for example, age and sex, but also time. In the Poisson framework, we can therefore consider time to be a covariate, as opposed to a response. Thus we can adjust for time just as we would for any other covariate. Time-dependent effects of a covariate of interest are then simply an interaction between time and the covariate.

4.4 Collapsing the data to speed up computation

It is well known that Poisson models can be fit either to individual-level data or to data collapsed over each covariate pattern, resulting in identical parameter estimates and SEs. The reason for this is that the sum of N independent Poisson distributions, each with parameter λ, is a Poisson distribution with parameter $N\lambda$. With very large datasets, collapsing the data over each covariate pattern can lead to major reductions in computing time, particularly with computationally intensive methods such as FPs. To collapse individual-level data to grouped data, the event indicator (`_d`) and the person-at-risk time (`risktime`) are summed over each covariate pattern. Each time interval is considered a covariate, as described above.

Collapsing is straightforward to implement in Stata using the `collapse` command. For example, because we are only including the effect of the 10 time intervals (years) and calendar period (`recent`), we can collapse over `split_time` (the variable defining the time intervals) and `recent`.

```
. collapse (min) start=_t0 (max) end = _t (count) n=_d (sum) risktime _d,
> by(split_time recent)

. sort recent split_time

. list recent start end n risktime _d, sepby(recent) noobs
```

recent	start	end	n	risktime	_d
1978-1987	0	1	1167	1123.398	107
1978-1987	1	2	1052	955.2923	163
1978-1987	2	3	881	825.6728	103
1978-1987	3	4	770	720.5927	69
1978-1987	4	5	686	648.3039	58
1978-1987	5	6	616	583.2704	46
1978-1987	6	7	553	535.3272	26
1978-1987	7	8	515	490.0992	27
1978-1987	8	9	465	436.2601	32
1978-1987	9	10	404	369.7166	23
1988-1993	0	1	1815	1757.723	145
1988-1993	1	2	1657	1541.631	199
1988-1993	2	3	1438	1336.553	155
1988-1993	3	4	1252	1178.201	105
1988-1993	4	5	1119	1043.457	77
1988-1993	5	6	955	868.9439	55
1988-1993	6	7	787	725.4497	28
1988-1993	7	8	650	550.2382	21
1988-1993	8	9	454	363.9062	24
1988-1993	9	10	275	208.0267	14

The result is a dataset with 20 observations—that is, 10 time intervals for each level of `recent`, as opposed to 17,511 observations in the individual-level data. The data resemble a life table, in which we have the start and end time of each interval, the number at risk at the start of the interval, the person-years of observation in each interval, and the number of deaths within each interval. The code for fitting the Poisson model is exactly as before:

```
. glm _d ibn.split_time recent, family(poisson) lnoffset(risktime) nocons nolog
> eform noheader
```

_d	IRR	OIM Std. Err.	z	P>|z|	[95% Conf.	Interval]
split_time						
0	.0967016	.0067456	-33.49	0.000	.0843445	.1108692
1	.1604905	.0097414	-30.14	0.000	.1424896	.1807654
2	.132105	.0091526	-29.22	0.000	.1153308	.1513189
3	.1014962	.0082949	-27.99	0.000	.0864738	.1191283
4	.088327	.0080601	-26.59	0.000	.0738616	.1056254
5	.076737	.0079604	-24.75	0.000	.0626188	.0940383
6	.0470707	.0065406	-21.99	0.000	.0358488	.0618055
7	.050304	.0073742	-20.39	0.000	.0377417	.0670475
8	.0753501	.0102016	-19.10	0.000	.0577883	.0982488
9	.0678678	.0112165	-16.28	0.000	.0490891	.0938301
recent	.843453	.0444216	-3.23	0.001	.7607311	.9351701
ln(risktime)	1	(exposure)				

The parameter estimates and their SEs are the same when fitting the model to the 20 observations in the collapsed data as when fitting the model to the 17,511 observations in the individual-level data. It is much quicker to fit the model to the collapsed data. Speed may become an issue when the original dataset is much larger or the time scale is split into more intervals (as occurs with splines and FPs in sections 4.8.3 and 4.9). However, the speed issue should not be overstated; running `glm` on the 17,511 observations took only 2.4 seconds on a rather old laptop computer.

4.5 Splitting at unique failure times

How many time intervals are required? The most we can have is the number of unique event times, so let us see what happens when we split the time scale at each of these times. We can apply the `at(failures)` option of `stsplit`.

The output below shows fitting a Cox model to the Rotterdam breast cancer data. We then split the time scale at each unique failure time and fit a Poisson model.

```
. stcox recent, nolog noshow
Cox regression -- Breslow method for ties
No. of subjects =         2982                  Number of obs   =       2982
No. of failures =         1477
Time at risk    =  16262.06298
                                                LR chi2(1)      =      10.39
Log likelihood  =   -11199.067                  Prob > chi2     =     0.0013

------------------------------------------------------------------------------
          _t | Haz. Ratio   Std. Err.      z    P>|z|     [95% Conf. Interval]
-------------+----------------------------------------------------------------
      recent |   .8432847   .0444234    -3.24   0.001     .7605606    .9350065
------------------------------------------------------------------------------

. stsplit, at(failures) riskset(riskset)
(1097 failure times)
(2206827 observations (episodes) created)
. gen y = _t - _t0
. glm _d ibn.riskset recent, family(poisson) lnoffset(y) nolog nocons eform
Generalized linear models                       No. of obs      =    2208480
Optimization     : ML                           Residual df     =    2207382
                                                Scale parameter =          1
Deviance         =  21240.76703                 (1/df) Deviance =   .0096226
Pearson          =  2208003.008                 (1/df) Pearson  =   1.000281
Variance function: V(u) = u                     [Poisson]
Link function    : g(u) = ln(u)                 [Log]
                                                AIC             =   .0119497
Log likelihood   = -12097.38351                 BIC             = -3.22e+07

------------------------------------------------------------------------------
             |                 OIM
          _d |        IRR   Std. Err.      z    P>|z|     [95% Conf. Interval]
-------------+----------------------------------------------------------------
     riskset |
          1  |   .0035643   .0035659    -5.63   0.000     .0005016    .0253252
          2  |   .0123214   .0123269    -4.39   0.000     .0017341    .0875468
  (output omitted)
       1096  |   .2582589   .2582893    -1.35   0.176     .0363708    1.833822
       1097  |   .0378215   .0378257    -3.27   0.001     .0053265    .2685552
             |
      recent |   .8432847   .0444234    -3.24   0.001     .7605606    .9350065
       ln(y) |          1  (exposure)
------------------------------------------------------------------------------
```

There are 1,097 unique failure times. Splitting at these times adds 2,206,827 observations, making a total of 2,207,924 observations. This is clearly a large dataset, and models are going to take longer to fit. The estimated hazard ratio for the Poisson model is identical to the estimates from the Cox model, as is its SE. However, for the Poisson model, 1,097 dummy variables (one for each of the intervals) were needed for the baseline hazard. This is a large number of parameters, and it is this, rather than the number of observations, that most increases the computing time. The equivalence between the Poisson and the Cox models always holds when using the Breslow method for handling ties in the Cox model. The main point we want to make here is that including such a large number of dummy variables results in a noisy estimate of the baseline hazard function. By using smoothing methods, such as splines or FPs, we can still fit PH models but also obtain a much more parsimonious and convincing estimate of the baseline hazard function.

4.5.1 Technical note: Why the Cox and Poisson approaches are equivalent*

This section mathematically shows why the Poisson approach with splitting at unique event times gives the same estimates as the Cox model. The section can be omitted if you are not interested in the details.

We define the number of intervals by the number of death times, and for the moment we assume that all survival times are unique—that is, there are no ties. We can write a model for the log hazard-rate for the ith subject in the jth time interval as

$$\ln h_i\left(t|\mathbf{x}_i\right) = \alpha_j + \mathbf{x}_i\boldsymbol{\beta}$$

The contribution to the log likelihood for a single subject at risk can be written as

$$\ln L(\alpha_j, \boldsymbol{\beta}) = \sum_{i\in R_j} d_i\left(\alpha_j + \mathbf{x}_i\boldsymbol{\beta}\right) - y_j \exp\left(\alpha_j + \mathbf{x}_i\boldsymbol{\beta}\right)$$

where R_j is the set of individuals still at risk of an event for the jth time interval. Because we are assuming unique death times, the first term is zero for all subjects except the single subject who experienced the event. The time at risk since the previous event, y_j, is the same for all subjects. Thus we can write the log likelihood as

$$\ln L(\alpha_j, \beta) = \alpha_j + \mathbf{x}_{i(j)}\boldsymbol{\beta} - y_j \exp\left(\alpha_j\right) \sum_{i\in R_j} \exp\left(\mathbf{x}_i\boldsymbol{\beta}\right) \tag{4.1}$$

where $\mathbf{x}_{i(j)}$ denotes the covariate vector for the subject who died at time j.

To obtain a maximum likelihood estimate, we differentiate and set to zero. Differentiating with respect to α_j,

$$\frac{d\ln L(\alpha_j, \beta)}{d\alpha_j} = 1 - y_j \exp\left(\alpha_j\right) \sum_{i\in R_j} \exp\left(\mathbf{x}_i\beta\right)$$

Setting this expression equal to zero and solving for α_j gives

$$\exp\left(\alpha_j\right) = \frac{1}{y_j \sum_{i\in R_j} \exp\left(\mathbf{x}_i\boldsymbol{\beta}\right)}$$

$$\alpha_j = -\ln(y_j) - \ln\left\{\sum_{i\in R_j} \exp\left(\mathbf{x}_i\boldsymbol{\beta}\right)\right\}$$

If we substitute this back into the log likelihood in (4.1) above, we get a *profile likelihood* for $\boldsymbol{\beta}$:

$$\ln L(\beta) = -\ln(y_j) - \ln\left\{\sum_{i \in R_j} \exp(\mathbf{x}_i\boldsymbol{\beta})\right\} + \mathbf{x}_{i(j)}\boldsymbol{\beta} - \frac{y_j \sum_{i \in R_j} \exp(\mathbf{x}_i\boldsymbol{\beta})}{y_j \sum_{i \in R_j} \exp(\mathbf{x}_i\boldsymbol{\beta})}$$

Terms that do not depend on the parameters, $\boldsymbol{\beta}$, can be dropped, and thus the profile likelihood above can be written as

$$\ln L(\boldsymbol{\beta}) = \ln\left[\frac{\exp\{\mathbf{x}_{i(j)}\boldsymbol{\beta}\}}{\sum_{i \in R_j} \exp(\mathbf{x}_i\boldsymbol{\beta})}\right]$$

This is exactly the same as the contribution of the jth failure time to the partial likelihood in a Cox model. Thus a Cox model can be estimated by splitting the time scale at each death time and fitting a Poisson model incorporating a dummy variable for every interval.

The strategy above covers the situation in which there are no ties. However, if there are time points with multiple failures, the Poisson approach is equivalent to the Cox model with the Breslow adjustment method (sometimes referred to as the Peto method). For more details of the equivalence of the Poisson and Cox models, see Whitehead (1980), Laird and Olivier (1981), and Carstensen (2006).

4.6 Comparing a different number of intervals

We have seen that the Poisson model with a split at each unique failure time gives the Cox model. However, we do not want to fit a model with so many parameters. An important question is, what is the effect of changing the number of time intervals on the parameters of interest (usually log hazard-ratios)? We can investigate this by looping over a number of different time intervals, using `stsplit`, fitting a Poisson model, and storing the results. We can also compare the results with those from a Cox model (equivalent to splitting at the unique failure times) and an exponential model (equivalent to no splitting of the time scale). The code below implements this plan.

```
use rott2, clear
local j 1
foreach split of numlist 0.25 0.5 0.75 1 {
   preserve
   quietly stsplit split_time, every(`split´)
   egen interval = group(split_time)
   generate risktime = _t - _t0
   collapse (min) start`j´=_t0 (max) end`j´ = _t (count) n=_d (sum) ///
      risktime _d, by(interval recent)
   glm _d ibn.interval recent, family(poisson) lnoffset(risktime) nocons
   estimates store  glm_`j´
   predict h`j´, nooffset mu
   replace h`j´ = h`j´*1000
   drop if recent == 1
   keep start`j´ end`i´ h`j´
   save split`j´, replace
   restore
   local j = `j´ + 1
}
quietly stcox recent
estimates store cox
quietly streg recent, dist(exp)
estimates store exp
```

Now we can compare the estimated log hazard-ratios and their SEs.

```
. estimates table cox glm_1 glm_2 glm_3 glm_4 exp, keep(recent) equations(1)
> varwidth(8) b(%6.4fc) se(%6.4fc) modelwidth(8)
```

Variable	cox	glm_1	glm_2	glm_3	glm_4	exp
recent	-0.1705	-0.1704	-0.1707	-0.1705	-0.1703	-0.1289
	0.0527	0.0527	0.0527	0.0527	0.0527	0.0524

legend: b/se

We have tabulated the estimated log hazard-ratio (top row) and its SE (bottom row). Model `glm_1` refers to split time of 0.25 years; `glm_2`, a split of 0.5 years; `glm_3`, a split of 0.75 years; and `glm_4`, a split of 1 year. The estimates of the log hazard-ratio are remarkably similar for all models except the exponential model, differing at the 4th decimal place. Similarly, the estimates of the SE of the log hazard-ratio are identical to 4 decimal places for all models except the exponential. Although the exponential model gives a different estimate, it is not much different; the hazard ratio for the exponential model is 0.88 compared to 0.84 for the other models.

If one is willing to assume PH, in many situations the baseline hazard can be modeled quite poorly without much affecting the estimate of the hazard ratio. There are some exceptions—for example, when follow-up time differs between any groups being compared or when PH is not a reasonable assumption. It is, of course, better to put some effort into modeling the baseline hazard adequately. As we have said already in this book and will say again, PH is often assumed when, in fact, it is not a reasonable assumption. One of our aims is to raise awareness of the issue.

An advantage of using Poisson models is that an estimate of the (log) baseline hazard function is obtained directly. We believe that the shape and the underlying values of the hazard function are of direct interest. Because the Cox model does not directly provide an estimate of the baseline hazard function, we believe that it becomes too easy to forget about the function's underlying shape. Thus it becomes too easy to forget about the impact of the estimated hazard ratios in terms of the absolute risk and differences in risk.

So far, with the Poisson approach we have used only a step function for the baseline hazard. We must decide how many time intervals to choose and where the break points should be located; the time intervals do not necessarily have to be of the same length. A plot of the estimated baseline hazard functions obtained from using different split points can be obtained using the following code:

```
use split1, clear
merge using split2 split3 split4
local h1 "Interval length: 0.25 years"
local h2 "Interval length: 0.5 years"
local h3 "Interval length: 0.75 years"
local h4 "Interval length: 1.0 years"
forvalues i = 1/4 {
   twoway  (pcspike h`i´ start`i´ h`i´ end`i´),  ///
      xtitle(Years from surgery)                 ///
      ytitle("Recurrence rate (1000 PYs)")       ///
      title(`h`i´´) yscale(range(0 200))         ///
      ylabel(0(50)200, angle(h))                 ///
      name(g`i´, replace)
}
graph combine g4 g3 g2 g1, nocopies
```

The resulting plot is shown in figure 4.3.

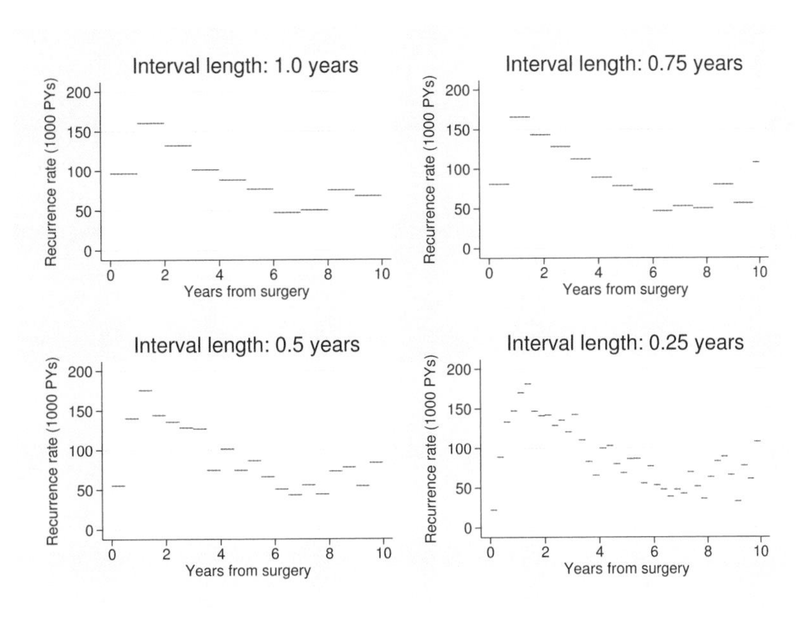

Figure 4.3. Rotterdam breast cancer data. Baseline hazard function estimated using Poisson models with different interval lengths. PYs stands for person-years.

The piecewise nature of the estimates of the hazard function can be clearly seen in these plots. The basic shape of the estimated hazard function is broadly similar in the four different models. However, as the intervals become wider, the shape is flattened. For example, for the intervals of 0.25 years there is considerable variation in the first year (from 22 to 147 recurrences per 1,000 person-years). The variation averages out to about 100 recurrences per 1,000 person-years when the interval length is one year.

Step functions are almost always biologically implausible, and so it makes sense to fit a continuous function, if possible. Categorization of continuous data is often criticized in medical research. Problems include a loss of power, residual confounding, and the inappropriate use of data-driven "optimal" cutpoints, leading to considerable bias (Royston, Altman, and Sauerbrei 2006).

We are initially interested in fitting a smooth function to the baseline hazard, and in chapter 7 we extend the methods to fit continuous time-dependent effects. The two approaches we use are regression splines and FPs.

4.7 Fine splitting of the time scale

We saw in section 4.6 that we can choose how many intervals to have, and thus we can choose how finely to split the time scale. The problem with the piecewise exponential model is that if we choose too few intervals we may miss important changes in the hazard rate; if we choose too many, we end up with too many parameters, and the underlying shape of the hazard rate is difficult to see because of random variation. This effect can be seen in the differing interval lengths in figure 4.3. In the next two sections, we choose very fine split points for the time intervals, but rather than estimating a parameter for each interval, we assume that we can fit a smooth function to approximate a continuous function for the (log) hazard rate. Two possible approaches to estimating smooth functions are splines and FPs. We will explain both of these approaches in detail, but first we show an example using splines to illustrate the basic ideas behind the approach.

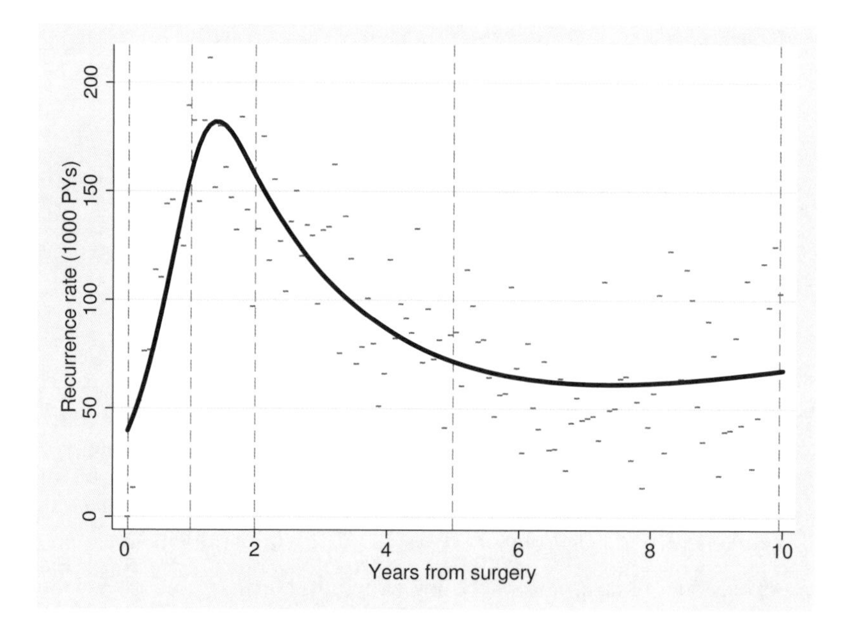

Figure 4.4. Rotterdam breast cancer data. Examples of the use of splines to model the baseline hazard rate with splits every month. The horizontal lines show the piecewise estimates. The vertical lines show the positions of the knots. PYs stands for person-years.

Figure 4.4 shows the baseline hazard rate where the time scale has been split into intervals of length 1 month (that is, 1/12 year), giving 120 intervals in total. Initially, a piecewise model was fit, and thus the estimate of the baseline hazard rate has 120 parameters—one for each interval. The estimates are shown as horizontal dashes in the figure. The dashes appear to indicate that the hazard rate increases to about 1.5

years and then decreases again. There seems to be greater variation in the estimated hazard rate as follow-up time increases, which is unsurprising because the number at risk decreases due to events and censoring. The smooth line is obtained using a restricted cubic spline (explained in more detail below) with only 5 parameters—that is, 115 fewer parameters. The smooth line gives a much more sensible fit from a biological perspective and smooths out most of the random variation seen in the piecewise model. The vertical lines show the position of the knots, which control the general shape and the degree of smoothness of the fitted function. There are more knots earlier on in follow-up because there are more events around this time. Choice of the number and location of knots is an important issue and is discussed further in sections 4.8.4 and 4.8.5.

4.8 Splines: Motivation and definition

We first use splines to model the baseline hazard rate. We assume familiarity with a cubic polynomial function—that is, $y = \beta_0 + \beta_1 x + \beta_2 x^2 + \beta_3 x^3$. We concentrate on cubic splines, which are piecewise cubic polynomials with a separate cubic polynomial fit in a predefined number of intervals. The number of intervals is chosen by the user, with the split points known as *knots*. These functions might be thought rather messy, especially if a large number of intervals was chosen. However, the nice thing about splines is that *continuity restrictions* can be imposed, leading to a smooth fitted function. We now briefly describe what we mean by continuity restrictions by fitting a spline function to estimate the baseline hazard rate to the Rotterdam breast cancer data. The details of these calculations are described in subsequent sections.

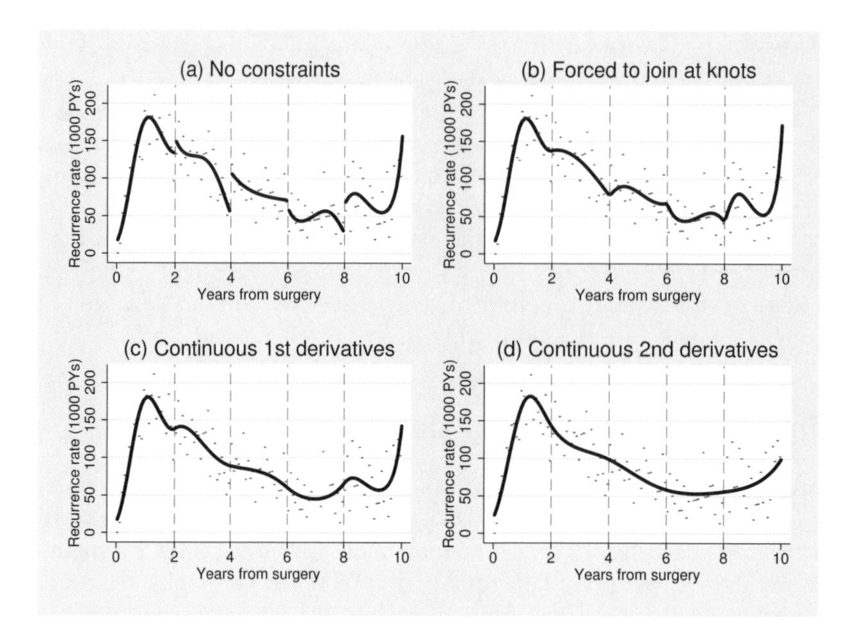

Figure 4.5. Rotterdam breast cancer data. Example of using cubic spline functions with increasingly stringent continuity restrictions. PYs stands for person-years.

Figure 4.5(a) shows the fit of a cubic spline function with no constraints—that is, no continuity restrictions. The vertical lines show the locations of four knots (at 2, 4, 6, and 8 years) that divide the time scale into five intervals. Within each interval, a cubic polynomial function has been fit. This is clearly not a sensible approach because in some intervals there is evidence of overfitting. If we believe that the function changes smoothly over time, we should ensure that our estimated functions join at the knots.

This introduces our first continuity restriction. We still fit cubic polynomials within each interval, but we force the functions to join at the knot locations. This can be seen in figure 4.5(b). There is a slight improvement because at least the function is now continuous. However, the function has a number of kinks and sharp turning points, and we do not really believe that the "true" function would have these kinks and turning points. By using a different number or different locations of the knots, the kinks and turning points are likely to occur in different places.

We thus introduce a second continuity restriction: as well as forcing the function to join at the knots, we also force the first derivative of the spline functions to agree at the knots. The first derivative is the gradient of the function, and thus we hope to remove the kinks and bumps. The fitted function that results from introducing this further continuity restriction can be seen in figure 4.5(c). The fitted function is much better and is clearly smoother. However, suppose that the vertical lines showing the knot positions were removed; one could probably guess where at least two of the knots were located. This is not desirable, and so we introduce a final continuity restriction.

As well as forcing the function and the first derivatives to agree at the knots, the final continuity restriction is to force the second derivative to agree at the knots. The second derivative is the rate of change in the gradient, and thus the function should become even smoother. We can see this in figure 4.5(d), where the fitted function is much smoother and truly does look continuous.

There are methods that treat both the number and the location of the knots as unknowns (DiMatteo, Genovese, and Kass 2001), but we consider only functions where the number and location of knots are specified in advance. The advantage is that one can estimate flexible nonlinear functions within any regression model that includes a linear predictor. We show that as long as there are enough knots, having a few extra knots or placing the knots in different places is generally not critical in the sense that it does not much alter the fitted curve.

4.8.1 Calculating splines*

We first describe calculating splines in general, but in what follows, we use restricted cubic splines, as discussed in section 4.8.2. When we use cubic splines to fit a continuous function, we have to calculate some new variables. This is analogous to creating x^2 and x^3 from x when fitting a cubic polynomial. With splines, the calculations of these transformed variables is more complex, but Stata commands already exist to do these calculations for you.

Let $s(x)$ denote a nonlinear spline function of order N for covariate x, with K knots at $k_1 < \cdots < k_K$. We can write the spline function, $s(x)$, with no continuity restrictions as follows:

$$s(x) = \sum_{j=0}^{n} \beta_{0j} x^j + \sum_{i=1}^{K} \sum_{j=0}^{N} \beta_{ij} (x - k_i)_+^j$$

Note the use of the "+" notation, where

$$u_+ = \begin{cases} u & \text{if } u > 0 \\ 0 & \text{if } u \leq 0 \end{cases}$$

If $s_{(j)}$ denotes the jth derivative of $s(x)$, then the presence of a $\beta_{ij} (x - k_i)_+^j$ term allows a discontinuity at knot k_i for $s_{(j)}$, and its absence forces the continuity of $s_{(j)}$ at k_i.

Cubic splines ($N = 3$) are the most common type of spline used in practice. Higher degree polynomials are generally not needed, because if there were a complicated shape between knots (for example, with more than two turning points), then further knots could be added rather than fitting a higher degree polynomial. A cubic spline can be written as

$$s(x) = \sum_{j=0}^{3} \beta_{0j} x^j + \sum_{i=1}^{K} \beta_{i3} (x - k_i)_+^3$$

Thus the number of parameters in a standard regression spline model is $K + 4$.

Regression splines are part of the large family of smoothing methods encompassed by the general term "splines". Sometimes regression splines are expressed using alternative formulations that are more computationally efficient. The most common of these are B-splines, which are described as being "nearly orthogonal" (de Boor 2001). A related nonparametric technique uses smoothing splines (Silverman 1985). The difference between regression splines and smoothing splines is mainly in the choice of knots. With regression splines, a fixed, relatively small number of knots is chosen; whereas with smoothing splines, each data point is taken as a knot, and a penalty term is included in the likelihood to control the smoothness of the fitted curve. Fitting smoothing splines requires relatively complex, nonstandard estimation algorithms. We favor the simplicity of regression splines because it is straightforward to incorporate them in the linear predictor of any regression model without special programming efforts.

4.8.2 Restricted cubic splines

In this book, we mainly use restricted cubic splines, which are a simple extension of the cubic splines defined above. The difference is that the function is forced (restricted) to be linear before the first knot and after the last knot. The first and last knots are known as the *boundary knots*. By default, when modeling survival time, we define the boundary knots as the minimum and maximum of the uncensored survival times. However, as we show, knot location is usually not particularly crucial. All we need to do to fit a restricted cubic spline function for a covariate x is to include new variables in the linear predictor. The new variables are transformations of x. Let $s(x)$ be the restricted cubic spline function. If we define m interior knots, $k_1, \ldots, k_m$, and also our two boundary knots, $k_{\min}$ and $k_{\max}$, we can write $s(x)$ as a function of parameters $\boldsymbol{\gamma}$ and some newly created variables $z_1, \ldots, z_{m+1}$, giving

$$s(x) = \gamma_0 + \gamma_1 z_1 + \gamma_2 z_2 + \cdots + \gamma_{m+1} z_{m+1}$$

We calculate the derived variables z_j (also known as the basis functions) as follows

$$\begin{aligned} z_1 &= x \\ z_j &= (x - k_j)_+^3 - \lambda_j (x - k_{\min})_+^3 - (1 - \lambda_j)(x - k_{\max})_+^3 \end{aligned}$$

where for $j = 2, \ldots, m+1$,

$$\lambda_j = \frac{k_{\max} - k_j}{k_{\max} - k_{\min}}$$

These functions are programmed in various Stata commands, including `mkspline`, `splinegen`, and `rcsgen`. `mkspline` is an official Stata command, while the other two are user-written commands. We make use of the `rcsgen` command because it can orthogonalize the derived spline variables. Orthogonalization can lead to more stable parameter estimates and quicker model convergence, and it can promote convergence in complex models. `rcsgen` is also the program used by `stpm2` when fitting the Royston–Parmar (RP) models described in chapter 5.

Figure 4.4 depicted restricted cubic splines. The boundary knots are at the minimum and maximum event times, and thus the linearity restriction is beyond the observed data. Restricted cubic splines tend to give more believable estimates in the tails of the distribution where data are often sparse. For example, compare the restricted cubic spline estimates in figure 4.4 with the standard spline estimates in figure 4.5(d). The restricted cubic splines are less influenced by the rise in the piecewise estimates in the last few intervals.

4.8.3 Splines: Application to the Rotterdam data

In this section, we apply restricted cubic splines within the Poisson approach to modeling the baseline hazard function for the Rotterdam breast cancer data. The extension from the piecewise models described in section 4.3.1 is simple. Rather than having a few wide intervals, we define a large number of narrow intervals and use a restricted cubic spline to model the baseline hazard function. Because we have a large number of intervals, we collapse the data as described in section 4.3. We start by defining the interval length to be 1 month. Because there are 10 years of follow-up, there is a maximum of 120 observations per subject, corresponding to an individual censored at 10 years. We can `stsplit` and `collapse` the data as follows:

```
. use rott2, clear
(Rotterdam breast cancer data, truncated at 10 years)
. stsplit split_time, every(`=1/12')
(193415 observations (episodes) created)
. generate risktime = _t - _t0
. collapse (min) start=_t0 (max) end = _t (count) n=_d (sum) risktime _d,
> by(split_time recent)
```

We use the option `every('=1/12')` in the `stsplit` command because the survival times are stored in years. We now generate the spline variables:

```
. generate midt = (start + end)/2
. rcsgen midt, df(4) gen(t_rcs) fw(_d) orthog
Variables t_rcs1 to t_rcs4 were created
. local knots `r(knots)'
```

We initially generated the midtime of each interval (`midt`) and then calculated the derived spline basis variables using `rcsgen`. We used four degrees of freedom (d.f.) by specifying the `df(4)` option, which equates to using five knots (three interior and two boundary knots). By default, these would be placed at the minimum and maximum and at the 25th, 50th, and 75th centiles of the variable `midt`. This is not sensible because we collapsed the data, and so we need to give appropriate weights. By using the `fw(_d)` option, we inform the `rcsgen` command how many deaths occurred in each interval. Thus the knots are located at the minimum and maximum and at the 25th, 50th, and 75th centiles of the uncensored survival times. We explore alternative knots in sections 4.8.4 and 4.8.5. Four new variables, `t_rcs1` through `t_rcs4`, are created.

We fit a Poisson model as before, but now we include the restricted cubic-spline basis variables:

```
. glm _d t_rcs1-t_rcs4 recent, family(poisson) lnoffset(risktime) nolog
> noheader
```

_d	Coef.	OIM Std. Err.	z	P>|z|	[95% Conf.	Interval]
t_rcs1	-.2591163	.037429	-6.92	0.000	-.3324758	-.1857567
t_rcs2	.0124319	.0338071	0.37	0.713	-.0538287	.0786926
t_rcs3	-.2459847	.0248115	-9.91	0.000	-.2946143	-.1973551
t_rcs4	.0139823	.0256243	0.55	0.585	-.0362405	.0642051
recent	-.1725334	.0526506	-3.28	0.001	-.2757267	-.06934
_cons	-2.484828	.0438392	-56.68	0.000	-2.570752	-2.398905
ln(risktime)	1	(exposure)				

We first look at the parameter estimate for `recent`. The hazard ratio is $\exp(-0.173)$, which gives 0.84, very similar to the number obtained from the Cox and the piecewise models. Although the coefficients for the individual spline terms are not interpretable, we can obtain an estimate of `lh1`, the predicted log baseline hazard function, as follows:

```
. generate lh1 = -2.485 + 0.259*t_rcs1 + 0.012*t_rcs2 - 0.246*t_rcs3 + 0.014*t_rcs4
```

However, it is much simpler to use the `predict` command. With the `predict` command, the offset is included by default in the linear predictor, so we need to include the `nooffset` option:

```
. predict lh2, xb nooffset
. predict lh2_se, stdp
. generate h = exp(lh2)*1000
. generate h_lci = exp(lh2 - 1.96*lh2_se)*1000
. generate h_uci = exp(lh2 + 1.96*lh2_se)*1000
```

We have also calculated the SE of the log hazard-rate, transformed to the hazard rate scale, and calculated a CI. We multiply the hazard rate by 1,000 to make interpretation easier, because this gives the rate of recurrence or death due to breast cancer per 1,000 person-years. Having obtained the hazard rate, we can now plot it (see figure 4.6).

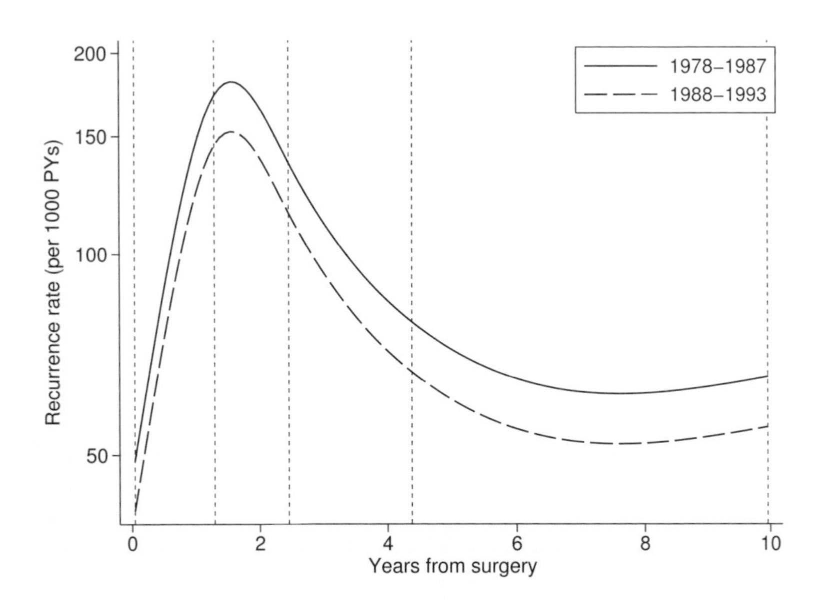

Figure 4.6. Rotterdam breast cancer data. Poisson PH model for `recent` with restricted cubic spline for the baseline hazard function. Knot positions are shown as vertical dashed lines. PYs stands for person-years.

We can now see the difference in the hazard rates between the two groups. There is a lower hazard rate in the more recent period. Also shown are the locations of the knots. The knot locations are closer together earlier in the time scale, which is indicative of the usual positively skewed distribution of survival data. Plotting the hazard function in both groups also demonstrates the assumption of PH in that the distance between the two lines (on the log scale) is the same throughout the time scale. We should not, of course, conclude that PH is a reasonable assumption from this plot because our model assumes PH, and thus predictions from the model force the hazard rates to be proportional.

It is also helpful to plot the hazard function with a CI to avoid potential overinterpretation in small datasets. The baseline hazard function (that is, at `recent==0`) with a 95% CI is shown in figure 4.7. The CI shows that the large rise and fall of the hazard rate is extremely unlikely to be due to chance, but that we should not necessarily believe the small rise in the hazard rate toward the end of follow-up.

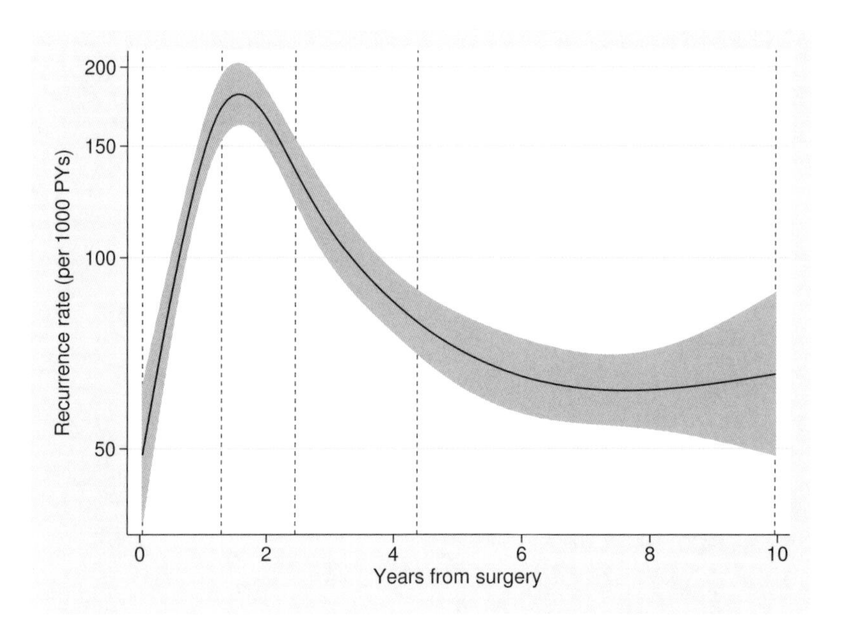

Figure 4.7. Rotterdam breast cancer data. Poisson PH model for `recent` with restricted cubic spline for the baseline hazard function. Knot positions are shown as vertical dashed lines. The curve is the estimated baseline hazard function with a 95% pointwise CI. PYs stands for person-years.

Let us review what we have done here. We have fit a PH survival model, which gives us the same estimate and 95% CI for `recent` as a Cox model. In addition, we have obtained an estimate of the baseline hazard rate, together with a 95% CI. Thus when estimating the hazard ratio, we can see directly what the relative increase or decrease is relative to. It is possible to estimate the fitted hazard rates after fitting a Cox model. For example, in Stata, you can use the `stcurve` command to plot the estimated hazard rate for any covariate pattern. The estimated hazard rate is obtained using a kernel-density smoothing method. Our view is that if you are interested in the estimated underlying hazard rate (and in most cases you should be), it makes more sense to estimate it directly in a parametric model. Further disadvantages of a nonparametric method, such as kernel density estimation, are that predictions are difficult to obtain and the model cannot be described succinctly.

4.8.4 Varying the number of knots

We have fit a spline function with four knots, but what happens if we choose a different number of knots? We can easily fit a number of different models with different d.f. using a loop. The following code does that:

```
forvalues i = 2 / 8 {
   rcsgen midt, df(`i') gen(t`i'_rcs) fw(_d) orthog
   local knots `r(knots)'
   glm _d t`i'_rcs* recent, family(poisson) lnoffset(risktime) nolog noheader
   estimates store df`i'
   estat ic, n(1477)
   local AIC`i': display %6.1f `= el(r(S),1,5)'
   predict h_df`i', mu nooffset
   replace h_df`i' = h_df`i'*1000
   local legend `legend' `=`i'-1' `"`i' df: AIC =  `AIC`i''"'
}
twoway (line h_df* midt if recent == 0, sort),          ///
   scheme(sj)                                           ///
   xtitle("Years from surgery")                         ///
   ytitle("Recurrence rate (per 1000 PYs)")             ///
   ylabel(0(50)200, angle(horizontal) format(%3.0f))    ///
   legend(order(`legend') ring(0) col(1) pos(1) size(*1))
```

Figure 4.8 shows the estimated baseline hazard function for the Rotterdam data with between 1 and 7 interior knots (2–8 d.f.) for follow-up time.

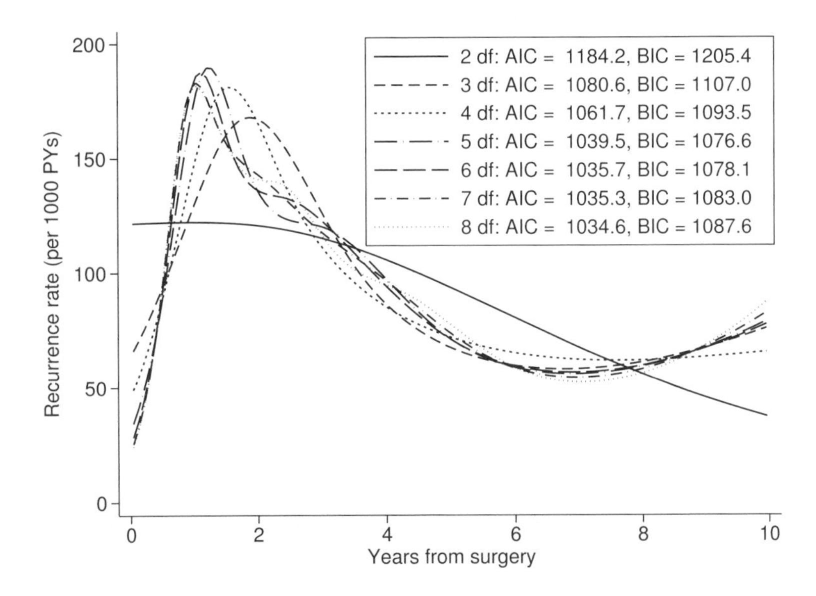

Figure 4.8. Rotterdam breast cancer data. Effect of varying the number of knots in the spline function on the estimated baseline hazard function. PYs stands for person-years.

The fitted curve for the model with 2 d.f. (1 interior knot) is noticeably different from that of the other models. The shape of the hazard function is similar for the other models, but there is some disagreement over the time at which the hazard function reaches its highest point. Two important questions are a) can (and should) we choose the "best-fitting" model?, and b) does model choice affect the estimate of the hazard ratio (and its SE)? The lowest AIC is for the model with 8 d.f. (7 interior knots). The parameters are many, and visually there is little difference among the estimated baseline hazard rates with 6 or more d.f. The BIC selects a simpler model with 6 d.f. because extra parameters carry a greater penalty. We can compare the parameter estimates and SEs for `recent` among different models using `estimates table` because we have stored the model estimates using `estimates store`.

```
. estimates table df*, keep(recent) b(%4.3f) se(%5.4f) varw(6)
```

Variable	df2	df3	df4	df5	df6	df7	df8
recent	-0.181 0.0526	-0.171 0.0527	-0.173 0.0527	-0.171 0.0527	-0.171 0.0527	-0.171 0.0527	-0.171 0.0527

```
legend: b/se
```

The estimated log hazard-ratios are very similar among the models, even for the model with 2 d.f.; the SE of the log hazard-ratios are identical for models with 3 or more d.f. If we are only interested in the hazard ratio, the complexity of the baseline hazard function does not appear to be crucial, at least in this example (and in many others we have encountered).

Often a better fitting model can be obtained by working with the log of follow-up time. Royston (2000) showed that when a variable is positively skewed (as survival time usually is), a spline function on the log transformed scale will generally provide a better fit than a spline function on the untransformed scale for models with the same number of d.f. The code is similar to that used for the splines on the untransformed scale above.

```
generate lnt = ln(midt)
forvalues i = 2 / 8 {
   rcsgen lnt, df(`i´) gen(lnt`i´_rcs) fw(_d) orthog
   glm _d lnt`i´_rcs* recent, family(poisson) lnoffset(risktime) nolog noheader
   estimates store ln_df`i´
   estat ic, n(1477)
   local AIC`i´: display %6.1f `= el(r(S),1,5)´
   local BIC`i´: display %6.1f `= el(r(S),1,6)´
   predict h_ln_df`i´, mu nooffset
   replace h_ln_df`i´ = h_ln_df`i´*1000
   local ln_legend `ln_legend´ `=`i´-1´ `"`i´ df: AIC =  `AIC`i´´, BIC = `BIC`i´´"´
}
```

Figure 4.9 shows the fitted values where splines have been calculated for ln(_t).

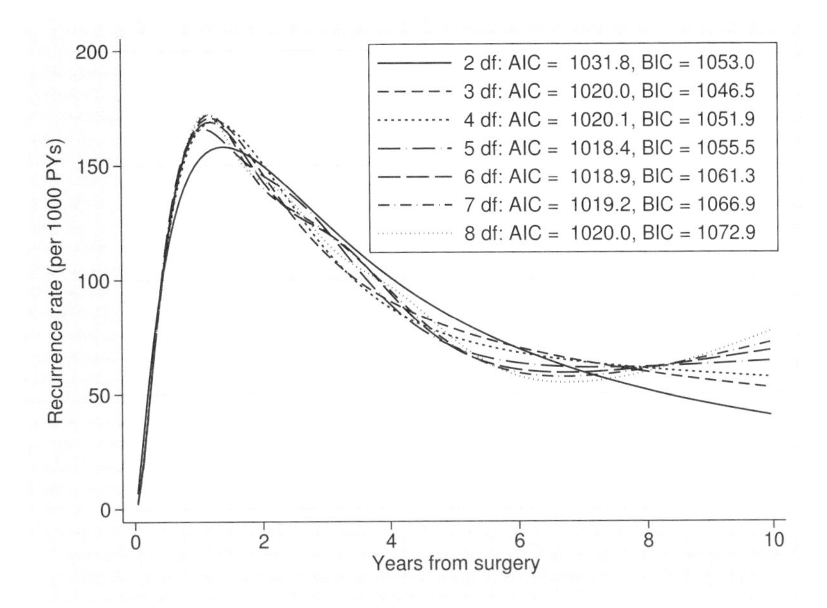

Figure 4.9. Rotterdam breast cancer data. Spline models for the baseline hazard fit on the scale of log time. PYs stands for person-years.

There is closer agreement among the models on the log transformed time scale. Even the model with only one interior knot (2 d.f.) agrees fairly well with the more complex models. There is less variation in the time at which the peak of the hazard rate occurs. The model with 5 d.f. for the baseline hazard has the lowest AIC, and it requires fewer parameters than when modeling on the untransformed scale. However, the AICs from 3 d.f. or more are all broadly similar. The lowest BIC is for the model with 3 d.f., compared with 6 d.f. for the untransformed time scale. We can use `estimates table` again to compare the log hazard-ratios.

```
. estimates table ln_df*, keep(recent) b(%4.3f) se(%5.4f) varw(6)
```

Variable	ln_df2	ln_df3	ln_df4	ln_df5	ln_df6	ln_df7	ln_df8
recent	-0.187 0.0525	-0.177 0.0526	-0.175 0.0526	-0.173 0.0526	-0.172 0.0527	-0.172 0.0527	-0.171 0.0527

legend: b/se

The estimate of the log hazard-ratio for `recent` and its SE are very similar to each other and to those in all the previous analyses. However, the models with fewer d.f. actually have a lower AIC and BIC than all of those obtained when fitting splines on the untransformed time scale. In fact, the spline model with only one interior knot on the log time scale gives a lower AIC and BIC than all of the spline models on the untransformed time scale. This behavior is consistent with the recommendation of Royston (2000) and is also one of the reasons why RP models (described in chapter 5) incorporate splines in $\ln t$ rather than in t.

4.8.5 Varying the location of the knots

A further important question is whether the location of knots has an impact on the shape of the estimated hazard function and the parameter estimates of interest. To investigate this question, we fit a model with 6 knots (4 interior and 2 boundary knots); each knot was selected randomly within a range of percentiles defined in table 4.1. We generate the restricted cubic splines variables in $\ln t$ because of the improved fit seen in the previous section. The following routine fits 10 different models where the percentiles are randomly sampled according to those knots defined in table 4.1.

```
forvalues i = 1 / 10 {
    local p1 = 0 + int(runiform()* 6)
    local p2 = 6 + int(runiform()*20)
    local p3 = 26 + int(runiform()*25)
    local p4 = 51 + int(runiform()*25)
    local p5 = 76 + int(runiform()*20)
    local p6 = 96 + int(runiform()*5)
    rcsgen lnt, p(`p1´ `p2´ `p3´ `p4´ `p5´ `p6´) gen(trnd`i´_rcs) ///
        orthog fw(_d)
    glm _d trnd`i´_rcs* recent, family(poisson) lnoffset(risktime)
    predict h_rnd`i´, mu nooffset
    replace h_rnd`i´ = h_rnd`i´*1000
}
```

Table 4.1. Locations of randomly selected knots. Range refers to the centiles of the uncensored log event times.

Knot	Range
1	0th–5th
2	6th–25th
3	26th–50th
4	51st–75th
5	76th–95th
6	96th–100th

Figure 4.10 shows the estimated hazard function from the 10 different models using these random knot locations. There is very little difference in the fitted values. The greatest difference is toward the end of follow-up, which is to be expected given there are fewer events in that region. The log hazard-ratios from the 10 different models were very similar, ranging between -0.1733 and -0.1708.

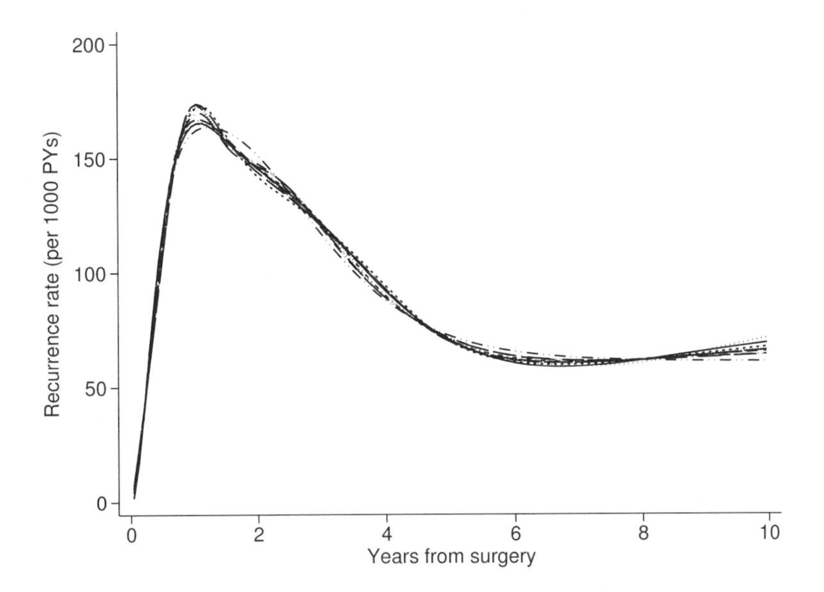

Figure 4.10. Rotterdam breast cancer data. Estimated hazard functions from 10 different models with random knot locations. PYs stands for person-years.

4.8.6 Estimating the survival function*

One of the advantages of modeling the baseline hazard function is that other useful functions can be obtained by transforming the model parameters. We often wish to obtain the predicted survival function for a particular covariate pattern. The approach we adopt to estimating the survival functions in Poisson models is based on that of Carstensen (2006) and can be summarized as follows:

1. Select the time points at which we want to calculate the survival function—for example, 200 equally spaced time points.
2. For a particular covariate pattern, predict the log hazard-rate at each of the above time points.
3. Exponentiate to obtain the estimated hazard function.
4. Compute the cumulative sum of the hazard function to get an estimate of the cumulative hazard function.
5. Use the relationship between the cumulative hazard and survival functions—that is, $S(t) = \exp\{-H(t)\}$—to estimate the survival function.

It is also possible to calculate a CI by applying the delta method to obtain an estimate of the variance of the cumulative hazard. We skip the mathematical details here and refer the reader to the work of Carstensen (2006).

The calculations make use of the matrix facilities in Mata. The code below calculates the survival function with a 95% CI for the Rotterdam breast cancer data when `recent=0`. The location of the knots is stored after using `rcsgen` in a macro using `local knots 'r(knots)'`.

```
preserve
drop _all
range plottime 0 5 200
rcsgen plottime, knots(`knots') gen(t_rcs)
mata
X = st_data((1,200), ("t_rcs1", "t_rcs2", "t_rcs3", "t_rcs4"))
X = X,J(200,1,0), J(200,1,1)
V = st_matrix("e(V)")
b = st_matrix("e(b)")'
h = exp(X*b)
L = lowertriangle(J(200,200,5/200),5/200)
ch = L*exp(X*b)
var_ch = L*(diag(h)*(b'*V*b)*diag(h)')*L'
st_store(., st_addvar("double", "predsurv"),exp(-ch))
st_store(., st_addvar("double", "predsurv_uci"), exp(-ch - sqrt(diagonal(var_ch))))
st_store(., st_addvar("double", "predsurv_lci"), exp(-ch + sqrt(diagonal(var_ch))))
end
twoway (rarea predsurv_lci predsurv_uci plottime, pstyle(ci)) ///
   (line predsurv plottime, clpattern(solid)),              ///
   legend(off)                                              ///
   xtitle("Years from surgery")                             ///
   ytitle("Survival")                                       ///
   ylabel(0(0.2)1, angle(h) format(%3.1f))
restore
```

The main trick in the code is to define a lower triangular matrix, `L`, which is used to sum the estimates of the hazard function and thus to obtain the cumulative hazard function. The resulting plot can be seen in figure 4.11.

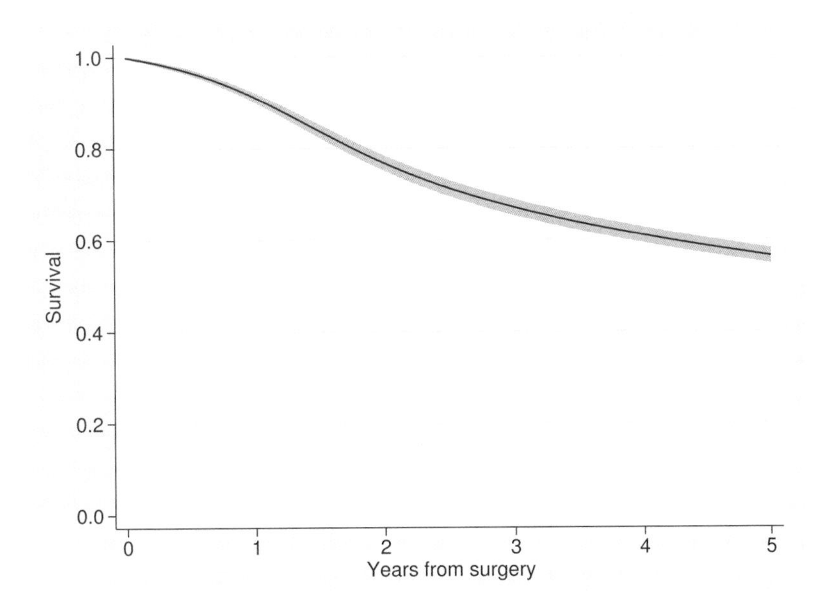

Figure 4.11. Rotterdam breast cancer data. Estimated relapse-free survival function with a 95% CI for `recent=0` from a Poisson model.

We acknowledge that the calculations are awkward for a novice user. Deriving the survival function and other useful functions is much easier for the RP models described in chapter 5.

4.9 FPs: Motivation and definition

An alternative to splines for modeling the baseline hazard function is FPs (Royston and Sauerbrei 2008). FPs are an extension of standard polynomials that greatly increase the flexibility available to model nonlinear relationships. The basic idea is to allow negative and noninteger powers, as well as the standard linear, quadratic, and cubic terms. Historically, analysts have either fitted quadratic or higher order polynomials; or they have applied a simple ad hoc transformation, such as $\log(x)$ or $\sqrt{x}$. Less often, they have used $1/x$ or, occasionally, some other power of x. The idea of a "ladder of powers" is to be found in the early works of John Tukey (Tukey 1957). With FPs, a set of powers, $S = \{-2, -1, -0.5, 0, 0.5, 1, 2, 3\}$, is defined. One or more of these power transformations of covariates are selected to include in the linear predictor. Power 0 means the natural log (ln) transformation in the present context. The set S is the set of powers originally defined by Royston and Altman (Royston and Altman 1994). Subsequent experience has confirmed that they are good enough for most practical situations, and a refinement or extension has not proved necessary.

First-order fractional polynomial (FP1) models include just one term, p_1, from the defined set S. Examples of FPs include standard polynomials—for example, a quadratic function

$$y = \beta_0 + \beta_1 x + \beta_2 x^2$$

Added flexibility is obtained by incorporating other powers—for example,

$$y = \beta_0 + \beta_1 x^{-2} + \beta_2 x^{0.5}$$

The functions above are both second-order fractional polynomial (FP2) models because they incorporate two fractional polynomials terms. A general FP2 model with powers p_1 and p_2 can be written as

$$y = \beta_0 + \beta_1 x^{p_1} + \beta_2 x^{p_2}$$

A further important refinement is the inclusion of "repeated powers"; by letting $p_1 = p_2 = p$, one arrives at the FP2 model

$$y = \beta_0 + \beta_1 x^p + \beta_2 x^p \ln x$$

An FPm model includes up to m powers from S, some or all of which may be repeated. For example, the function third-order fractional polynomial FP3$(-1, 2, 2)$ involves two powers from S (that is, -1 and 2), one of which (that is, 2) is repeated:

$$y = \beta_0 + \beta_1 x^{-1} + \beta_2 x^2 + \beta_2 x^2 \ln x$$

The flexibility of FP2 functions is illustrated schematically in figure 4.12. Four different FP2 functions demonstrate the variety of shapes available with a few combinations of p_1 and p_2.

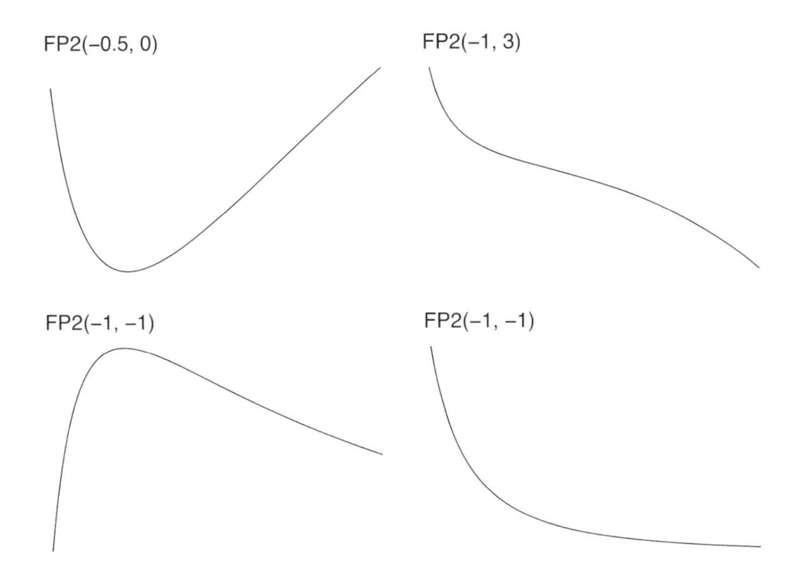

Figure 4.12. Schematic plots of possible curve shapes of four FP2 functions.

The best-fitting FPm model is the one that minimizes the deviance. It is possible to compare FP models of a different complexity using a likelihood-ratio test or by comparison of AIC or BIC. For more details of FPs, see Royston and Sauerbrei (2008).

Like splines, FP can be used for any statistical model with a linear predictor. Thus FPs are an extremely powerful tool for modeling nonlinear relationships for a wide range of models used in practice.

4.9.1 Application to Rotterdam data

We first need to split and collapse the data in the same way as for the restricted cubic spline models.

```
. use rott2
(Rotterdam breast cancer data, truncated at 10 years)
. stsplit split_time, every(`=1/12')
(193415 observations (episodes) created)
. generate risktime = _t - _t0
. collapse (min) start=_t0 (max) end = _t (count) n=_d (sum) risktime _d,
> by(split_time recent)
. generate midt = (start + end)/2
```

We start by fitting an FP3 model, which can be implemented using the `fracpoly` command as shown below:

```
. fracpoly, degree(3) compare: glm _d midt recent, family(poisson)
> lnoffset(risktime) noheader
.............................................
-> gen double Imidt__1 = midt^-1-.1999999944 if e(sample)
-> gen double Imidt__2 = midt^2-25.0000014 if e(sample)
-> gen double Imidt__3 = midt^2*ln(midt)-40.23595077 if e(sample)
Iteration 0:   log likelihood = -523.39834
Iteration 1:   log likelihood = -500.74292
Iteration 2:   log likelihood = -499.41425
Iteration 3:   log likelihood = -499.40544
Iteration 4:   log likelihood = -499.40544
```

_d	Coef.	OIM Std. Err.	z	P>|z|	[95% Conf.	Interval]
Imidt__1	-.3758894	.0452224	-8.31	0.000	-.4645237	-.2872551
Imidt__2	-.1372148	.0137249	-10.00	0.000	-.1641152	-.1103144
Imidt__3	.0548142	.006137	8.93	0.000	.0427859	.0668425
recent	-.1707984	.0526714	-3.24	0.001	-.2740325	-.0675644
_cons	-2.619828	.0571856	-45.81	0.000	-2.73191	-2.507746
ln(risktime)	1	(exposure)				

```
Deviance:   998.81. Best powers of midt among 164 models fit: -1 2 2.
Fractional polynomial model comparisons:
```

midt	df	Deviance	Dev. dif.	P (*)	Powers
Not in model	0	1279.124	280.313	0.000	
Linear	1	1188.712	189.901	0.000	1
m = 1	2	1180.153	181.342	0.000	2
m = 2	4	1014.713	15.902	0.000	-.5 0
m = 3	6	998.811	—	—	-1 2 2

```
(*) P-value from deviance difference comparing reported model with m = 3 model
```

The `fracpoly` command is a prefix command. The `degree(3)` option of `fracpoly` requests an FP3 model to be fit, and the `compare` option also shows the best-fitting FP1 and FP2 models, as well as formally testing for differences between the models. The output shows that the best-fitting FP3 model has powers $(-1, 2, 2)$. This is the best-fitting of 164 different FP models. Three new derived variables have been created (`Imidt__1`, `Imidt__2`, and `Imidt__3`), one for each of the three power terms. These variables are then included in the final model. Because 2 is a repeated power, `Imidt__3` is a combination of a squared and a ln function of `midt`, as explained in section 4.9. Also the derived powers have a constant subtracted. This constant is actually the mean of the derived variable because this is the default behavior of `fracpoly` (see also section 4.11 of Royston and Sauerbrei [2008]). The next part of the output shows the parameter estimates, SEs, etc., of the best fitting model. The log hazard-ratio for `recent` is the same as we observed with the spline models in section 4.8.3. This is not surprising, because all we are doing is modeling the baseline hazard function in a different way.

The final table in the output shows the deviances of the null, linear, FP1, FP2, and FP3 models. The best fitting of the 8 FP1 model has power (2), and the best fitting of the 36 FP2 model has powers $(-0.5, 0)$. All p-values in the comparison table relate to a comparison with the FP3 model. The d.f. for the FP models is double the number of power terms included. The reason is that there is 1 d.f. for the variable and there is 1 d.f. for the selected power. See section 4.9.1 of Royston and Sauerbrei (2008) for more details. Informally, it is clear that the FP3 model gives the best fit; its deviance is 15.90 lower than that of the best FP2 model ($P < 0.001$, according to a χ^2 test on 2 d.f.). See section 4.9.3 for discussion of how an FP model is formally chosen.

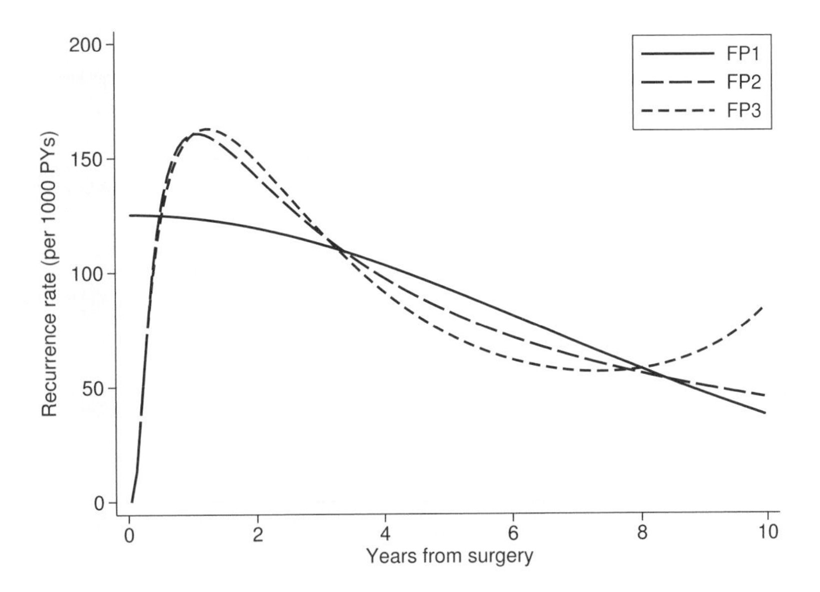

Figure 4.13. Rotterdam breast cancer data. Estimated baseline hazard function for best-fitting FP1, FP2, and FP3 models. PYs stands for person-years.

To plot the baseline hazard for the FP3 model, we need to obtain predictions, which can be done in a similar way to using splines, as shown in the code below:

```
. predict lh_fp3, nooffset xb
. predict lh_fp3_se, nooffset stdp
. generate h_fp3 = exp(lh_fp3)*1000
. generate h_fp3_lci = exp(lh_fp3 - 1.96*lh_fp3_se)*1000
. generate h_fp3_uci = exp(lh_fp3 + 1.96*lh_fp3_se)*1000
```

If we want to compare the fitted values of the FP3 model with the best-fitting FP2 and FP1 models, then we need to refit these latter two models. Specific FP models with predefined power can be fit using `fracpoly` by listing the power terms after the covariate. This is done in the code below:

```
. fracpoly: glm _d midt -0.5 0 recent, family(poisson) lnoffset(risktime)
> noheader
-> gen double Imidt__1 = midt^-0.5-.4472135892 if e(sample)
-> gen double Imidt__2 = ln(midt)-1.609437941 if e(sample)
Iteration 0:   log likelihood = -529.61883
Iteration 1:   log likelihood = -507.95839
Iteration 2:   log likelihood = -507.35691
Iteration 3:   log likelihood = -507.35636
Iteration 4:   log likelihood = -507.35636

------------------------------------------------------------------------------
             |                 OIM
          _d |      Coef.   Std. Err.      z    P>|z|     [95% Conf. Interval]
-------------+----------------------------------------------------------------
    Imidt__1 |   -3.01495   .2683118   -11.24   0.000    -3.540832   -2.489069
    Imidt__2 |  -1.446375   .1111769   -13.01   0.000    -1.664278   -1.228473
      recent |  -.1819141    .052479    -3.47   0.001     -.284771   -.0790572
       _cons |  -2.492186   .0458393   -54.37   0.000    -2.582029   -2.402343
ln(risktime) |          1  (exposure)
------------------------------------------------------------------------------
Deviance:  1014.71.
. predict lh_fp2, nooffset xb
. generate h_fp2 = exp(lh_fp2)*1000
. fracpoly: glm _d midt 2 recent, family(poisson) lnoffset(risktime) noheader
-> gen double Imidt__1 = midt^2-25.0000014 if e(sample)
Iteration 0:   log likelihood = -603.65168
Iteration 1:   log likelihood = -590.09734
Iteration 2:   log likelihood = -590.07637
Iteration 3:   log likelihood = -590.07637

------------------------------------------------------------------------------
             |                 OIM
          _d |      Coef.   Std. Err.      z    P>|z|     [95% Conf. Interval]
-------------+----------------------------------------------------------------
    Imidt__1 |  -.0121371   .0013116    -9.25   0.000    -.0147078   -.0095665
      recent |  -.1793875   .0525381    -3.41   0.001    -.2823602   -.0764147
       _cons |  -2.380886   .0404796   -58.82   0.000    -2.460225   -2.301548
ln(risktime) |          1  (exposure)
------------------------------------------------------------------------------
Deviance:  1180.15.
. predict lh_fp1, nooffset xb
. generate h_fp1 = exp(lh_fp1)*1000
```

Figure 4.13 shows the estimated baseline hazard rate from the best-fitting FP1, FP2, and FP3 models. The fit of the FP3 model is similar to that obtained with splines (see figure 4.7). The FP1 model is clearly inadequate.

The estimated baseline hazard with 95% pointwise CIs is plotted in figure 4.14. It shows a curve resembling that from a restricted cubic spline function for the baseline hazard (as shown in figure 4.7), but with a more noticeable upturn toward the end of the follow-up period.

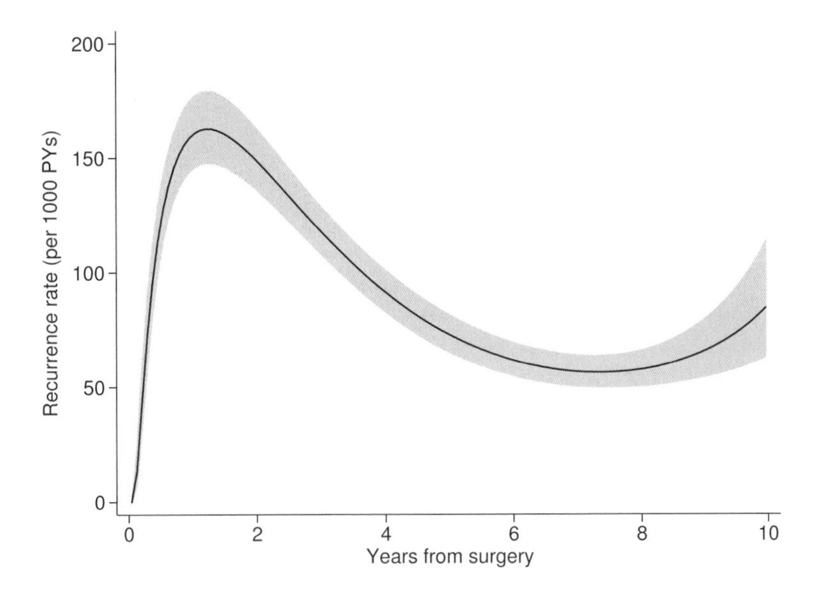

Figure 4.14. Rotterdam breast cancer data. Fitted baseline hazard function with pointwise 95% CI from an FP3 model. PYs stands for person-years.

4.9.2 Higher order FP models

It is, of course, possible to fit higher order FP models, but our experience of modeling the baseline hazard is that it is rarely necessary to go beyond an FP3 model. An FP4 model can be fit using the `degree(4)` when using `fracpoly` as shown below:

```
. fracpoly, degree(4): glm _d midt recent, family(poisson) lnoffset(risktime)
> noheader
.....................................................................
> ..................................................................
> .......
-> gen double Imidt__1 = midt^-.5-.4472135892 if e(sample)
-> gen double Imidt__2 = ln(midt)-1.609437941 if e(sample)
-> gen double Imidt__3 = midt^3-125.0000105 if e(sample)
-> gen double Imidt__4 = midt^3*ln(midt)-201.1797595 if e(sample)
Iteration 0:   log likelihood = -513.38173
Iteration 1:   log likelihood = -499.85372
Iteration 2:   log likelihood = -499.13723
Iteration 3:   log likelihood = -499.13564
Iteration 4:   log likelihood = -499.13564
```

_d	Coef.	OIM Std. Err.	z	P>|z|	[95% Conf.	Interval]
Imidt__1	-2.600424	.4687359	-5.55	0.000	-3.519129	-1.681718
Imidt__2	-1.132209	.2634774	-4.30	0.000	-1.648615	-.6158024
Imidt__3	-.0112465	.0039164	-2.87	0.004	-.0189224	-.0035705
Imidt__4	.0050288	.0016444	3.06	0.002	.0018059	.0082518
recent	-.1705701	.0526809	-3.24	0.001	-.2738229	-.0673174
_cons	-2.604785	.0557502	-46.72	0.000	-2.714054	-2.495517
ln(risktime)	1	(exposure)				

```
Deviance:   998.27. Best powers of midt among 494 models fit: -.5 0 3 3.
```

There are 494 different FP4 models fit with the best-fitting model having powers $(-0.5,\ 0,\ 3,\ 3)$. Figure 4.15 shows the estimates from FP3 and FP4 models for the Rotterdam breast cancer data. The fits are very similar and the reduction in deviance is only 0.54. An FP3 model is clearly sufficient here.

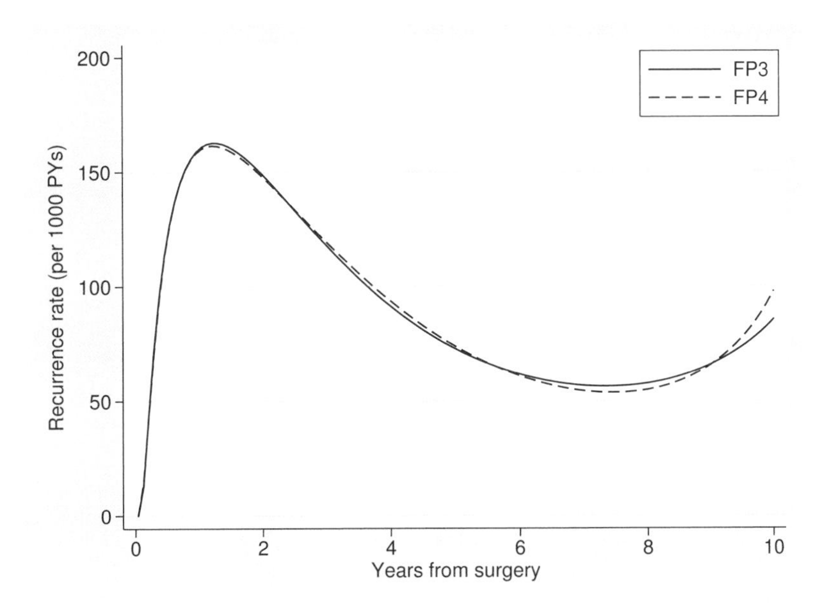

Figure 4.15. Rotterdam breast cancer data. Comparison of FP3 and FP4 functions for the baseline hazard rate. PYs stands for person-years.

4.9.3 FP function selection procedure

The procedure to select an FP function is described in detail in section 4.10 of Royston and Sauerbrei (2008). In outline, it goes as follows: We have a predictor x and seek the "best" FP function for it, not knowing in advance what degree of FP is required. Suppose that the most complex model we allow is FP2. (This restriction is easily relaxed; the procedure is general for any FP degree, but we do have to fix the maximum degree at the start). The best-fitting FP2 model is the one with the lowest deviance over all FP2 models. Starting with the best-fitting FP2 model, the overall significance of x is tested by comparing the FP2 model with one from which only x has been removed (the "null model"). The p-value from this test determines whether x should enter the model at all. If the test is not significant, the procedure terminates and x is not selected. Otherwise, possible nonlinearity of the effect of x is tested by comparing the FP2 model with a straight line (linear function). If the test is not significant, the linear model is accepted; otherwise, the final test is performed—that of FP2 versus FP1. A significant result here indicates the need for a more complex function, FP2; with a nonsignificant outcome, the simpler FP1 function is chosen.

CIs obtained for nonlinear functions from RP models may be too narrow because they are calculated assuming that the final model is the "true model". Recent work on model averaging may provide more realistic CIs (Faes et al. 2007).

4.10 Discussion

In this chapter, we have demonstrated how to set up and fit Poisson models for censored survival data. One can obtain exactly the same parameter estimates using a Cox model and its equivalent Poisson model. Computational time is greater for the Poisson model, but in the era of fast, cheap computers this is likely to be a problem only with very large datasets. In any case, computational time can be dramatically reduced by collapsing the data over covariate patterns.

Poisson models are used extensively to model rates in epidemiology. Usual practice is to split the time scale into a small number of large intervals and to obtain a piecewise-constant estimate of the hazard function (that is, a step function). A step function is biologically unrealistic, but if the analyst is interested only in the relative effect of a covariate under the PH assumption, such an approach is unlikely to lead to severely biased estimates. However, the extension to modeling the baseline hazard as a continuous function of time with splines or FPs is simple, and in general leads to a greater understanding of the disease under study. In addition, the modeling of time-dependent effects is more appealing when time is treated as continuous, as we discuss in detail in chapter 7.

Poisson models still present some difficulties. For piecewise models, the number of intervals is chosen subjectively, although under PH, moderate variations are unlikely to lead to dramatic changes in inference for regression parameters. There is also some subjectivity in deciding how finely to split the time scale for use with splines or FPs. If there are sufficient intervals, dramatic differences are unlikely. One option is to split at the unique failure times, although computational problems may occur with large datasets.

We have advocated collapsing the data over covariate patterns. However, collapsing is not possible with continuous data unless one is willing to round or group the continuous covariates. For example, age could be rounded to the nearest year, as is done in age–period–cohort modeling (Carstensen 2007).

We hope we have shown that the Poisson approach to modeling survival data can be extremely flexible. The advantage of fitting a model in the GLM framework is that one can use GLM methodology. For example, it is relatively easy to extend the models to deal with clustering, through either a random-effects model or by utilizing sandwich-type estimators of SEs (Stata's `vce(robust)` and `vce(cluster` *clustvar*`)` options).

The main issues with Poisson modeling are deciding on how to split the time scale and the potential computational problems with large datasets. In chapter 5, we discuss another alternative to the Cox model where it is not necessary to split the time scale. The approach overcomes most of the limitations of Poisson modeling.

5 Royston–Parmar models

Summary

1. Well-known standard parametric survival models are the starting point for generalizations we call Royston–Parmar (RP) models, which have considerably greater flexibility with respect to the shapes of the survival distributions they can model.
2. Weibull, loglogistic, and lognormal models are generalized to proportional hazards (PH), proportional odds (PO), and probit-scaled RP models, respectively.
3. The additional flexibility of RP models arises because we represent the baseline distribution function as a restricted cubic spline function of log time instead of simply as a linear function of log time.
4. Modeling with spline functions requires us to choose their complexity. The complexity is determined by the number and the positions of the connection points in log time, known as *knots*, of the spline's cubic polynomial segments.
5. Spline models may be chosen informally by the appearance of the fitted survival functions, hazard functions, etc., or more formally, by minimizing the value of an information criterion [Akaike (AIC) or Bayes (BIC)].
6. Estimation of parameters is by maximum likelihood.
7. Quite often, the characteristics of the fitted model are rather insensitive to the number and particularly the position of the knots, lending a certain robustness to the process of model selection.

In this chapter, we describe a parametric approach to survival analysis that introduces flexibility in the shapes of survival functions that can be modeled. The resulting classes of models have many applications. The principal advantages over the Poisson models we describe in chapter 4 are that we do not need to split the time scale, we model at the individual level (no grouping is required), and we can obtain predictions and confidence intervals (CIs) more easily.

We describe RP models more formally in section 5.6, motivating them by way of familiar parametric survival models in sections 5.1, 5.2, 5.4, and 5.5. To start with, we give a flavor of what RP models are about. They are an extension of the Weibull, loglogistic, and lognormal models. In all of the latter, we assume that the effect of covariates is proportional on the appropriate scale (hazard, odds of failure, or probit of failure probability, respectively). We show that the proportionality assumption implies linearity between a particular transformation of the survival function and the logarithm of the survival time. For the Weibull distribution, for example, the log cumulative-hazard function, $\ln H(t)$, is a linear function of $\ln t$ (see section 5.1.2). Because $H(t) = -\ln S(t)$ (see section 1.7), in the Weibull we find that $\ln\{-\ln S(t)\}$ is a linear function of $\ln t$. We require different transformations of $S(t)$ for the loglogistic (section 5.4.2) and lognormal (section 5.5) models.

The restriction that the transformed survival function be linear in $\ln t$ is, in practice, severely limiting and is not really necessary. In RP models, we relax linearity and allow nonlinear functions. There are, of course, many possible families of nonlinear functions that we could use. Because cubic splines are very flexible yet relatively simple to work with and understand, Royston and Parmar (2002) chose them as their preferred tool to extend standard models. As we aim to show in our book, the result is a major advance in the practical usefulness of parametric survival analysis and in the range of applications that can be tackled.

In this chapter, we use the Rotterdam breast cancer dataset in essentially all the example analyses. We assume, therefore, that the file `rott2.dta` has been loaded (that is, `use rott2, clear`) before each of the examples is run.

5.1 Motivation and introduction

5.1.1 The exponential distribution

The simplest parametric survival model is the exponential, which is distinguished by being the only such model with a constant hazard function:

$$h(t) = \lambda$$

We can check graphically whether the exponential distribution fits the data by plotting the empirical and fitted cumulative hazard functions against t. The cumulative hazard function is proportional to t:

$$H(t) = \int_0^t \lambda du = \lambda t$$

A much-used empirical approximation to $H(t)$ is the Nelson–Aalen estimator,

$$H_{\mathrm{NA}}(t) = \sum_{j=1}^{k} \frac{d_j}{n_j}$$

for $t_{(k)} \le t < t_{(k+1)}$, where $k = 1, \ldots, r$, and where $t_{(1)}, \ldots, t_{(r)}$ are the r ordered event times, with $t_{(r+1)} = \infty$ (see Collett [2003, 33]). Here n_j and d_j are the number at risk and number of deaths at time $t_{(j)}$, respectively. We can estimate $H_{\rm NA}(t)$ and its 95% CI in Stata using **sts generate** *newvar* = **na**, **lb(na)**, and **ub(na)**.

We can fit the exponential model (without covariates) to the Rotterdam data using the **streg** command:

```
. streg, distribution(exponential) nohr nolog noshow noheader
```

_t	Coef.	Std. Err.	z	P>|z|	[95% Conf.	Interval]
_cons	-2.398822	.0260201	-92.19	0.000	-2.449821	-2.347823

The option **nohr** produces estimates on the log-hazard scale, and **nolog** suppresses the iteration log. The estimate **_cons** is the constant log hazard function. The hazard and its 95% CI may be displayed by replaying the results of **streg**, this time without option **nohr**:

```
. streg, noheader
```

_t	Haz. Ratio	Std. Err.	z	P>|z|	[95% Conf.	Interval]
_cons	.0908249	.0023633	-92.19	0.000	.0863091	.095577

That **streg** shows the baseline hazard under the the column labeled **Haz. Ratio** is a new feature of Stata 12. Users of previous versions of Stata can obtain similar output by typing

```
. lincom _cons, eform
 ( 1)  [_t]_cons = 0
```

_t	exp(b)	Std. Err.	z	P>|z|	[95% Conf.	Interval]
(1)	.0908249	.0023633	-92.19	0.000	.0863091	.095577

The cumulative hazard function (H) is just t times the hazard. We calculate it in an obvious way:

```
. generate H = exp(_b[_cons]) * _t
```

The survival function is given by $S(t) = \exp(-\lambda t)$, as we can also see from the standard identity $S(t) = \exp\{-H(t)\}$.

In figure 5.1, we graphically compare the two estimates of the cumulative hazard and survival functions using the Rotterdam breast cancer data as an example.

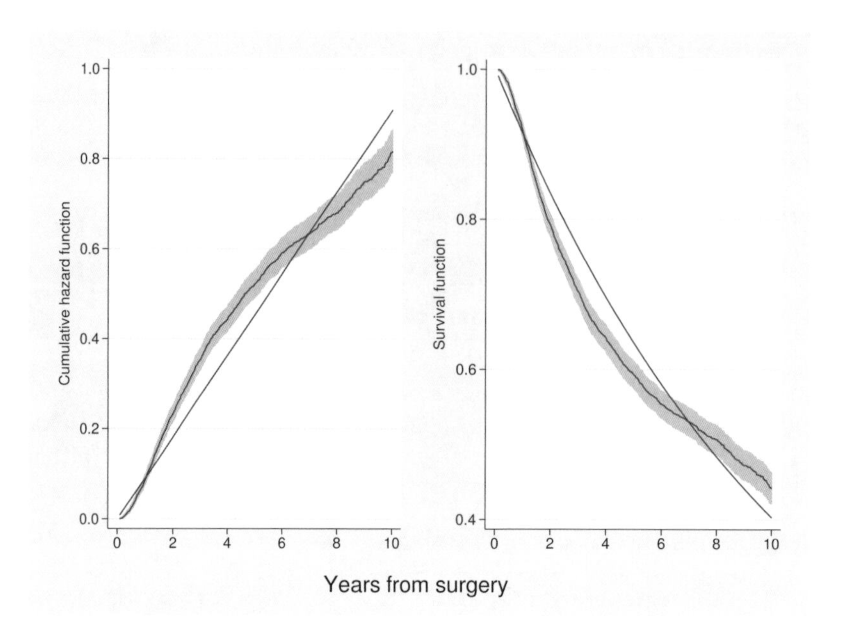

Figure 5.1. Rotterdam breast cancer data. Left panel: Nelson–Aalen estimator of the cumulative hazard function (jagged lines) with 95% CI (shading) compared with the estimate from the exponential model (diagonal line). Right panel: similar comparison between Kaplan–Meier and exponential estimates of the survival function.

The code for the graph is as follows:

```
. // Generate nonparametric estimates
. sts gen Hna = na
. sts gen Hlb = lb(na)
. sts gen Hub = ub(na)
. sts gen S = s
. sts gen Slb = lb(s)
. sts gen Sub = ub(s)
. // Fit -streg- exponential model
. quietly streg, distribution(exponential)
. generate Hexp = exp(_b[_cons]) * _t
. generate Sexp = exp(-Hexp)
. // Plot results
. quietly bysort _t: drop if _n > 1
. twoway (rarea Hlb Hub _t, pstyle(ci) sort)
> (line Hna Hexp _t, sort lstyle(refline ..) pstyle(p2 ..)),
> leg(off) ytitle("Cumulative hazard function") xtitle("")
> ylab(, angle(h) format(%4.1f)) name(g1, replace) nodraw
```

```
. twoway (rarea Slb Sub _t, pstyle(ci) sort)
> (line S Sexp _t, sort lstyle(refline ..) pstyle(p2 ..)),
> leg(off) ytitle("Survival function") xtitle("")
> ylab(, angle(h) format(%4.1f)) name(g2, replace) nodraw
. graph combine g1 g2, b2title("Years from surgery")
```

The exponential distribution is clearly a poor fit. Except for $t < 1$ year, the cumulative hazard is higher for $t < 7$ years and lower for $t \geq 7$ years than the model predicts.

5.1.2 The Weibull distribution

The Weibull distribution is a natural generalization of the exponential. In terms of the cumulative hazard function, we have

$$H(t) = \lambda t^{\gamma_1}$$

for some $\gamma_1 > 0$, where γ_1 is a shape parameter (Although we do not really need the subscript 1 in γ_1, we use it in section 5.1.3 and later on, and we include it here for consistency.) The Weibull hazard function

$$h(t) = dH(t)/dt = \lambda\gamma_1 t^{\gamma_1 - 1}$$

is constant when $\gamma_1 = 1$ (that is, the exponential subcase), monotonic increasing when $\gamma_1 > 1$, and monotonic decreasing when $\gamma_1 < 1$.

The Weibull may be fit using `streg, distribution(weibull)`:

```
. streg, distribution(weibull) nohr nolog noshow noheader
```

_t	Coef.	Std. Err.	z	P>|z|	[95% Conf.	Interval]
_cons	-2.277565	.0484468	-47.01	0.000	-2.372519	-2.182611
/ln_p	-.0659574	.0230952	-2.86	0.004	-.1112231	-.0206917
p	.9361707	.021621			.8947391	.9795209
1/p	1.068181	.0246698			1.020907	1.117644

In the output from `streg`, the shape parameter is called p. In the Rotterdam breast cancer data, we estimate p (that is, γ_1) as 0.94 (95% CI; [0.89, 0.98]). Because γ_1 is close to 1, we would not expect a Weibull to offer much improvement in fit compared with the exponential. Figure 5.2, which corresponds to figure 5.1 except for the Weibull distribution, confirms this expectation.

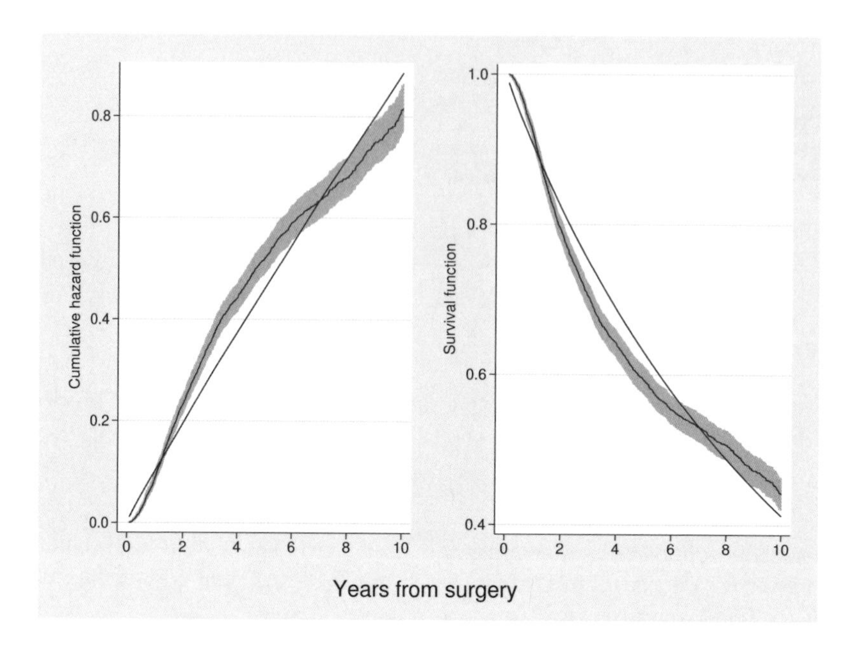

Figure 5.2. Rotterdam breast cancer data. Left panel: Nelson–Aalen estimator of the cumulative hazard function (jagged lines) with 95% CI (shading) compared with estimate from the Weibull model (diagonal line). Right panel: similar comparison between Kaplan–Meier and Weibull estimates of the survival function.

The cumulative hazard function for the Weibull distribution is close to a straight line in t, reflecting the nearness of p to 1.

Part of the reason the Weibull does not fit the Rotterdam breast cancer data well is what we already know from figure 4.3—that the hazard function is nonmonotonic, whereas the hazard function for a Weibull model is monotonic. We obviously need a more complex functional form.

For a comprehensive account of the Weibull and other parametric survival distributions, see chapters 12 and 13 of Cleves et al. (2010).

5.1.3 Generalizing the Weibull

As we just discussed, the Weibull fails to fit the distribution of time to recurrence in the Rotterdam breast cancer data. How should we proceed to arrive at a more reasonable model? One approach begins by writing the Weibull cumulative hazard function in logarithmic form as

$$\ln H(t) = \ln \lambda + \gamma_1 \ln t = \gamma_0 + \gamma_1 \ln t \tag{5.1}$$

We see that $\ln H(t)$ is a sum of two components: a constant (γ_0) and a linear function of log time ($\gamma_1 \ln t$). We can deduce from figure 5.2 that $\gamma_1 \ln t$ does not correctly capture the shape of the (log) cumulative hazard function for the Rotterdam breast cancer data. Therefore, we need a more flexible family of functions that extend (5.1).

Suppose that $f(t;\boldsymbol{\gamma})$ represents some general family of nonlinear functions of time t, having some parameter vector $\boldsymbol{\gamma}$. We can extend (5.1) as follows:

$$\ln H(t) = f(t;\boldsymbol{\gamma})$$

Because cumulative hazard functions are monotonic in t, so also must $f(t;\boldsymbol{\gamma})$ be. Many families of functions are potentially suitable. Two particularly useful ones are fractional polynomials (Royston and Altman 1994) and splines (de Boor 2001). Here we concentrate mostly on splines. Cubic splines are made up of cubic polynomial segments smoothly joined at ordinate values known as knots. Our preferred form is the restricted cubic regression spline; we give details in section 4.8. The restricted cubic spline function always includes a term that is linear in the argument, and its additional terms involve cubic polynomials.

We write a restricted cubic spline function as $s(\ln t;\boldsymbol{\gamma})$ rather than as $f(t;\boldsymbol{\gamma})$, with s standing for spline and $\ln t$ to emphasize that we are working on the scale of log time. We may generalize (5.1) using spline functions as

$$\ln H(t) = s(\ln t;\boldsymbol{\gamma}) = \gamma_0 + \gamma_1 \ln t + \gamma_2 z_1(\ln t) + \gamma_3 z_2(\ln t) + \cdots \tag{5.2}$$

where $\ln t$, $z_1(\ln t)$, $z_2(\ln t)$, and so on, are the basis functions of the restricted cubic spline (see section 4.8.2). When we specify one or more knots, the spline function includes a constant (γ_0), a linear function of $\ln t$ with parameter γ_1, and a basis function of $\ln t$ for each knot, which also has a regression parameter, γ_i. By convention, the "no knots" case corresponds to the linear function, $s(\ln t;\gamma_0,\gamma_1) = \gamma_0 + \gamma_1 \ln t$—that is, the Weibull model.

An additional point about (5.2) is worth making. As we have already noted, with a standard survival distribution, $H(t)$ is a monotonic increasing function of t. However, spline functions are not necessarily monotonic. In practical datasets, we rarely find examples in which the monotonicity condition is breached. The reason is that most datasets contain considerable information about the shape of the cumulative hazard function, and splines are sufficiently flexible to accommodate the shape accurately. In the relative survival context (chapter 8), nonmonotonicity may actually be an advantage because it allows us to model negative excess hazards, which are medically interpretable.

We estimate the parameters $\boldsymbol{\gamma}$ of model (5.2) by maximum likelihood using the routine `stpm2` (Lambert and Royston 2009), a further development of Royston's (2001) `stpm` command. We gave a brief introduction to `stpm2` in section 1.6; for further details, please see Lambert and Royston (2009) and the many examples of its usage throughout the present book. Because the `stpm2` command is easy to use, we give an idea of the necessary computations as we go along.

It turns out that a spline with 2 interior knots and 2 boundary knots provides an adequate approximation to the distribution of time to recurrence in the Rotterdam breast cancer data (although 1 interior knot is nearly as good). We fit model (5.2) as follows:

```
. stpm2, df(3) scale(hazard) noorthog nolog
Log likelihood = -3673.5469                     Number of obs   =       2982

------------------------------------------------------------------------------
             |      Coef.   Std. Err.      z    P>|z|     [95% Conf. Interval]
-------------+----------------------------------------------------------------
xb           |
       _rcs1 |   2.511366   .1682784    14.92   0.000     2.181546    2.841185
       _rcs2 |   .1557798   .0433252     3.60   0.000     .0708641    .2406956
       _rcs3 |  -.0391964   .0492701    -0.80   0.426    -.1357641    .0573712
       _cons |  -1.786363   .0957299   -18.66   0.000     -1.97399   -1.598736
------------------------------------------------------------------------------
```

`df(3)` specifies 2 interior knots (because the degrees of freedom (d.f.) are one more than the number of interior knots, see section 4.8) and `scale(hazard)` calls for hazards scaling (more on this later). The regression coefficients for `_cons`, `_rcs1`, `_rcs2`, and `_rcs3` correspond to the parameters γ_0, γ_1, γ_2, and γ_3 in (5.2), respectively.

We make two specific points about `stpm2` here. First, the `nolog` option suppresses the "iteration log", which shows the progress of the iterative fitting routine toward convergence at the maximum likelihood estimate. Typically, the iteration log is of little interest, but is traditionally displayed by most Stata regression commands. Second, the `noorthog` option prevents the default "orthogonalization" of the spline basis functions (here `_rcs1`, `_rcs2`, and `_rcs3`). Orthogonalization (or more precisely, orthonormalization) linearly transforms the basis functions to be uncorrelated and to have mean 0 and standard deviation (SD) 1. Untransformed spline basis functions can be highly correlated. We apply orthogonalization to improve numerical stability when fitting the model. We have used `noorthog` here because in section 5.3.1 we illustrate how the spline variables are calculated.

Figure 5.3 shows the resulting fit to the cumulative hazard function for the Rotterdam breast cancer data.

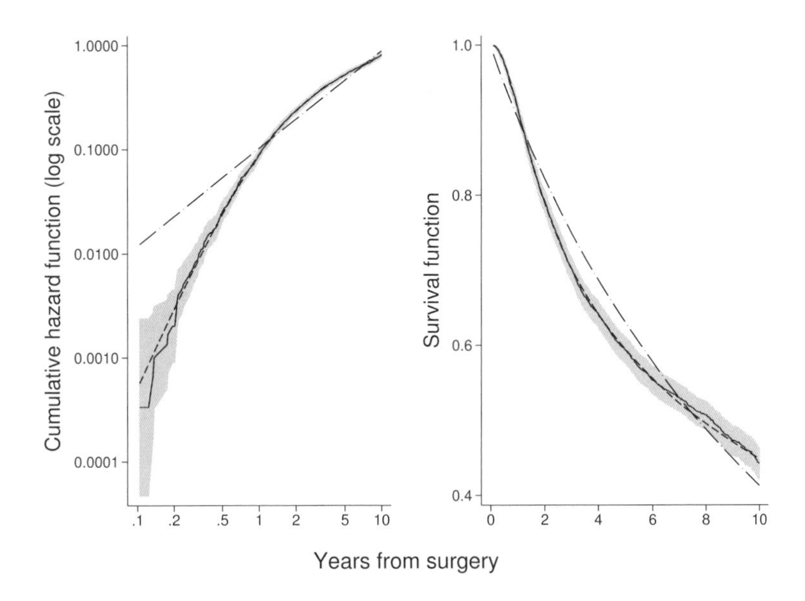

Figure 5.3. Rotterdam breast cancer data. Left panel: Nelson–Aalen estimator of the cumulative hazard function (jagged lines) with 95% CI (shading) compared with estimates from the spline based model with 2 interior knots (dashed line) and a Weibull model (dash-dotted line). Horizontal and vertical scales are logarithmic. Right panel: same comparison for the survival function.

The fit is now excellent—compare figure 5.3 with figures 5.1 and 5.2. We calculated the predicted cumulative hazard and survival functions using `stpm2`'s postestimation `predict` function, as follows:

```
. predict H, cumhazard
. predict S, survival
```

SEs and CIs are also available.

Figure 5.3 includes the corresponding fitted functions for a Weibull distribution. The poor fit is obvious. We have plotted the cumulative hazard function on a log scale against time on a log scale. On these scales, the Weibull cumulative hazard function is a straight line. In many datasets, such a log–log plot reveals a simple relationship. The Weibull gives the simplest possible relationship (that is, linearity).

5.1.4 Estimating the hazard function

One of Royston and Parmar's (2002) aims was to develop models that enable researchers to investigate the hazard function. The hazard function is important because it is a trace in time of the intensity of the disease or condition under study. In general, it is less stable and harder to estimate than the cumulative distribution functions (survival, cumulative hazard, cumulative incidence, etc.). After fitting a RP model with `stpm2`, we can easily compute the hazard function and its CI by using the postestimation command `predict` *hazard_var*`, hazard ci`.

As an example, we compare the hazard function from the spline model having two knots (that was introduced in section 5.1.3) with the hazard functions from two other methods. First, `sts graph, hazard` gives a kernel-smoothed plot of the hazard contributions (see [ST] **sts graph** for details). The second method is an ad hoc analysis with fractional polynomial (FP) functions. For several reasons, we do not claim this is a serious method, but it is interesting for illustrative purposes. Let $H_{\mathrm{NA}}(t)$ be the Nelson–Aalen estimate of the cumulative hazard function ([ST] **sts generate**). This estimate is too noisy for us to use it directly to estimate its first derivative, which is the hazard function; it needs to be smoothed first. Suppose that $\widetilde{H}(t)$ is a smoothed version of $H_{\mathrm{NA}}(t)$ that we obtained by FP regression of $\ln H_{\mathrm{NA}}(t)$ on t. To get a corresponding estimate, $\widetilde{h}(t)$, of the hazard function, we see

$$\widetilde{h}(t) = \frac{d\widetilde{H}(t)}{dt} = \widetilde{H}(t)\,\frac{d\ln \widetilde{H}(t)}{dt}$$

Code to do the necessary calculations using a third-order FP (or FP3) function is as follows:

```
sts generate Hna = na
generate lnHna = ln(Hna)
fracpoly, degree(3): regress lnHna _t
predict lnHtilde
fracdydx, gen(hazard_FP)
replace hazard_FP = hazard_FP * exp(lnHtilde)
```

The command `fracdydx` is not part of standard Stata. It computes derivatives (by default, the first derivative) of the most recently fitted FP function, which is what we need here.

The results from the three approaches are illustrated in figure 5.4.

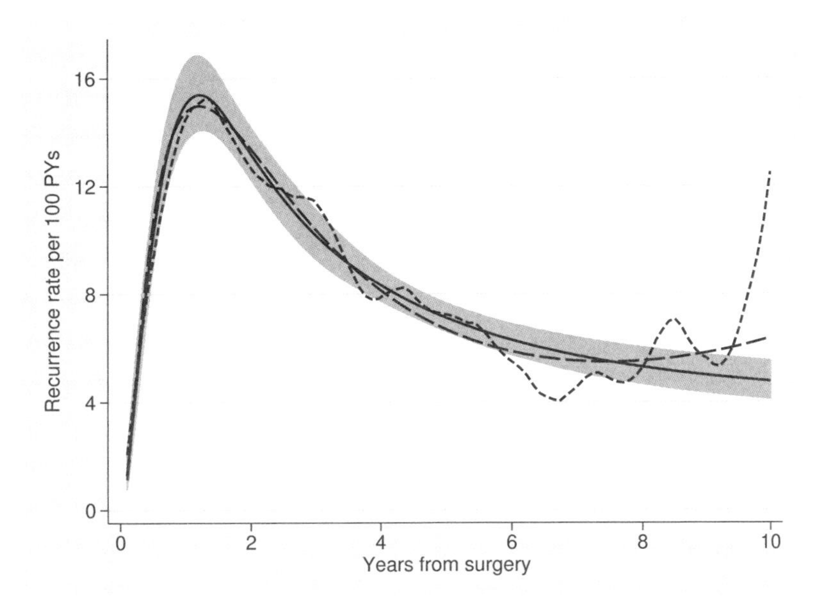

Figure 5.4. Rotterdam breast cancer data. Three approaches to estimating the hazard function. Solid lines, spline model with 2 knots; short dashes, kernel smooth using `sts graph, hazard`; long dashes, based on smoothing the log of the Nelson–Aalen cumulative hazard function with an FP3 model. Shaded area is a 95% pointwise CI for the spline-based hazard estimate. PYs stands for person-years.

The kernel estimate is rather unstable (note the "humps and bumps"), which is typical of such a method. The other two methods agree quite closely, the main difference being that the FP3 function and the kernel estimate suggest a small increase in the hazard at long follow-up times, which may or may not be sensible. All three methods agree on the time of the maximum hazard, which appears to occur about 1.5 years after surgery.

5.2 Proportional hazards models

5.2.1 Generalizing the Weibull

Suppose that we want to include a covariate vector, $\mathbf{x}$, in the survival model. If we write the basic Weibull model (5.1) as

$$\ln H(t) = \ln H_0(t) = \gamma_0 + \gamma_1 \ln t$$

then we can write the Weibull model with covariates $\mathbf{x} = (x_1, \ldots x_k)$ and parameter vector $\boldsymbol{\beta} = (\beta_1, \ldots \beta_k)^T$ as

$$\ln H(t; \mathbf{x}) = \ln H_0(t) + \mathbf{x}\boldsymbol{\beta} = \gamma_0 + \gamma_1 \ln t + \mathbf{x}\boldsymbol{\beta} \tag{5.3}$$

Because $\mathbf{x}\boldsymbol{\beta}$ does not depend on time, we can describe (5.3) as a proportional cumulative hazards model, or as we see by differentiating $H(t; \mathbf{x}) = H_0(t) \exp(\mathbf{x}\boldsymbol{\beta})$ with respect to t to get $h(t; \mathbf{x}) = h_0(t) \exp(\mathbf{x}\boldsymbol{\beta})$, as a PH model. For example, for a single, binary covariate x taking values 0 and 1, we can write (5.3) as

$$H(t; x = 1) = H(t; x = 0)\, \beta$$

showing that the cumulative hazards are proportional.

Now suppose that we extend the baseline cumulative hazard function of the Weibull model, in the manner of (5.2), to $\ln H_0(t) = s(\ln t; \boldsymbol{\gamma})$, a restricted cubic spline function of $\ln t$. The extension of (5.3) to a more general PH model is then

$$\ln H(t; \mathbf{x}) = \ln H_0(t) + \mathbf{x}\boldsymbol{\beta} = s(\ln t; \boldsymbol{\gamma}) + \mathbf{x}\boldsymbol{\beta} \tag{5.4}$$

Equation (5.4) is a generalization of the standard Weibull model with covariates. Exponentiating and then differentiating with respect to t gives the hazard function,

$$h(t; \mathbf{x}) = \frac{ds(\ln t; \boldsymbol{\gamma})}{dt} \exp\{s(\ln t; \boldsymbol{\gamma}) + \mathbf{x}\boldsymbol{\beta}\}$$

and thus the log hazard function,

$$\ln h(t; \mathbf{x}) = \ln\left\{\frac{ds(\ln t; \boldsymbol{\gamma})}{dt}\right\} + s(\ln t; \boldsymbol{\gamma}) + \mathbf{x}\boldsymbol{\beta}$$

showing that (5.4) is also a PH model. The $\boldsymbol{\beta}$ vector is identical between the two forms of the model. By virtue of the flexibility of spline functions, we can consider (5.4) to be a (flexible) parametric version of the Cox PH model. By convention, $H_0(t) = H(t; \mathbf{0})$.

To see what the log hazard function looks like mathematically, we need to evaluate $ds(\ln t; \boldsymbol{\gamma})/dt = t^{-1} ds(\ln t; \boldsymbol{\gamma})/d\ln t$. Because $z_1 = z_1(\ln t) = \ln t$, we have

$$\begin{aligned}
\frac{ds(\ln t; \boldsymbol{\gamma})}{d\ln t} &= \frac{d}{d\ln t}(\gamma_0 + \gamma_1 z_1 + \gamma_2 z_2 + \cdots + \gamma_{m+1} z_{m+1}) \\
&= \gamma_1 + \gamma_2 \frac{dz_2(\ln t)}{d\ln t} + \ldots + \gamma_{m+1} \frac{dz_{m+1}(\ln t)}{d\ln t}
\end{aligned}$$

We have, for $j = 2, \ldots, m+1$,

$$z_j(\ln t) = (\ln t - k_j)^3_+ - \lambda_j (\ln t - k_{\min})^3_+ - (1 - \lambda_j)(\ln t - k_{\max})^3_+$$

so that

$$\frac{dz_j}{d\ln t} = z'_j = 3(\ln t - k_j)^2_+ - 3\lambda_j (\ln t - k_{\min})^2_+ - 3(1 - \lambda_j)(\ln t - k_{\max})^2_+$$

Putting it all together,

$$\ln h(t; \mathbf{x}) = -\ln t + \ln\left(\gamma_1 + \gamma_2 z_2' + \ldots + \gamma_{m+1} z_{m+1}'\right) + \gamma_0 + \gamma_1 z_1 + \gamma_2 z_2 + \ldots + \gamma_{m+1} z_{m+1} + \mathbf{x}\boldsymbol{\beta}$$

We refer to a PH model whose spline function has d d.f. (that is, $d - 1$ interior knots and when $d > 1$, two boundary knots) as a PH(d) model.

5.2.2 Example

The Rotterdam breast cancer dataset includes a predefined binary covariate, `recent`, which takes the values 0 and 1 for patients registered between 1978–1987 and those registered between 1988–1993, respectively. According to a Cox model for `recent`, $\widehat{\beta} = -0.170$ (95% CI; $[-0.274, -0.067]$). Ignoring possible confounding by other factors, we infer that the hazard of recurrence for more recent patients is about $1 - e^{-0.170} =$ 15.6% lower than for earlier patients. If we fit a PH(3) model, we find that $\widehat{\beta} = -0.179$ (95% CI; $[-0.282, -0.076]$), which is very similar to the Cox model. The effect of `recent` is to reduce the cumulative hazard function for the `recent==1` subclass by $1 - e^{-0.179} = 16.4\%$, compared with `recent==0`. We illustrate the good fit of the PH model in the two subclasses in figure 5.5.

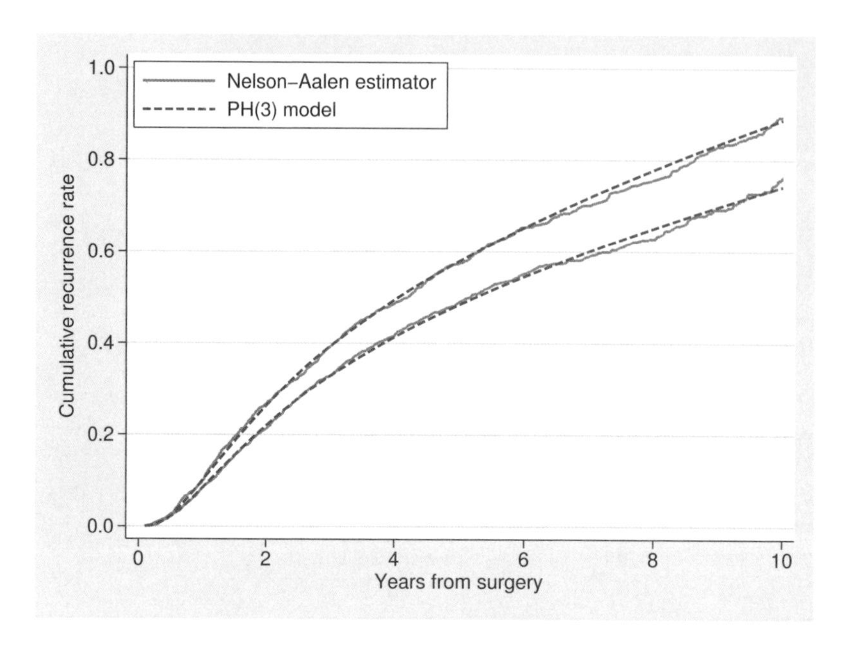

Figure 5.5. Rotterdam breast cancer data. Cumulative recurrence rate (hazard function) in two groups according to the binary covariate `recent`, estimated from a PH(3) model. Upper pair of lines, earlier patients (`recent==0`); lower pair, more recent patients (`recent==1`).

We see no obvious indication of a failure of the PH assumption in this example.

The code to use the `stpm2` command to fit the RP PH model and estimate the cumulative hazard functions in the two subgroups is included in the code that produced figure 5.5:

```
stpm2 recent, df(3) scale(hazard)
predict H0, cumhazard zeros
predict H1, cumhazard at(recent 1)
```

The `zeros` option of `predict` computes baseline values for which all covariates equal zero (here, values at `recent==0`). The option `at(recent 1)` evaluates the hazard function at the value 1 of `recent`. This approach gives out-of-sample estimates of the cumulative hazard function; that is, the functions `H0` and `H1` are each calculated for all observations. We could compute the cumulative hazard function at the observed times and covariate values for all patients by using `predict H, cumhazard`.

5.2.3 Comparing parameters of PH(1) and Weibull models

We have described PH(d) models with $d > 1$ as generalizations of Weibull models; and we noted that PH(1) is the same as the Weibull, albeit with a different parameterization.

We use `stpm2` to fit a PH(1) model to the covariate `recent` in the Rotterdam breast cancer data, and we compare its parameters with those of the Weibull. We include the `noorthog` option to ensure that $\ln t$ (that is, `_rcs1`) is fit in raw form rather than standardized to have mean 0 and SD 1:

```
. stpm2 recent, df(1) scale(hazard) nolog noorthog
Log likelihood = -3798.4791                    Number of obs   =       2982

              |      Coef.   Std. Err.      z    P>|z|     [95% Conf. Interval]
--------------+----------------------------------------------------------------
xb            |
       recent |   -.137097   .0524498    -2.61   0.009    -.2398967   -.0342972
        _rcs1 |   .9333692   .0215781    43.26   0.000     .8910768    .9756616
        _cons |  -2.193575   .0576154   -38.07   0.000    -2.306499    -2.08065
```

Provided we remember to specify `nohr` to report the regression coefficients on a log scale, the results from `streg, distribution(weibull)` are similar:

```
. streg recent, distribution(weibull) nolog nohr noheader noshow

           _t |      Coef.   Std. Err.      z    P>|z|     [95% Conf. Interval]
--------------+----------------------------------------------------------------
       recent |   -.137097   .0524498    -2.61   0.009    -.2398967   -.0342972
        _cons |  -2.193575   .0576154   -38.07   0.000    -2.306499    -2.08065
--------------+----------------------------------------------------------------
        /ln_p |  -.0689545   .0231185    -2.98   0.003     -.114266   -.0236429
--------------+----------------------------------------------------------------
            p |   .9333692   .0215781                      .8920207    .9766344
          1/p |   1.071387   .0247689                      1.023925     1.12105
```

The Weibull parameters that `streg` reports as `_cons` and `p` are γ_0 and γ_1 in a PH(1) model, and they are reported by `stpm2` as `_b[_cons]` and `_b[_rcs1]`, respectively. The full names (that is, including the equation name) of the three `streg` parameters are `[_t]_b[_cons]`, `[_t]_b[recent]`, and `[ln_p]_b[_cons]`—the last-named being $\ln \gamma_1$. One minor difference is that `streg` estimates $\ln p$ and its CI and back-transforms it, whereas `stpm2` estimates γ_1 and its CI directly. The estimates of γ_1 and p are identical, but estimates of their CIs differ slightly because of back-transformation from the log scale of p, as we just mentioned. In the example, `streg` reports a CI of $[0.892, 0.977]$ for p, whereas `stpm2` gives $[0.891, 0.976]$ for γ_1.

We now consider the extent to which generalizing a Weibull model with PH(d) models with increasing d improves the fit, and how it affects the parameter estimate ($\widehat{\beta}$) for `recent`. Table 5.1 shows the AIC and BIC for models with $d = 1$ (Weibull) up to $d = 6$ (in which the baseline log cumulative hazard is a spline function with 5 interior knots).

Table 5.1. Rotterdam breast cancer data. Variations in parameter estimates for `recent` and goodness of fit (measured by AIC or BIC) of PH(d) models fit by `stpm2` as d increases. The model that minimizes the AIC is shown in italics.

Model	d.f. (d)	$\widehat{\beta}$	standard error (SE)	AIC	BIC
Weibull	1	−0.137	0.052	7602.96	7620.96
PH(2)	2	−0.182	0.052	7348.46	7372.46
PH(3)	*3*	*−0.179*	*0.053*	*7345.60*	*7375.60*
PH(4)	4	−0.179	0.053	7347.45	7383.45
PH(5)	5	−0.178	0.053	7349.04	7391.04
PH(6)	6	−0.177	0.053	7349.13	7397.13

The model that minimizes the AIC (shown in italics) is PH(3), whereas a slightly simpler model, PH(2), minimizes the BIC. $\widehat{\beta}$ for the Weibull model is markedly lower than for the PH(2) model, but it changes little for higher d.f. ($d > 2$). We might equally well choose PH(2) or PH(3) as our preferred model here.

In the left panel of figure 5.6, we compare the baseline hazard functions for the Weibull, PH(2), PH(3), and PH(6) models.

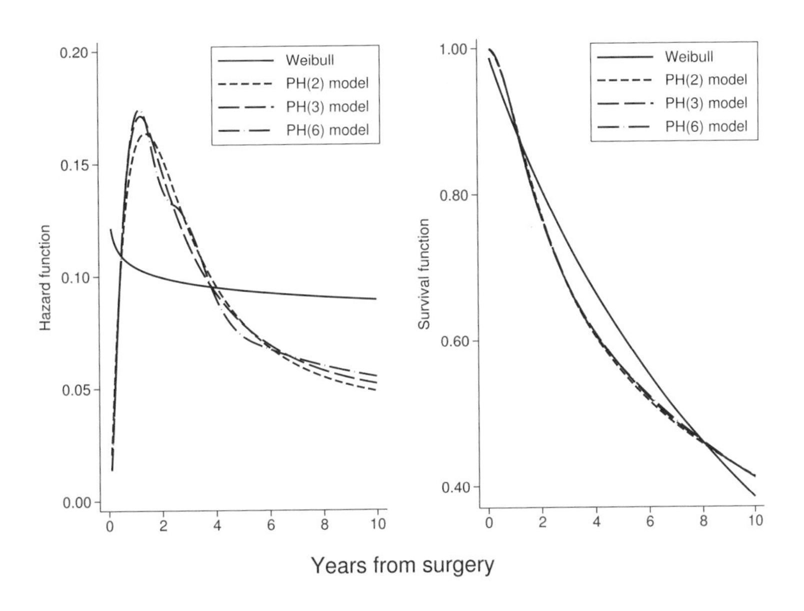

Figure 5.6. Rotterdam breast cancer data. Baseline distribution functions after fitting Weibull, PH(2), PH(3), and PH(6) models with covariate `recent`. Left panel, hazard function; right panel, survival function.

The code for figure 5.6 is as follows:

```
. forval j = 1 / 4 {
  2.        if (`j´ < 4) local df `j´
  3.        else local df 6
  4.        quietly stpm2 recent, df(`df´) scale(hazard)
  5.        predict h`j´, hazard zero
  6.        predict s`j´, surv zero
  7. }
. line h1 h2 h3 h4 _t, sort lpattern(l - _ _.) lwidth(medthick ..)
> legend(label(1 "Weibull") label(2 "PH(2) model") label(3 "PH(3) model")
> label(4 "PH(6) model") ring(0) pos(1) col(1))
> ytitle("Hazard function") xtitle("")
> yla(, angle(h) format(%4.2f)) name(g1, replace)
. line s1 s2 s3 s4 _t, sort lpattern(l - _ _.) lwidth(medthick ..)
> legend(label(1 "Weibull") label(2 "PH(2) model") label(3 "PH(3) model")
> label(4 "PH(6) model") ring(0) pos(1) col(1))
> ytitle("Survival function") xtitle("")
> yla(, angle(h) format(%4.2f)) name(g2, replace)
. graph combine g1 g2, b2title("Years from surgery")
```

The baseline hazard function for the Weibull model is dramatically different from those of the PH models, confirming the poor fit of the Weibull. Using d.f. greater than 2 hardly changes the shape of the baseline hazard function. However, the baseline hazard function for the PH(6) model is noticeably more wiggly than the others, which suggests (as is apparent in table 5.1) that it is overfitted. We can hardly distinguish between the survival functions of the three PH models (see the right panel); only the function for the Weibull is different.

5.3 Selecting a spline function

We wish to extend Weibull models to PH(d) models by representing the baseline log cumulative-hazard function as a spline in $\ln t$. We must therefore choose a spline function. We need to decide the position of the knots and how many of them to use. We discuss knot positions next. Identical considerations apply to the additional types of models that we introduce later in the chapter.

5.3.1 Knot positions

We introduced restricted cubic splines with m interior knots and 2 boundary knots in section 4.8.2. To fit a PH model, we must preselect knots on the log survival-time scale. As we have already mentioned, a sensible choice for the boundary knots k_{min}, k_{max} is the smallest and largest uncensored log survival-times. How we place the interior knots is an issue (see, for example, section 4.8.5 and the discussion by Durrleman and Simon [1989]). Fortunately, optimal (optimized) knot positioning does not appear to be critical for a good fit and may even be undesirable in that the fitted curve may follow small-scale features of the data too closely. Furthermore, if we employ data-driven knot selection, knots become additional model parameters. We should then make sure that uncertainty in parameter estimates due to knot optimization is reflected in enlarged SEs and CIs. However, this is not straightforward to do.

Royston and Parmar (2002) suggested knot positions based on empirical centiles of the distribution of log time, as given in the first four rows of table 5.2. Here we augment the values with a few higher d.f.

Table 5.2. Positions of internal knots for modeling the baseline distribution function in RP models. Knots are positions on the distribution of uncensored log event-times.

Knots	d.f.	Centiles
1	2	50
2	3	33, 67
3	4	25, 50, 75
4	5	20, 40, 60, 80
5	6	17, 33, 50, 67, 83
6	7	14, 29, 43, 57, 71, 86
7	8	12.5, 25, 37.5, 50, 62.5, 75, 87.5
8	9	11.1, 22.2, 33.3, 44.4, 55.6, 66.7, 77.8, 88.9
9	10	10, 20, 30, 40, 50, 60, 70, 80, 90

The positions are essentially those recommended by Durrleman and Simon (1989) for restricted cubic splines. The reason we choose knots not too far from the median uncensored log survival-time is to allow the data to be most closely modeled in the region of greatest density. In many applications, we do not need and do not recommend models with more than 3 knots (that is, with more than 4 d.f.), because the resulting curves are potentially unstable (wiggly). If we desire, however, we can use `stpm2` with as many as 9 knots at the positions given in table 5.2. Other numbers and positions of knots are available through the `knots()` option.

Example

To show how spline functions are computed, we deconstruct the example illustrated in figure 5.3. The number of interior knots is $m = 2$. The smallest and largest uncensored event times in the Rotterdam breast cancer data are 0.104 and 9.99 years, so the boundary knots are $k_{\min} = \ln(0.104) = -2.26$ and $k_{\max} = \ln(9.99) = 2.30$. The 33rd and 67th centiles of the uncensored event times are 1.577 and 3.571 years, so $k_1 = 0.46$, $k_2 = 1.27$. From this we find that $\lambda_1 = (k_{\max} - k_1) / (k_{\max} - k_{\min}) = 0.404$, $\lambda_2 = (k_{\max} - k_2) / (k_{\max} - k_{\min}) = 0.226$. We give crude Stata code to calculate the spline basis functions $z_1(\ln t)$ and $z_2(\ln t)$ below:

```
. scalar kmin = -2.26
. scalar kmax = 2.30
. scalar k1 = 0.46
. scalar k2 = 1.27
. scalar lambda1 = 0.404
. scalar lambda2 = 0.226
. generate lnt = ln(_t)
. generate z0 = cond(lnt > kmin, (lnt-kmin)^3, 0)
. generate z3 = cond(lnt > kmax, (lnt-kmax)^3, 0)
. generate z1 = cond(lnt > k1, (lnt-k1)^3, 0) - lambda1*z0 - (1-lambda1)*z3
. generate z2 = cond(lnt > k2, (lnt-k2)^3, 0) - lambda2*z0 - (1-lambda2)*z3
```

The maximum likelihood estimates of the parameters γ_0, γ_1, γ_2, and γ_3 are -1.7864, 2.5114, 0.158, and -0.0392, respectively:

```
. stpm2, df(3) scale(hazard) nolog noorthog
Log likelihood = -3673.5469                     Number of obs   =       2982

------------------------------------------------------------------------------
             |      Coef.   Std. Err.      z    P>|z|     [95% Conf. Interval]
-------------+----------------------------------------------------------------
xb           |
       _rcs1 |   2.511366   .1682784    14.92   0.000     2.181546    2.841185
       _rcs2 |   .1557798   .0433252     3.60   0.000     .0708641    .2406956
       _rcs3 |  -.0391964   .0492701    -0.80   0.426    -.1357641    .0573712
       _cons |  -1.786363   .0957299   -18.66   0.000     -1.97399   -1.598736
------------------------------------------------------------------------------
```

Use of the `noorthog` option prevents orthogonalization of the spline functions to ensure that the estimates of γ_0, γ_1, γ_2, and γ_3 agree with those calculated from first principles. In practice, we would not normally apply the `noorthog` option, because it tends to make the estimates of the spline model parameters slower to compute and numerically less stable.

As we already indicated, the model has three predictors, `_rcs1`, `_rcs2`, and `_rcs3`, the spline basis functions whose estimated regression coefficients are $\widehat{\gamma}_1$, $\widehat{\gamma}_2$, and $\widehat{\gamma}_3$, respectively. `stpm2` also leaves behind variables `_d_rcs1`, `_d_rcs2`, and `_d_rcs3`, which contain the first derivatives of the spline basis functions with respect to ln(`_t`). We use these variables in fitting the model but constrain their coefficients to equal those of the spline basis functions, so `stpm2` does not report them. We can calculate the estimated log cumulative-hazard function as

```
. generate lnH = -1.7864 + 2.5114 * lnt + 0.1558 * z1 - 0.0392 * z2
```

The variables `lnt`, `z1`, and `z2` correspond to `_rcs1`, `_rcs2`, and `_rcs3`, respectively. In the example, we could also obtain the log cumulative-hazard function using

```
. generate lnH = _b[_cons] + _rcs1 * _b[_rcs1] + _rcs2 * _b[_rcs2] +
> _rcs3 * _b[_rcs3]
```

Of course, such hard work is unnecessary, because `predict lnH, xb` will provide us with the log cumulative hazard function directly.

5.3.2 How many knots?

With datasets of modest size, we can get a worthwhile improvement in fit over the "no knots" case by using a spline model with a single interior knot (that is, 2 d.f.), but often we gain little by adding further knots. For that reason, with smaller datasets we suggest a 2 d.f. or 3 d.f. spline model as a reasonable initial or default choice. With larger datasets, we may find we need a larger number of knots—say 5 or 6. For further guidance, we suggest looking informally at the AIC, or if we prefer a more stringent criterion, the BIC of models with between 1 and 6 d.f. (that is, between 0 and 5 interior knots). The AIC is defined to be the deviance (minus twice the maximized log likelihood) plus a penalty of twice the number of model parameters, whereas the BIC has a penalty of $\ln n$ times the number of model parameters, where n is the number of events. Formally, the preferred model is the one with minimum AIC (or BIC). However, in the interests of parsimony and of reducing overfitting, we should not apply the criterion mechanically. Because the smaller sets of knots given in table 5.2 are not generally subsets of the larger sets, not all the models of a given type are nested within those with higher d.f. Formal significance testing between the models is therefore not always appropriate.

With large datasets (tens of thousands of observations and more), formal inference using AIC or even BIC may not much help us to choose the number of knots. We often find that adding knots to an already reasonably adequate model produces a highly significant reduction in deviance and an apparently worthwhile reduction in AIC or BIC, but we see virtually no difference in plots of the estimated hazard function or (particularly) the survival function. Our advice in such cases is to be guided by the "feel" of the model fit, rather than by formal statistics. We are aiming to capture the essence of how the data behaves, rather than trying to find an optimal fit in some theoretical sense.

5.4 PO models

5.4.1 Introduction

The odds ratio (OR) is familiar from epidemiological studies as an approximate measure of the change in risk of an event, such as death, occurring in the presence of some factor of interest. In a 2×2 table of status (dead or alive) versus a risk factor (present or absent), the OR summarizes the status of subjects at the conclusion of the investigation. In a long-term follow-up study, we need a measure of risk that incorporates the survival times of all individuals, not simply whether they were dead or alive at a particular time point. Repeated evaluation and pooling (for example, using the Mantel–Haenszel method) of a sequence of 2×2 tables at successive time points to obtain a single estimate of the OR is incorrect, because the tables are highly correlated.

Building on the work of others, Bennett (1983) proposed an extension of the logistic regression model to censored survival data. The model is structurally similar to a Cox model, but with the feature that the hazard ratio for a covariate converges to 1 as $t \to \infty$. We may be able to exploit converging hazard functions when modeling a prognostic factor with a short- or medium-term effect.

We define the OR in a 2×2 table by

$$\mathrm{OR} = \frac{p_1}{1 - p_1} \Big/ \frac{p_2}{1 - p_2} \tag{5.5}$$

where p_1 and p_2 are the proportions of individuals with an event in groups 1 and 2, respectively. Generalizing (5.5) to the case where failure occurs with probabilities $F_1(t)$ and $F_2(t)$ by time $t > 0$, we obtain

$$\text{OR}(t) = \frac{F_1(t)}{1 - F_1(t)} \Big/ \frac{F_2(t)}{1 - F_2(t)}$$

or equivalently

$$\frac{F_1(t)}{1 - F_1(t)} = \frac{F_2(t)}{1 - F_2(t)} \text{OR}(t)$$

If $\text{OR}(t)$ is constant, the model implies that the odds of an event occurring up to time t (for any t) are proportional across levels of the covariate—that is, what we call the proportional (cumulative) odds or PO assumption.

We can easily generalize the PO model to the situation where individual i has a covariate vector $\mathbf{x}_i$ with parameter vector $\boldsymbol{\beta}$. We let $\text{OR}_i = \exp(\mathbf{x}_i\boldsymbol{\beta})$ and write

$$\frac{F(t; \mathbf{x}_i)}{1 - F(t; \mathbf{x}_i)} = \frac{F_0(t)}{1 - F_0(t)} \exp(\mathbf{x}_i\boldsymbol{\beta})$$

where $F(t; \mathbf{x}_i)$ is the cumulative distribution (incidence) function at time t and $F_0(t) = F(t; \mathbf{0})$ is the baseline distribution function. By writing the survival function $S(t; \mathbf{x}_i) = 1 - F(t; \mathbf{x}_i)$, writing the logistic function $\text{logit}(x) = \ln\{x/(1-x)\}$, and taking logarithms of both sides, we can express the PO model as

$$\text{logit}\{1 - S(t; \mathbf{x}_i)\} = \text{logit}\{1 - S_0(t)\} + \mathbf{x}_i\boldsymbol{\beta} \tag{5.6}$$

5.4.2 The loglogistic model

The best-known parametric PO model is the loglogistic model, for which the baseline survival function is

$$S_0(t) = \left[1 + \{\exp(-\beta_0)\, t\}^{\frac{1}{\gamma}}\right]^{-1}$$

where $\gamma > 0$ (see Cleves et al. [2010, 241]). After a little algebra, we find that

$$\text{logit}\{1 - S_0(t)\} = (-\beta_0 + \ln t)/\gamma = \gamma_0 + \gamma_1 \ln t$$

where $\gamma_0 = -\beta_0/\gamma$, $\gamma_1 = 1/\gamma$, and $\text{logit}\{1 - S_0(t)\} = \ln[\{1 - S_0(t)\}/S_0(t)]$. The loglogistic is an accelerated failure-time (AFT) model with parameter vector $\boldsymbol{\beta}^*$, defined by

$$S(t; \mathbf{x}_i) = S_0\{\exp(-\mathbf{x}_i\boldsymbol{\beta}^*)\, t\}$$

so that

$$\begin{aligned}
\text{logit}\{1 - S(t; \mathbf{x}_i)\} &= \text{logit}[1 - S_0\{\exp(-\mathbf{x}_i\boldsymbol{\beta}^*)\, t\}] \\
&= \gamma_0 + \gamma_1 \ln\{t \exp(-\mathbf{x}_i\boldsymbol{\beta}^*)\} \\
&= \gamma_0 + \gamma_1 \ln t - \mathbf{x}_i\boldsymbol{\beta}^*
\end{aligned}$$

Thus

$$\text{logit}\left\{1 - S\left(t; \mathbf{x}_i\right)\right\} = \text{logit}\left\{1 - S_0\left(t\right)\right\} - \mathbf{x}_i \boldsymbol{\beta}^* \tag{5.7}$$

By writing $\boldsymbol{\beta} = -\boldsymbol{\beta}^*$, we see that (5.7) and (5.6) are identical, showing that the loglogistic is a PO model.

5.4.3 Generalizing the loglogistic model

Equations (5.7) and (5.3) are similar in structure. To increase flexibility, we extended the Weibull model by using spline functions of $\ln t$, as we indicated in (5.4). We can extend the loglogistic model in a similar way by writing

$$\text{logit}\left\{1 - S\left(t; \mathbf{x}\right)\right\} = \text{logit}\left\{1 - S_0\left(t\right)\right\} + \mathbf{x}\boldsymbol{\beta} = \boldsymbol{s}\left(\ln t; \boldsymbol{\gamma}\right) + \mathbf{x}\boldsymbol{\beta} \tag{5.8}$$

We model the logit of the baseline distribution function as a restricted cubic spline in $\ln t$. We call a model with d d.f. (or $d-1$ interior knots) that satisfies (5.8) a PO(d) model.

5.4.4 Comparing parameters of PO(1) and loglogistic models

The PO(1) model—that is, with 1 d.f.—is identical to the loglogistic model, albeit with a different parameterization. The survival function (see the *Lognormal and loglogistic models* section in [ST] **streg**) for the loglogistic distribution with predictors $\mathbf{x}$, parameter vector $\boldsymbol{\beta}^*$, and constant β_0, and as fit by `streg, distribution(llogistic)`, can be written as

$$S\left(t\right) = \left\{1 + \left(\lambda t\right)^{1/\gamma}\right\}^{-1} = \left[1 + \exp\left\{-\left(\beta_0 + \mathbf{x}\boldsymbol{\beta}^*\right)/\gamma\right\} t^{1/\gamma}\right]^{-1} \tag{5.9}$$

`streg` reports the maximum likelihood estimates of the scale parameter, γ, and the regression parameters, β_0 and $\boldsymbol{\beta}^*$. We may compare (5.9) with that for the PO(1) model,

$$S\left(t\right) = \left\{1 + \exp\left(\gamma_0 + \mathbf{x}\boldsymbol{\beta} + \boldsymbol{\gamma}_1 \ln t\right)\right\}^{-1} = \left\{1 + \exp\left(\gamma_0 + \mathbf{x}\boldsymbol{\beta}\right) t^{\gamma_1}\right\}^{-1}$$

from which we see that $\gamma_1 = 1/\gamma$, $\gamma_0 = -\beta_0/\gamma$, and $\boldsymbol{\beta} = -\boldsymbol{\beta}^*/\gamma$. We interpret the parameters $\boldsymbol{\beta}$ of the PO(1) model as log odds-ratios, with a positive value of a regression coefficient indicating an increased risk of an event and hence diminished survival. By contrast, we interpret the parameters $\boldsymbol{\beta}^*$ of the loglogistic model that `streg` presents as those of an AFT model; the covariates impact the log survival-time. For example, $\beta^* = -0.1$ denotes a reduction of approximately 10% in the survival time for a unit change in the associated covariate value. Only the PO(1) model is susceptible to both the AFT and the log odds-ratio interpretation of its parameters. PO(d) models with $d > 1$ include spline terms in t that destroy the AFT interpretation. Similar remarks about the AFT interpretation apply to the PH(1) and Weibull models, substituting “hazard ratio” for “odds ratio”.

Example

To demonstrate the relationship between the parameters, we fit the covariate `recent` in the Rotterdam breast cancer data using PO(1) and loglogistic models. We display the parameters $\gamma_1 = 1/\gamma$, $\gamma_0 = -\beta_0/\gamma$, and $\beta_1 = \beta_1^*/\gamma$ by direct calculation from those of the `streg` model:

```
. stpm2 recent, df(1) scale(odds) noorthog nolog
Log likelihood = -3747.2718                     Number of obs   =       2982

------------------------------------------------------------------------------
             |      Coef.   Std. Err.      z    P>|z|     [95% Conf. Interval]
-------------+----------------------------------------------------------------
xb           |
      recent |  -.2125921   .0702564    -3.03   0.002    -.3502921   -.0748922
       _rcs1 |   1.135033   .0252106    45.02   0.000     1.085621    1.184445
       _cons |  -2.139772   .0662093   -32.32   0.000     -2.26954   -2.010004
------------------------------------------------------------------------------

. streg recent, distribution(llogistic) noshow noheader nolog

------------------------------------------------------------------------------
          _t |      Coef.   Std. Err.      z    P>|z|     [95% Conf. Interval]
-------------+----------------------------------------------------------------
      recent |   .1873004   .0620361     3.02   0.003     .0657119     .308889
       _cons |   1.885207   .0480622    39.22   0.000     1.791007    1.979407
-------------+----------------------------------------------------------------
     /ln_gam |  -.1266616   .0222114    -5.70   0.000     -.170195   -.0831281
-------------+----------------------------------------------------------------
       gamma |   .8810318   .0195689                      .8435003    .9202333
------------------------------------------------------------------------------

. display "gamma_1 = " 1 / exp([ln_gam]_b[_cons])
gamma_1 = 1.1350328

. display "gamma_0 = " -_b[_cons] / exp([ln_gam]_b[_cons])
gamma_0 = -2.139772

. display "beta_1 = " -_b[recent] / exp([ln_gam]_b[_cons])
beta_1 = -.21259214
```

There is agreement to at least 6 decimal places.

5.5 Probit models

5.5.1 Motivation

We can most naturally introduce probit models and their generalizations in the survival context through linear regression on log time—that is, the lognormal survival model, written as

$$\ln t = \beta_0 + \mathbf{x}\boldsymbol{\beta}^* + \varepsilon$$

where $\varepsilon \sim N(0, \sigma^2)$ is a normally distributed residual. We write $\boldsymbol{\beta}^*$ for the vector of regression coefficients rather than the usual $\boldsymbol{\beta}$, for reasons that will become clear shortly. It follows that $\ln t \sim N(\beta_0 + \mathbf{x}\boldsymbol{\beta}^*, \sigma^2)$ has distribution and survival functions

$$F(\ln t) = \Phi\left(\frac{\ln t - \beta_0 - \mathbf{x}\boldsymbol{\beta}^*}{\sigma}\right)$$
$$S(\ln t) = 1 - F(\ln t) = \Phi\left(-\frac{\ln t - \beta_0 - \mathbf{x}\boldsymbol{\beta}^*}{\sigma}\right)$$

respectively. Hence

$$-\Phi^{-1}\{S(\ln t)\} = \frac{\ln t - \beta_0 - \mathbf{x}\boldsymbol{\beta}^*}{\sigma} = \frac{\ln t - \beta_0}{\sigma} + \mathbf{x}\boldsymbol{\beta}$$

where $\boldsymbol{\beta} = -\boldsymbol{\beta}^*/\sigma$. When $\mathbf{x} = \mathbf{0}$ (the baseline condition), the random variable $(\ln t - \beta_0)/\sigma$ equals ε/σ and so has a standard normal distribution. Thus the baseline survival function is given by

$$S_0(\ln t) = \Phi\left(-\frac{\ln t - \beta_0}{\sigma}\right)$$

implying that

$$-\Phi^{-1}\{S_0(\ln t)\} = \frac{\ln t - \beta_0}{\sigma}$$

and finally

$$-\Phi^{-1}\{S(\ln t)\} = -\Phi^{-1}\{S_0(\ln t)\} + \mathbf{x}\boldsymbol{\beta} \tag{5.10}$$

We can describe a model satisfying (5.10) as a probit model on the survival-probability scale. To make the connection clear, we can write the more familiar probit model for a binary outcome y with covariates $\mathbf{x}$ as

$$-\Phi^{-1}\{\Pr(y = 1|\mathbf{x})\} = \beta_0 + \mathbf{x}\boldsymbol{\beta}$$

with the constant β_0 substituting for the transformed baseline survival function, $-\Phi^{-1}\{S_0(\ln t)\}$.

5.5.2 Generalizing the probit model

If we write $\gamma_1 = 1/\sigma$ and $\gamma_0 = -\beta_0/\sigma$, then (5.10) becomes

$$-\Phi^{-1}\{S(\ln t)\} = \gamma_0 + \gamma_1 \ln t + \mathbf{x}\boldsymbol{\beta}$$

inviting us to generalize in a fashion similar to (5.8):

$$-\Phi^{-1}\{S(\ln t)\} = \mathbf{s}(\ln t; \boldsymbol{\gamma}) + \mathbf{x}\boldsymbol{\beta}$$

We model the probit of the baseline survival distribution as a restricted cubic spline with $d > 1$ d.f. We denote such a model by probit(d). In `stpm2`, we specify probit(d) models by using the `scale(normal)` and `df(`d`)` options.

As an example, a probit(3) model for `recent`, fit using `stpm2 recent, df(3) scale(normal)`, gives the estimate $\widehat{\beta} = -0.133$ (SE 0.042). The interpretation is that `recent==1` is associated with a reduction of 0.133 on the probit scale compared with `recent==0`. Let us write $S_1(t) = S(t;1)$. At $t = 2$ years, for example, we find the predicted survival functions as follows:

```
. stpm2 recent, df(3) scale(normal) nolog
Log likelihood =  -3669.044                        Number of obs    =        2982

------------------------------------------------------------------------------
             |
-------------+----------------------------------------------------------------
xb           |
      recent |   -.132748   .0415023    -3.20   0.001    -.2140911   -.0514048
       _rcs1 |   .6125795   .0124476    49.21   0.000     .5881828    .6369763
       _rcs2 |   .0742954   .0096501     7.70   0.000     .0553816    .0932092
       _rcs3 |   .0089784   .0065179     1.38   0.168    -.0037965    .0217533
       _cons |  -.3446513   .0318649   -10.82   0.000    -.4071055   -.2821972
------------------------------------------------------------------------------

. generate t2 = 2
. predict s, timevar(t2) survival
. tabulate s

          s |      Freq.     Percent        Cum.
------------+-----------------------------------
   .7688745 |      1,167       39.13       39.13
   .8072736 |      1,815       60.87      100.00
------------+-----------------------------------
      Total |      2,982      100.00
```

If we inspect the difference between $-\Phi^{-1}\{S_1(t)\}$ and $-\Phi^{-1}\{S_0(t)\}$, we find

```
. display  (-invnormal(.8072736)) - (-invnormal(.7688745))
-.13274789
```

—that is, $\widehat{\beta}$. We interpret $\widehat{\beta}$ in a similar fashion to that in Stata's `probit` command for binary outcomes.

5.5.3 Comparing parameters of probit(1) and lognormal models

As with the PH(1) and Weibull and the PO(1) and loglogistic models, although the probit(1) and lognormal models are identical, their parameterizations differ. We can compare their parameters as follows. The lognormal model may be fit by using `streg, distribution(lnormal)`. Alternatively, we could fit this model by using `intreg` with $\ln t$ as the left endpoint and a right endpoint that is equal to missing for censoring observations and $\ln t$ for uncensored ones.

```
. streg recent, distribution(lnormal) nolog noheader
        failure _d:  rfi == 1
  analysis time _t:  rf/12
 exit on or before:  time 10 * 12
                id:  pid
```

_t	Coef.	Std. Err.	z	P>|z|	[95% Conf.	Interval]
recent	.1814727	.0618445	2.93	0.003	.0602597	.3026858
_cons	1.910411	.0489092	39.06	0.000	1.814551	2.006271
/ln_sig	.3990617	.0204162	19.55	0.000	.3590468	.4390767
sigma	1.490426	.0304288			1.431964	1.551274

With stpm2, we have

```
. stpm2 recent, df(1) scale(normal) noorthog nolog
Log likelihood = -3703.7629                    Number of obs   =       2982
```

	Coef.	Std. Err.	z	P>|z|	[95% Conf.	Interval]
xb						
recent	-.121759	.0413958	-2.94	0.003	-.2028932	-.0406248
_rcs1	.6709493	.0136982	48.98	0.000	.6441013	.6977973
_cons	-1.281789	.0364696	-35.15	0.000	-1.353268	-1.21031

The reason the parameter estimates are different is that γ_1^{-1} in the probit(1) model is the SD of the lognormal distribution (see above):

```
. display 1 / _b[_rcs1]
1.4904256
```

We need to divide the coefficients $\widehat{\gamma}_0$ and $\widehat{\beta}$ (that is, _b[_cons] and _b[recent]) from stpm2 by $-\widehat{\gamma}_1$ to give _b[_cons] and _b[recent] in the streg model:

```
. display -_b[_cons] / _b[_rcs1]
1.9104108
. display -_b[recent] / _b[_rcs1]
.18147273
```

An advantage of the stpm2 parameterization is that we take into account uncertainty in the estimate of the lognormal variance in estimating the SEs of $\widehat{\gamma}_0$ and $\widehat{\beta}$.

5.5.4 Comments on probit and POs models

The density functions underlying the lognormal and loglogistic models are similar. On the log scale, both distributions are symmetric, but the loglogistic has longer tails (a coefficient of kurtosis of 4.2 compared with 3). With a given dataset, the hazard functions are usually similar in shape and tend to zero as $t \rightarrow \infty$. Depending on γ_1, the hazard function of the loglogistic may decrease monotonically, whereas that for the lognormal is always unimodal. Also the hazard ratio for a binary variable tends to 1 as $t \to \infty$; nonproportional hazards for covariate effects is built in. As we already pointed out, this feature can be useful, because assuming that hazards converge may often be sensible when modeling certain phenomena. An example is prognosis in cancer, where the effect of a prognostic factor (covariate) on the hazard is typically greatest near $t = 0$ and fades gradually over time.

5.6 Royston–Parmar (RP) models

The well-known mathematical formula $H(t) = -\ln S(t)$ relating the survival function, $S(t)$, to the cumulative hazard function allows us to rewrite (5.3) in the following equivalent form:

$$\ln\{-\ln S(t)\} = \ln\{-\ln S_0(t)\} + \mathbf{x}\boldsymbol{\beta} \tag{5.11}$$

We may generalize (5.11) to

$$g_\theta\{S(t)\} = g_\theta\{S_0(t)\} + \mathbf{x}\boldsymbol{\beta} \tag{5.12}$$

where $g_\theta(.)$ is a monotonic increasing function, depending on a parameter θ. Royston and Parmar (2002) took $g_\theta(.)$ to be Aranda-Ordaz's (1981) function

$$g_\theta(x) = \ln\left(\frac{x^{-\theta} - 1}{\theta}\right) \tag{5.13}$$

where $\theta > 0$. We can show that the limit of $g_\theta(x)$ as θ tends to 0 is $\ln(-\ln x)$, so that with $\theta = 0$ we get the PH model (5.3).

When $\theta = 1$, then $g_\theta(x) = \ln\left(x^{-1} - 1\right) = \ln\{(1-x)/x\}$. Writing $x = S(t)$, we see that $g_1\{S(t)\} = \ln[\{1 - S(t)\}/S(t)] = \ln[F(t)/\{1 - F(t)\}]$, where $F(t) = 1 - S(t)$ is the cumulative distribution function—that is, the probability of failure in the interval $(0, t)$. Thus $g_1\{S(t)\}$ is the logit of the cumulative distribution function, and the covariate effects are proportional on the scale of the cumulative odds of an event. We can write such a PO model as

$$\text{logit}\{1 - S(t)\} = \text{logit}\{1 - S_0(t)\} + \mathbf{x}\boldsymbol{\beta}$$

In `stpm2`, we specify PO(#) models by using the `scale(odds)` and `df(#)` options.

The RP family of survival models is defined by (5.12). We estimate the transformed baseline survival function, $g_\theta\{S_0(t)\}$, by a restricted cubic spline. As we explained in section 5.5.2, the family of distributions described by Royston and Parmar (2002) is completed by adding the probit class of models. Here the parameter θ is redundant and we define $g_\theta(.)$ as minus the probit or inverse normal cumulative distribution function, $-\Phi^{-1}(.)$, or `-invnormal()` in Stata. The resulting model is

$$g_\theta\{S(t;\mathbf{x})\} = -\Phi^{-1}\{S(t;\mathbf{x})\} = -\Phi^{-1}\{S_0(t)\} + \mathbf{x}\boldsymbol{\beta}$$

In principle, many other generalizations of (5.12) are possible, depending only on an appropriate choice of $g_\theta(.)$. However, we are not aware of proposals for further generalizations.

5.6.1 Models with θ not equal to 0 or 1

With the Aranda-Ordaz definition of $g_\theta\{S(t)\}$, (5.12) is valid for any nonnegative value of θ, thereby providing a rich class of potential models. Because models with θ not equal to 0 or 1 have no natural scale for covariate effects, their interpretation is difficult, and therefore Royston and Parmar (2002) downweighted their importance. In some datasets, however, a model with $\theta \neq 0$ or 1 may provide a better fit than either $\theta = 0$ or $\theta = 1$. Further, by estimating θ and its 95% CI from the data, we can judge informally whether the model is closer to satisfying the PH or the PO assumption. Whether to consider models with θ not equal to 0 or 1 depends on whether we must have interpretable covariate effects or whether we simply want a good predictor, irrespective of the interpretation of its component parts.

5.6.2 Example

In the Rotterdam breast cancer data, we define a variable **np** (node positive) to be 0 if a patient is node negative and 1 if node positive. We fit RP models on the single covariate **np** with two interior knots for the baseline spline function, allowing θ in (5.13) to vary. We fit the model using the **scale(theta)** option of **stpm2**, as follows:

```
. generate byte np = (nodes > 0)
. stpm2 np, df(3) scale(theta) nolog
Log likelihood = -3545.1757                    Number of obs   =       2982

              Coef.    Std. Err.       z    P>|z|     [95% Conf. Interval]

xb
         np   1.120418   .1203344     9.31   0.000     .8845671    1.356269
      _rcs1   1.160949    .066155    17.55   0.000     1.031287     1.29061
      _rcs2   .2297915   .0267035     8.61   0.000     .1774536    .2821294
      _rcs3  -.0104059    .012556    -0.83   0.407    -.0350151    .0142034
      _cons  -1.367053   .0701706   -19.48   0.000    -1.504585   -1.229521

ln_theta
      _cons  -.0389786   .3652229    -0.11   0.915    -.7548023     .676845

. lincom [ln_theta]_cons, eform
 ( 1)  [ln_theta]_cons = 0

             exp(b)   Std. Err.       z    P>|z|     [95% Conf. Interval]

        (1)  .9617713   .3512609    -0.11   0.915     .4701036     1.96766
```

Because we have estimated $\ln\theta$ rather than θ, we obtain $\widehat{\theta}$ and its 95% CI using **lincom**. We find $\widehat{\theta} = 0.96$ (95% CI; [0.47, 1.97]). The result has two implications. First, $\widehat{\theta}$ is very close to 1, suggesting that a PO model is best; second, $\widehat{\theta}$ is far from 0, suggesting that a PH model does not fit satisfactorily.

5.6.3 Likelihood function and parameter estimation*

Suppose that the sample comprises n independent observations $\{t_i, \delta_i, \mathbf{x}_i\}$, where δ_i is 0 for a right-censored observation and 1 for an observed event. Let the likelihood for the ith observation be l_i, so that the likelihood for the whole sample is $\Pi_{i=1}^n l_i$. As already stated in (1.1), for all models the contribution, l_i, of the ith observation to the total log likelihood is $\delta_i \ln h(t_i) + \ln S(t_i)$; with late entry at t_{0i}, it becomes $\delta_i \ln h(t_i) + \ln S(t_i) - \ln S(t_{0i})$. Let $\eta_i = s(\ln t_i; \boldsymbol{\gamma}) + \mathbf{x}_i \boldsymbol{\beta}$ and its first derivative be $\eta_i' = d\eta_i/dt_i = ds(\ln t_i; \boldsymbol{\gamma})/dt_i = t_i^{-1} ds(\ln t_i; \boldsymbol{\gamma})/d(\ln t_i)$. In detail, (1.1) becomes the following:

For PH models,

$$l_i = \begin{cases} \eta_i' \exp(\eta_i - \exp \eta_i) & \text{for an observed event,} \\ \exp(-\exp \eta_i) & \text{for a censored observation} \end{cases}$$

For PO models,

$$l_i = \begin{cases} \eta_i' \exp(\eta_i)(1 + \exp \eta_i)^{-2} & \text{for an observed event,} \\ (1 + \exp \eta_i)^{-1} & \text{for a censored observation} \end{cases}$$

For probit models,

$$l_i = \begin{cases} \eta_i' \phi(\eta_i) & \text{for an observed event,} \\ \Phi(-\eta_i) & \text{for a censored observation} \end{cases}$$

where $\phi(.)$ is the standard normal density function (`normalden()` in Stata). The expressions for l_i are the density function at t_i for observed events and the estimated survival probability at t_i for censored observations. Also

$$\begin{aligned} \frac{ds(\ln t_i; \boldsymbol{\gamma})}{d(\ln t_i)} &= \gamma_1 + \sum_{j=2}^{m} \gamma_j \frac{dz_j(\ln t_i)}{d(\ln t_i)} \\ &= \gamma_1 + \sum_{j=2}^{m} \gamma_j \left\{ 3(\ln t_i - k_j)_+^2 - 3\lambda_j (\ln t_i - k_{\min})_+^2 \right. \\ &\quad \left. -3(1 - \lambda_j)(\ln t_i - k_{\max})_+^2 \right\} \end{aligned}$$

We can readily extend the expressions for the likelihood to allow for late entry, but the details are not given here.

Estimation is by maximum likelihood. To obtain estimates of $\boldsymbol{\gamma}$ and $\boldsymbol{\beta}$, we need suitable starting values. We make initial guesses by fitting a Cox model with covariates $\mathbf{x}$. We estimate the survival function $\widehat{S}(t_i; \mathbf{x}_i)$ at the ith observation from the Cox model as the baseline survival function at t_i raised to the power of the estimated relative hazard, $\exp\left(\mathbf{x}_i \widehat{\boldsymbol{\beta}}\right)$. The initial guesses are $\ln\left\{-\ln \widehat{S}(t_i; \mathbf{x}_i)\right\}$ for $\ln H(t_i; \mathbf{x}_i)$ in the PH model, $\text{logit}\left\{1 - \widehat{S}(t_i; \mathbf{x}_i)\right\}$ for the log cumulative odds of an event in the PO model, and $-\Phi^{-1}\left\{\widehat{S}\left(t_i;\mathbf{x}_i\right)\right\}$ for the probit of the cumulative incidence in the probit model. We determine starting values for $\boldsymbol{\gamma}$ and $\boldsymbol{\beta}$ by ordinary least-squares regression of these functions on $\ln t_i$, $\mathbf{x}_i$ and the spline basis functions with the desired number of knots. We use only the observed event times in the initial computations. We then perform full maximum likelihood estimation by using the `ml` routine. Typically, convergence occurs in about 3 to 10 iterations.

5.6.4 Comparing regression coefficients

The number of positive lymph nodes (`nodes`) is the strongest predictor in the Rotterdam breast cancer dataset. In table 5.3, we compare the estimated regression coefficients for the effect of three dummy variables (`n1`, 1–3 nodes; `n2`, 4–9 nodes; `n3`, 10 or more nodes) with 0 nodes as the baseline in a number of PH models.

Table 5.3. Rotterdam breast cancer data. Estimated regression coefficients for three dummy variables representing the number of positive lymph nodes. PH(d) denotes a proportional cumulative hazards model with $d-1$ interior knots.

Model	n1		n2		n3	
	$\widehat{\beta}$	SE	$\widehat{\beta}$	SE	$\widehat{\beta}$	SE
Exponential	0.452	0.068	1.155	0.068	1.616	0.081
Weibull	0.452	0.068	1.157	0.069	1.619	0.082
PH(2)	0.432	0.068	1.101	0.069	1.575	0.082
PH(3)	0.433	0.068	1.101	0.069	1.572	0.082
PH(4)	0.433	0.068	1.101	0.069	1.572	0.082
Cox	0.432	0.067	1.099	0.069	1.569	0.082

The values of $\widehat{\beta}$ for a given variable are generally similar among models, and the SEs are almost identical. The values of $\widehat{\beta}$ hardly vary among PH models, and are very close to those from the Cox model.

5.6.5 Model selection

Here we give a simple example of choosing a model from the RP class with given covariates, leaving the more complex issue of selecting variables and functional forms for continuous variables to chapter 6. Table 5.4 shows the AIC values for models including `n1`, `n2`, and `n3` (see section 5.6.4).

Table 5.4. Rotterdam breast cancer data. AIC values for 12 models. For legibility, 6,900 has been subtracted from all AIC values.

Interior knots	PH	PO	probit
0	249.8	134.4	83.2
1	31.0	9.1	18.6
2	28.5	8.9	20.4
3	30.4	10.8	21.5

Recalling that a smaller AIC indicates a better fit (penalized for model complexity), the best of the 12 models appears to be PO(2). However, the AIC for the PO(1) model is barely inferior, and we might prefer the latter model on grounds of parsimony.

5.6.6 Sensitivity to number of knots

Figure 5.7 compares the estimated baseline survival functions from PO models with 0, 1, 2, and 3 interior knots (1, 2, 3, and 4 d.f.), with covariates `n1`, `n2`, and `n3`.

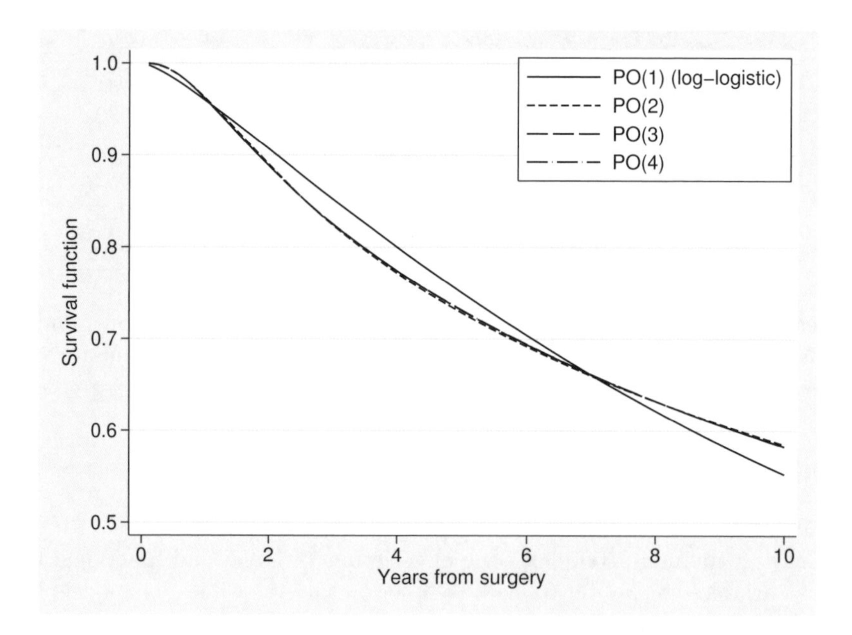

Figure 5.7. Rotterdam breast cancer data. Estimated baseline survival functions for three models, with covariates `n1`, `n2`, and `n3`.

We can barely distinguish among the survival functions for 1 to 3 knots. In this example, the simplest model, PO(1) (that is, loglogistic) is a poor fit, failing to capture the shape of the survival function. The results tie in nicely with the AIC values given in table 5.4.

5.6.7 Sensitivity to location of knots

By default, we choose knot positions for models with 2 interior knots at the 33rd and 67th centiles of the log observed event times. How critical is the choice? To investigate this, we selected knot centile positions to be 10 random pairs of integers in the range $[1, 99]$. The following sets of numbers were selected: $(67, 93)$, $(47, 48)$, $(56, 97)$, $(82, 84)$, $(38, 58)$, $(12, 51)$, $(3, 57)$, $(50, 84)$, $(59, 72)$, and $(1, 2)$. None of these is particularly close to $(33, 67)$. Figure 5.8 shows the resulting estimated survival curves.

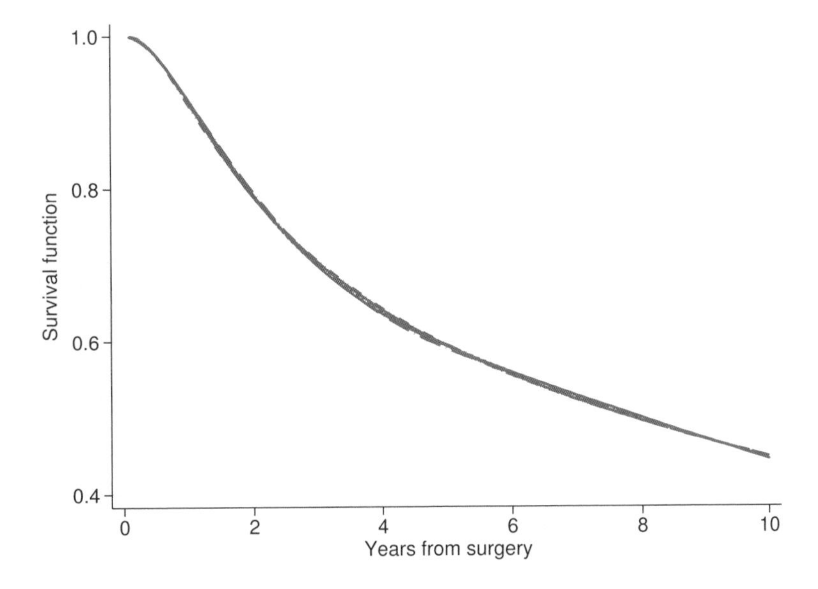

Figure 5.8. Rotterdam breast cancer data. Effect of varying knot positions in two-knot PH models. See text for details.

The curves are very similar, even when the extreme knot positions $(1, 2)$ are used. We would not wish to claim that knot positioning is always as uncritical as in this example. It pays to try a few variations.

5.7 Concluding remarks

In this chapter, we introduced RP survival models as generalizations of the exponential, Weibull, loglogistic, and lognormal models. We showed that RP models reproduce familiar parametric models (Weibull, loglogistic, and lognormal) when the d.f. are set to 1, although with a different parameterization. So far, we have explored only simple models with essentially one covariate at most. In subsequent chapters, we demonstrate the power and flexibility of the models in more complex cases. For example, we consider multivariable models for prognosis, models to accommodate time-varying effects of time-fixed covariates, and models for relative survival, in which the force of mortality from background causes competes with risk from the disease or condition of principal interest.

6 Prognostic models

Summary

1. Prognostic models are multiple regression models that predict future outcomes given values of several covariates measured at the time origin $t = 0$.
2. It is important to exercise care in choosing a meaningful baseline survival function for a prognostic model. This requires appropriate arithmetic centering of covariates, for example, on their mean, median, or mode.
3. Selection of influential covariates can be done on subject-matter grounds, or by applying statistical selection criteria such as backward elimination of variables whose p-values are not sufficiently low, or by a combination of both approaches.
4. Parametric prognostic models (including Royston–Parmar [RP] models) have many advantages, such as the ability to predict a wide range of relevant outputs, which include several different types of survival curves.
5. Goodness of fit may be assessed by using smoothed martingale residuals.
6. It is useful to assess the discrimination and variation explained by a prognostic model.
7. Full validation of prognostic models requires external data and out-of-sample prediction of relevant quantities.
8. Survival times may be visualized using imputation of right-censored observation times.

6.1 Introduction

Prognostic models are multiple regression models that are intended to enable prediction of future outcomes given values of several covariates measured at or before the time origin $t = 0$. They are widely used in medicine, particularly in common, serious disorders such as cancer and heart disease. Although we are often interested in the prognostic ability of specific single markers of disease progression or mortality, statistical prognostication is typically multifactorial. See Moons et al. (2009) for further background on prognostic modeling.

What outputs are needed from a prognostic model? Purely from the point of view of prediction, we require survival probabilities at given covariate values—or often, for entire prognostic groups. Also important are the baseline hazard function and conditional survival probabilities. The latter are probabilities of the form $S(t|t_a;\mathbf{x})$ where $t_a > 0$ is some time point of interest. They provide answers to the question "given that I have survived to such-and-such a time, what is the chance of an event in future?" In some diseases, the hazard peaks early on, and provided the patient gets beyond that point in time without an event, their prospects improve considerably.

Usually, prognostic models are derived from data with long-term follow-up. Often the effect of a covariate on the hazard scale is most marked near $t = 0$ but wanes with time (a so-called time-dependent effect), as opposed to having a constant multiplicative effect (for example, on the hazard function). We need to be able to extend a prognostic model with time-dependent effects as necessary.

Flexible parametric prognostic survival models, which we describe in the present chapter, provide a good workable solution to the problem of developing useful prognostic models. Although in principle we could have used Poisson models (see chapter 4), in practice RP models are easier to work with.

In this chapter, we use the Rotterdam breast cancer dataset in essentially all the example analyses. Unless stated otherwise, we assume that the file `rott2.dta` has been loaded (that is, `use rott2, clear`) before each of the examples is run.

6.2 Developing and reporting a prognostic model

A good example of developing and reporting a prognostic model is Clark et al. (2001). The disease is ovarian cancer and the (partially censored) outcome of interest is time from diagnosis to death from any cause (that is, overall survival time).

Typically, authors of articles in the medical literature on prognostic modeling of a time-to-event outcome adopt the following sequence:

1. Describe the background (disease, past research, prognostic factors of interest and why they are thought to be prognostic).
2. Describe the statistical distribution of the potential prognostic factors.
3. Describe the univariate association between each covariate and the outcome (usually, relative hazard from a Cox model). The aim is to get a feel for the importance (or otherwise) of each factor on its own and its association with the outcome.
4. Build a multivariable Cox model from some or all the available factors, usually by a stepwise selection method eliminating factors not statistically significant at, say, the 5% level.
5. Form the resulting prognostic index (linear predictor) $\mathbf{x}\widehat{\beta}$ and categorize it into a number (usually 3–5) of equal- or unequal-sized prognostic groups.

6. Compute and plot the Kaplan–Meier survival curve for each group. A typical example using 4 groups is figure 1 of Clark et al. (2001).
7. Discuss the results.

The prognostic index is sometimes known as a risk score. Some authors provide a nomogram, based on the prognostic index, to assist the computation of predicted outcomes. For example, the nomogram in figure 2 of Clark et al. (2001) provides an estimate of the predicted 2 year and 5 year survival probability for an individual with ovarian cancer, given the values of her prognostic factors. With modern computing facilities and the widespread use of Internet tools, nomograms are rather outdated now.

In this chapter, we focus on selecting a suitable RP model and presenting its results in different ways, using the Rotterdam breast cancer data for the sake of example.

6.3 What does the baseline hazard function mean?

As noted in section 1.2, the term baseline hazard means "the hazard function when all covariates are equal to zero" in the context of the Cox model. In a randomized trial, for example, the control arm (standard treatment) is often coded 0, and the experimental arm (new treatment) is coded 1. The baseline hazard (and survival) functions then quite naturally refer to the control arm. In the more general context of multivariable models, though, we see three problems with the definition:

1. The terminology is misleading. "Baseline" may suggest "low(est) risk", which is not always the case when $\mathbf{x} = 0$. For example, if a covariate is negatively associated with the hazard rate, a lower value means higher risk.
2. The subpopulation with $\mathbf{x} = 0$ may be irrelevant or even nonexistent. For example, age is a strong prognostic factor in many adult diseases. If age is included in the model, the strict definition of baseline age implies reference to a subpopulation of newborn babies (age $= 0$). If hemoglobin (a key component of red blood cells) were in the model, a baseline with hemoglobin $= 0$ would apply to no living human being.
3. Multivariable models typically comprise a mixture of binary, categorical, and continuous predictors, sometimes with transformations of the latter. It is not obvious what to take as a sensible baseline value for each predictor.

In a multivariable model that includes continuous variables, for the baseline $\mathbf{x} = 0$ to make sense, some form of centering of the covariates is needed. The fractional polynomial (FP) commands in Stata (that is, `fracpoly` and `mfp`) automatically center a continuous covariate x on its mean, $\overline{x}$, such that the partial predictor for x evaluates to zero at $\overline{x}$. An option (`adjust()` in Stata 10, `center()` in Stata 11 or later) is available for the user to choose centering value(s). If necessary, `fracpoly` and `mfp` also recode binary variables by subtracting the value corresponding to the lower category if that value is not zero. Multicategory variables are typically handled by way of dummy variables, with one dummy omitted corresponding to the chosen baseline level. Dummy variables automatically provide a reasonable base category.

A simple alternative to explicit centering or referencing is computing the prognostic index ($\mathbf{x}\widehat{\beta}$) from uncentered covariates, subtracting a central value (c, say) such as the mean or median of $\mathbf{x}\widehat{\beta}$, and refitting the model to $\mathbf{x}\widehat{\beta} - c$.

For the model to be used in a different setting, we must record details of the centering carried out on the predictors. Then someone else can recover all the information necessary to construct predictions and prognostic groups.

6.3.1 Example

To illustrate what may go wrong with baseline calculation, we consider the predictor `nodes` in the Rotterdam breast cancer data. As we note in section 6.4.2, the transformation `enodes` $= \exp(-0.12 \times$ `nodes`$)$ represents the functional form for this variable in a proportional hazards (PH) model quite well. We use `stpm2` to fit a RP PH model with 2 degrees of freedom (d.f.) for the baseline log cumulative hazard, first without centering of `enodes` and then centering on the mean of `enodes`. We predict the baseline survival function in each case and compare the resulting estimates with the Kaplan–Meier curve for the entire dataset. The results are shown in figure 6.1.

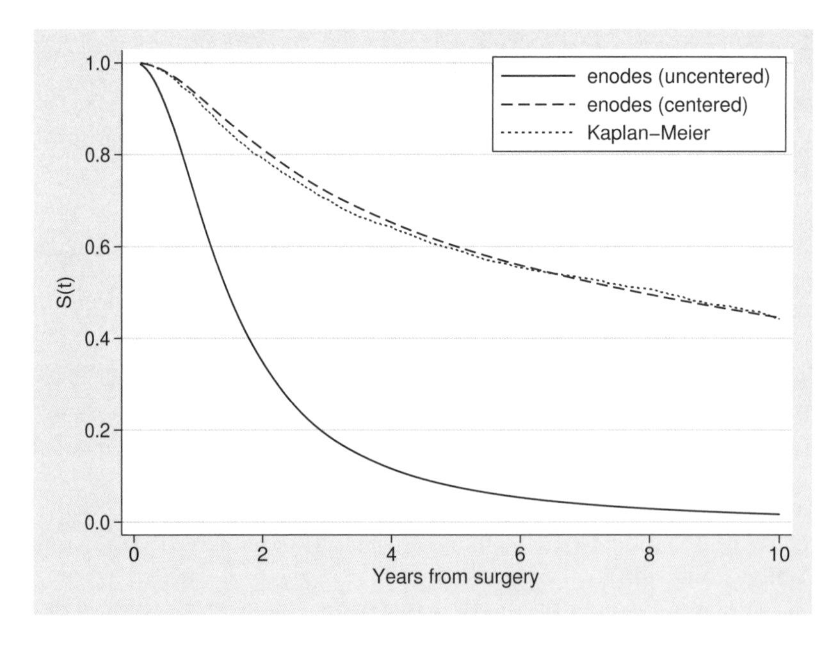

Figure 6.1. Rotterdam breast cancer data. Comparison of baseline survival curves for two RP PH models, each with 2 d.f. and a single covariate (`enodes` uncentered or centered) and the Kaplan–Meier estimate for the entire dataset.

The Stata code for the task is as follows:

```
. // Center enodes on mean
. summarize enodes
    Variable |       Obs        Mean    Std. Dev.       Min        Max
-------------+--------------------------------------------------------
      enodes |      2982    .7958886    .2638654   .0169075          1
. generate enodes_cent = enodes - r(mean)
. // Fit uncentered covariate
. quietly stpm2 enodes, df(2) scale(hazard)
. predict s0, survival zeros
. // Fit centered covariate
. quietly stpm2 enodes_cent, df(2) scale(hazard)
. predict s1, survival zeros
. // Kaplan-Meier
. sts gen s = s
. line s0 s1 s _t, sort xtitle("Years from surgery")
> ytitle("S(t)") connect(l l J) ylabel(, angle(h) format(%4.1f))
> legend(label(1 "enodes (uncentered)") label(2 "enodes (centered)")
> label(3 "Kaplan-Meier") ring(0) pos(1) col(1))
```

The baseline survival curve for `enodes` (uncentered) represents far worse relapse-free survival than the overall (Kaplan–Meier) curve. By contrast, the baseline survival curve for `enodes` (centered) quite closely matches the Kaplan–Meier estimate and well represents the "average" survival curve in the dataset. The mean of `enodes` is 0.80, corresponding to `nodes` = 1.9. Because `nodes` is always whole number, for descriptive purposes we should have centered the curve on two nodes—that is, on `enodes` = 0.79.

We have evaluated the survival curve for `enodes` (uncentered) at `enodes` = 0—that is, at `nodes` = $\ln(0)/(-0.12) = \infty$. A large number of nodes predicts poor survival, so the curve for `enodes` = 0 represents the worst survival imaginable for this variable. Of course, `nodes` = ∞ is infeasible, anyway; the largest value in the dataset is 34.

6.4 Model selection

An important issue in developing a prognostic model is how to build a multivariable RP model from a number of candidate predictors. We must consider four key issues:

1. Choice of scale (hazards, odds, or probit) and baseline complexity (d.f. for the spline function)
2. Selection of influential variables
3. Dealing with possible nonlinearity of continuous covariates
4. Assessing the need to extend the model for time-dependent effects

In this chapter, we address issues 1–3, leaving a discussion of modeling time-dependent effects for chapter 7.

6.4.1 Choice of scale and baseline complexity

To choose a suitable scale for the model, we need a preliminary model that roughly fits the data. A perfect fit of the covariates with maximal explanatory power is not needed when we are concerned only with choice of scale; we are mainly concerned with identifying the best (or perhaps least bad!) proportionality assumption about the covariate effects. We may obtain a simple preliminary model by categorizing all continuous covariates into, say, five equal groups and then creating 4 dummy variables per covariate. We represent categorical variables by their dummy variables in the usual way. As an alternative, we may assume linear effects for continuous covariates, but if there are major nonlinearities, imposing linearity may be a dangerous strategy. We perform no variable selection, but fit the full model (without interactions). We assess choice of scale and number of knots for the baseline spline function by inspecting the Akaike information criterion (AIC) or Bayes information criterion (BIC) statistics, as described in section 5.6.5.

Example

As mentioned above, we use the Rotterdam breast cancer data. The variables we wish to fit are `size`, `meno`, and `grade`, and categorized versions of `age`, `nodes`, `pr`, `er`, and `year`. Code for computing the AIC and BIC values for PH, proportional odds (PO), probit, and Aranda-Ordaz (AO) models each with 1–5 d.f. for the baseline spline function is as follows:

```
// Categorize continuous predictors in 5 groups
foreach v of varlist age nodes pr er year {
     xtile `v´c5 = `v´, n(5)
}
foreach scale in hazard odds normal theta {
     display _n "Scale = `scale´"
     forvalues j = 1 / 5 {
           quietly xi: stpm2 i.agec5 i.nodesc5 i.prc5 i.erc5 i.yearc5 i.size ///
               i.grade meno chemo hormon, df(`j´) scale(`scale´)
           display "df = `j´, AIC = " %7.2f e(AIC) " BIC = " %7.2f e(BIC)
     }
}
```

The results are given in table 6.1.

Table 6.1. Rotterdam breast cancer data. Choice of scale and baseline complexity for a simplified multivariable prognostic model. For legibility, 6,000 has been subtracted from all AIC and BIC values.

d.f.	PH		PO		probit		AO	
	AIC	BIC	AIC	BIC	AIC	BIC	AIC	BIC
1	986.25	1129.29	821.57	964.61	782.78	925.82	772.12	920.46
2	768.85	917.19	700.58	848.92	716.37	864.71	699.96	853.60
3	767.72	921.35	701.71	855.34	717.26	870.90	701.42	860.35
4	769.67	928.60	703.79	862.72	718.29	877.22	703.46	867.69
5	771.43	935.66	705.44	869.67	719.43	883.66	705.05	874.58

We have underlined the best (lowest) values of AIC and BIC for each scale. Except for PH with AIC, a model with 2 d.f. optimizes both AIC and BIC. The scale minimizing the AIC is AO, but it is trivially better than the more parsimonious PO, which also minimizes the BIC. The preliminary analysis therefore indicates that PO(2) is a suitable family of RP models for this dataset. Recall that in the PO model, we assume that the relative effect of a covariate on the hazard scale diminishes with time.

The AO model has $\widehat{\theta} = 1.34$ (95% confidence interval [CI]: $[0.96, 1.85]$), so in any case the model does not fit significantly better than the PO model (for which $\theta = 1$).

We reach the same conclusions if we fit models that assume linear covariate effects (data not shown).

We may repeat the exercise without covariates; that is, we look for the best way to model the overall log cumulative hazard, log cumulative odds, or probit functions. We find that according to AIC, the PH, PO, and probit models with 2 d.f. all give about the same fit. Perhaps not surprisingly, excluding covariates largely removes our ability to distinguish among scales.

6.4.2 Selection of variables and functional forms

Royston and Sauerbrei (2008, 32–34) argue for backward elimination of weakly influential variables in regression models. Starting from the full model including all predictors, we identify the least significant variable by applying either a Wald test or a likelihood-ratio test. If the variable is not significant at some predetermined significance level, α, we drop it. We assess the next least important variable in the same way and continue the process until no further variables can be removed. A variant (backward stepwise) is to consider reincluding variables that have been dropped already. We may consider variables that are linked (for example, dummy variables for a categorical predictor or transformations of a continuous variable) jointly for exclusion *en bloc*.

The other important issue is possible nonlinearity of continuous predictors. Royston and Sauerbrei (2008) describe the multivariable FP procedure, which is implemented in Stata's mfp command (see [R] **mfp**). We again apply a type of backward elimination to select FP transformations of continuous predictors, which involves a closed test procedure. We preselect the most complex model permitted for each continuous predictor; by default, this is a second-order fractional polynomial (FP2). We perform the following sequence of nested tests: FP2 versus null, FP2 versus linear, and FP2 versus first-order fractional polynomial (FP1). We stop when a given test is nonsignificant at the predetermined significance level, α.

We wish to point out that although selection of variables on statistical criteria was described as long ago as the 1960s, it is still a controversial topic. The main reason is that selecting variables in this way can incur biases of different types: a) selection bias when a regression coefficient just happens to be larger than its true value and more significant by chance than it should be; and b) omission bias when inappropriate omission of a variable biases the regression coefficients of other, correlated variables that remain. Some people complain that p-values arising within selection procedures are not honest—that is, they exaggerate the true statistical significance of a selected variable and downplay that of an omitted variable. To try to circumvent these issues, some statisticians, notably Frank Harrell, advocate fitting the full model comprising all available covariates (Harrell 2001). However, the full model is not an adequately defined entity in many studies. For example, does it include transformations of variables or interactions between variables to improve fit? What about variables that we measured but discarded in the early stages of data appraisal, never to be mentioned again—an aspect of Mallows's (1998) "zeroth problem"?. In practice, Harrell would prune some predictors from the list, specifically, he says, by *not* looking at the strength of their relationship with the outcome variable.

Of course, we should not ignore the principle of including a variable in a model, irrespective of its statistical significance, when subject matter knowledge or other convincing evidence suggests its prior importance.

Our view is that the statistical ills discussed above are largely the province of small samples, weak covariate effects, and too many predictors. In substantial datasets with adequately prognostic variables and a reasonable number of predictors (for example, 5 to 30), we see selection and omission bias as no serious issue. In the context of variable selection, we regard p-values more as tools for screening for important variables than as accurate reflections of statistical significance. See Sauerbrei, Royston, and Binder (2007a) for a further discussion of the issues. In particular, practical recommendations may be found in their tables 1 and 3.

Example

We introduced FPs in section 4.9. We apply mfp to construct a prognostic model of type PO(2) for the Rotterdam breast cancer data. We use a significance level of $\alpha = 0.05$ for selecting variables and FP functional forms. (Occasionally, it makes sense to use different α-values to select variables and functions.) First, as proposed by Sauerbrei and Royston (1999), we apply a preliminary negative exponential transformation, `enodes = exp(-0.12* nodes)`, where `nodes` is the number of positive lymph nodes. The variable `enodes` has already been created in `rott2.dta`. To ensure that an FP1 (not an FP2) model is fit to `enodes`, we specify 2 d.f. for it; we thereby make sure we get a monotonic function for `nodes`. The results are as follows:

```
. xi: mfp, select(0.05) df(enodes:2): stpm2 age enodes pr er year
> (i.size) i.grade meno chemo hormon, df(2) scale(odds)
i.size            _Isize_1-3         (naturally coded; _Isize_1 omitted)
i.grade           _Igrade_2-3        (naturally coded; _Igrade_2 omitted)
Deviance for model with all terms untransformed =  6692.184, 2982 observations
  (output omitted)
Fractional polynomial fitting algorithm converged after 3 cycles.
Transformations of covariates:
-> gen double Iage__1 = age-55.0583501 if e(sample)
-> gen double Ienod__1 = enodes^2-.6334386427 if e(sample)
-> gen double Ipr__1 = ln(X)+1.815040453 if e(sample)
   (where: X = (pr+1)/1000)
Final multivariable fractional polynomial model for _t
```

Variable	Initial df	Initial Select	Initial Alpha	Final Status	Final df	Final Powers
age	4	0.0500	0.0500	in	1	1
enodes	2	0.0500	0.0500	in	2	2
pr	4	0.0500	0.0500	in	2	0
er	4	0.0500	0.0500	out	0	
year	4	0.0500	0.0500	out	0	
_Isize_2 ...	1	0.0500	0.0500	in	1	1
_Igrade_3	1	0.0500	0.0500	in	1	1
meno	1	0.0500	0.0500	out	0	
chemo	1	0.0500	0.0500	in	1	1
hormon	1	0.0500	0.0500	in	1	1

```
Log likelihood = -3330.6375                    Number of obs   =       2982
```

	Coef.	Std. Err.	z	P>|z|	[95% Conf.	Interval]
xb						
Iage__1	-.0190175	.0031803	-5.98	0.000	-.0252507	-.0127843
Ienod__1	-2.469988	.1262644	-19.56	0.000	-2.717462	-2.222515
Ipr__1	-.0831007	.0164349	-5.06	0.000	-.1153125	-.0508888
_Isize_2	.3873098	.0786168	4.93	0.000	.2332237	.5413958
_Isize_3	.6630704	.1288065	5.15	0.000	.4106143	.9155265
_Igrade_3	.4909539	.0853156	5.75	0.000	.3237384	.6581693
chemo	-.7075086	.102732	-6.89	0.000	-.9088597	-.5061576
hormon	-.6668108	.1200258	-5.56	0.000	-.902057	-.4315647
_rcs1	1.287639	.0292011	44.10	0.000	1.230406	1.344872
_rcs2	.2205794	.0208198	10.59	0.000	.1797733	.2613854
_cons	-1.167841	.0894271	-13.06	0.000	-1.343115	-.9925673

```
Deviance: 6661.275.
```

A linear function is selected for `age`. FP1 transformations are selected for `enodes` (power 2) and `pr` (power 0—that is, log transformation). The variables `year`, `meno`, and `er` are eliminated. Each of the selected variables appears to be highly significant, each z-value (that is, regression coefficient divided by standard error [SE]) being no less than 4.9 in absolute value.

6.5 Quantitative outputs from the model

We treat the multivariable FP model reported in section 6.4.2 as final for present purposes. The results we describe below are all based on the final model.

6.5.1 Survival probabilities for individuals

It is easy to obtain estimated survival probabilities following use of `stpm2`. Figure 6.2 shows the distribution of $\widehat{S}(t|\mathbf{x})$ for $t = 2$ years and $t = 5$ years from the model fit in section 6.4.2.

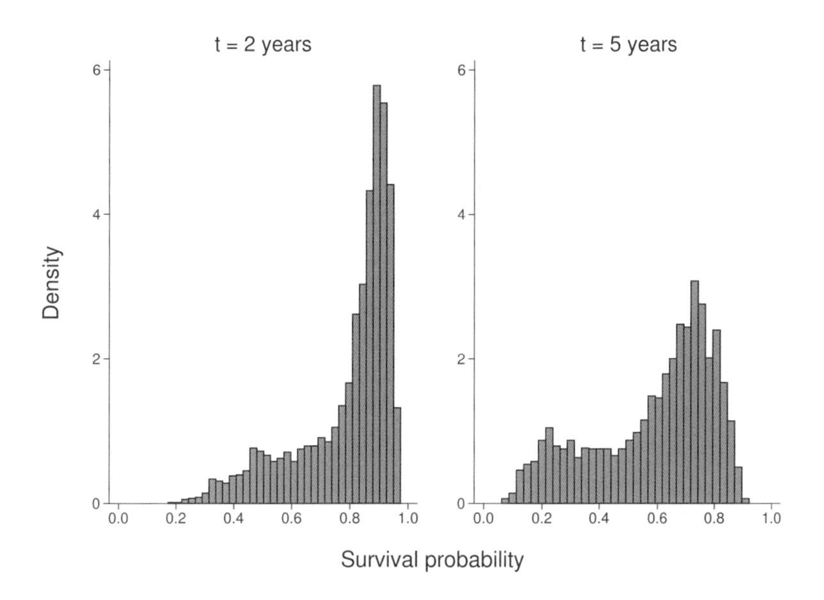

Figure 6.2. Rotterdam breast cancer data. Predicted survival probabilities of all patients at $t = 2$ and $t = 5$ years.

We created the plot from the commands

```
. // Fit MFP model and predict prognostic index
. quietly xi: stpm2 age enodes_1 pr_1 i.size grade chemo hormon,
> scale(odds) df(2)
. generate t2 = 2
. generate t5 = 5
. predict s2, timevar(t2) survival
. predict s5, timevar(t5) survival
. global stuff ytitle("") ylabel(, angle(horizontal))
> xtitle("") xlabel(, format(%4.1f))
. histogram s2, $stuff name(g1, replace) title("t = 2 years")
(bin=34, start=.17290842, width=.02355452)
. histogram s5, $stuff name(g2, replace) title("t = 5 years")
(bin=34, start=.0611941, width=.0252724)
. graph combine g1 g2, xcommon ycommon b2title("Survival probability")
> l1title("Density")
```

The median relapse-free survival probabilities are 0.86 and 0.65 at two and five years, respectively. We interpret the value of 0.86, for example, by saying that half the individuals in the sample had at least an 86% chance of surviving two years without an event. Note the wide range of probabilities at both time points, suggesting that the disease has a very variable clinical course.

An additional quantity of prognostic interest is conditional survival, which answers questions like "I have survived two years without a recurrence; what are my chances of surviving to five years without one?" We can easily estimate such probabilities with `stpm2`. Mathematically, we have

$$\begin{aligned}\Pr(T > 5 | T > 2; \mathbf{x}) &= \Pr(T > 5 \text{ and } \; T > 2; \mathbf{x}) / \Pr(T > 2; \mathbf{x}) \\ &= \Pr(T > 5; \mathbf{x}) / \Pr(T > 2; \mathbf{x}) \\ &= S(5; \mathbf{x}) / S(2; \mathbf{x})\end{aligned}$$

—that is, the survival probability at five years divided by that at two years. Using the data in figure 6.2, we simply divide the individual values in the right panel by those in the left panel.

```
. generate s52 = s5/s2
```

The result is shown in figure 6.3.

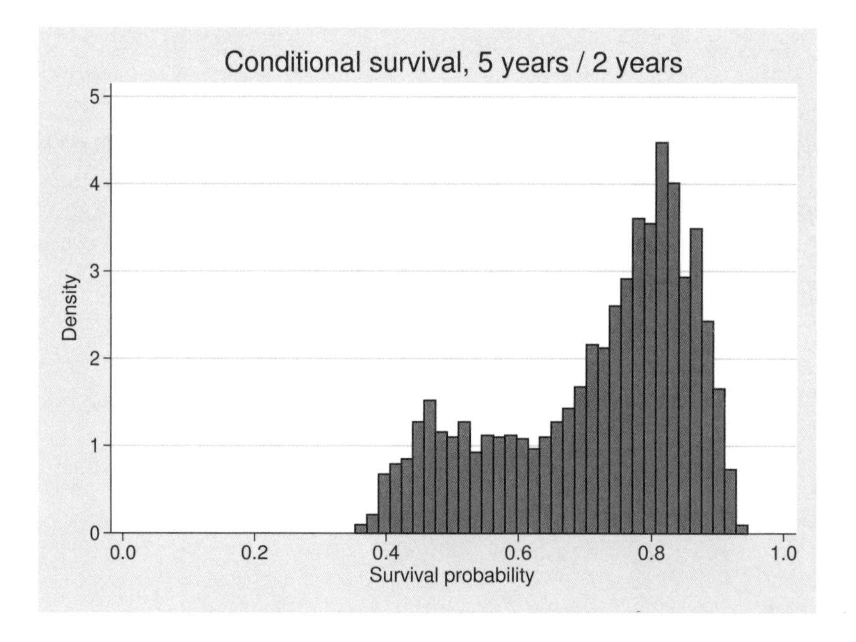

Figure 6.3. Rotterdam breast cancer data. Conditional survival probabilities at five years, given no relapse up to two years.

The conditional prognosis at five years, given two years, is much better than the unconditional prognosis at $t = 5$ years. The median conditional five-year probability is 0.76. The 10th centile is 0.48, double the unconditional value of 0.24.

6.5.2 Survival probabilities across the risk spectrum

Rather than fixing times of interest and examining the distribution of survival probabilities, an alternative is to plot estimated survival probabilities against t at specified centiles of the distribution of the prognostic index—for example, at the 10th, 20th, ..., 90th centiles. The plot gives an impression of the available range of discrimination, showing what may happen to individuals at the extremes of the risk spectrum and in the middle. We show an example of such a plot in figure 6.4.

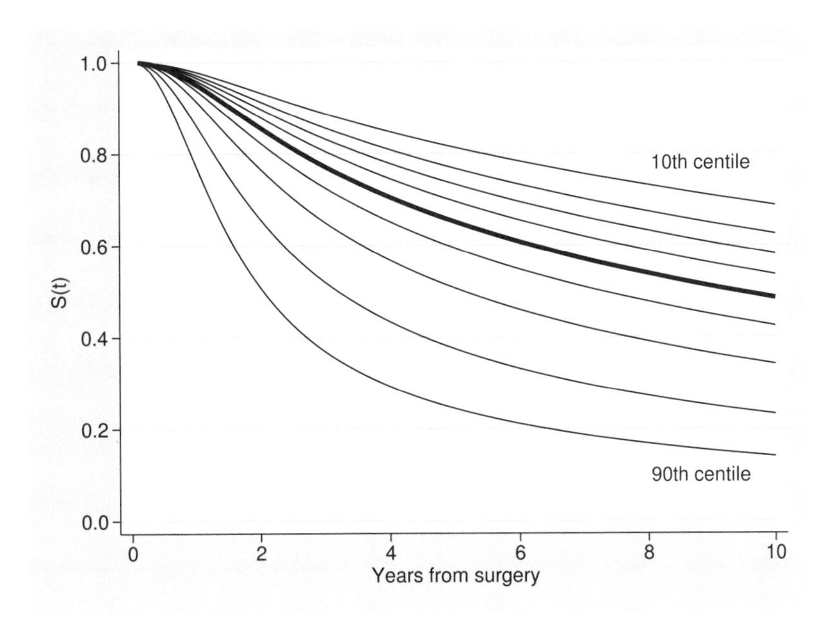

Figure 6.4. Rotterdam breast cancer data. Survival probabilities at the 10th, 20th, ..., 90th centiles of the prognostic index. The uppermost line corresponds to the 10th centile of $\mathbf{x}\widehat{\beta}$ (that is, low risk) and the lowermost line, to the 90th centile (high risk). The bold line represents the 50th centile.

Again we can observe a wide spread of prognoses.

The code we used to generate figure 6.4 is shown below:

```
. // Fit MFP model and predict prognostic index
. quietly xi: stpm2 age enodes_1 pr_1 i.size grade chemo hormon,
> scale(odds) df(2)
. predict xb, xbnobaseline // excludes the spline terms
. // Refit model to xb and estimate survival probabilities
. quietly stpm2 xb, scale(odds) df(2)
. // Compute survival curves at 10th,...,90th centiles of index
. generate timevar = _n / 10 in 1 / 100
(2882 missing values generated)
```

```
. forvalues j = 1 / 9 {
  2.         local centile = `j´ * 10
  3.         quietly centile xb, centile(`centile´)
  4.         local cxb = r(c_1)
  5.         predict s`j´, at (xb `cxb´) survival timevar(timevar)
  6. }
. line s1 s2 s3 s4 s5 s6 s7 s8 s9 timevar, sort legend(off) lpattern(l ..)
> lwidth(medthin medthin medthin medthin thick medthin  ..)
> xtitle("Years from surgery") ytitle("S(t)")
> ylabel(0(0.2)1, angle(h) format(%4.1f)) yscale(r(0 1))
> text(0.78 8 "10th centile", place(e)) text(0.1 8 "90th centile", place(e))
```

For convenience, the variables `pr_1` and `enodes_1` are predefined in `rott2.dta`. They equal $\ln(\texttt{pr} + 1)$ and $\exp(-0.12 \times \texttt{nodes})^2$, respectively.

In the code above, we have used the `xbnobaseline` option of `stpm2`. This option obtains the linear predictor without the spline terms. The model is then refit with the new variable, `xb`, as a covariate. The parameter estimates for the spline terms, the fitted values, and the log likelihood are the same in the two models, but refitting makes it simpler to obtain predicted values for centiles of the linear predictor.

6.5.3 Survival probabilities at given covariate values

Sometimes, we want to compare survival curves across the levels of an influential covariate (prognostic factor), at fixed values of the other covariates. We illustrate such a comparison for the Rotterdam breast cancer data.

The most important covariate is `nodes`. Figure 6.5 shows the survival curves for `nodes` = 0, 1, 2, 3, 5, 10, and 25.

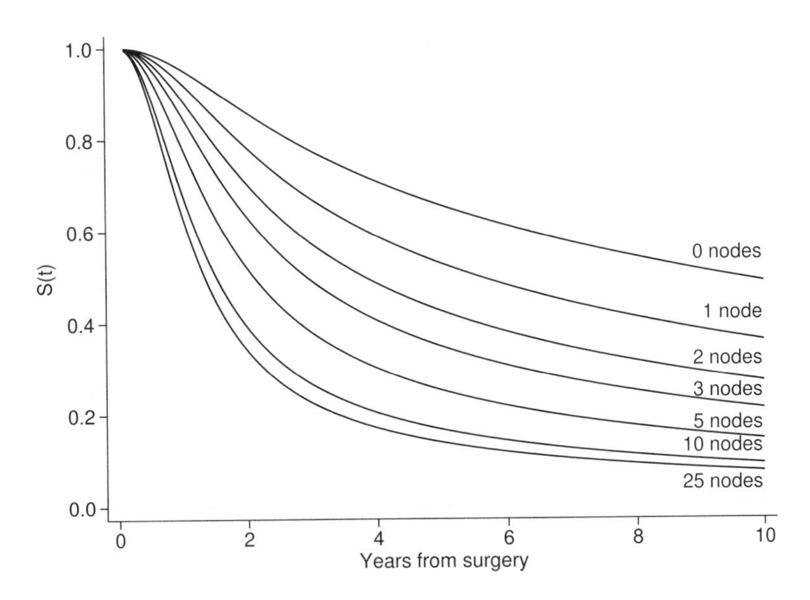

Figure 6.5. Rotterdam breast cancer data. Influence of `nodes`, the number of positive lymph nodes, on prognosis. Survival curves are adjusted for the other prognostic factors, as explained in the text.

We adjusted the values to the medians of the continuous predictors and to the most populous category for the binary ones. The adjustments are to `age` 54 years, `pr` 41 fmol/l, `size` 2 (20−50 mm), `chemo` 0, `hormon` 0 (no chemotherapy or hormonal therapy), and `grade` 3. The strong influence of `nodes` is obvious. Note also, quite reasonably, how (according to the model) the prognosis with 25 nodes is little different from that with 10.

The code to generate figure 6.5 is as follows:

```
. // Compute adjustment values for covariates other than nodes
. local at _Isize_2 1 _Isize_3 0 grade 3 chemo 0 hormon 0
. foreach var of varlist age pr_1 {
  2.         quietly centile `var´, centile(50)
  3.         local at `at´ `var´ `=r(c_1)´
  4. }
. // Fit Royston-Parmar model
. quietly xi: stpm2 age enodes_1 pr_1 i.size grade chemo hormon,
> scale(odds) df(2)
```

```
. // Predict survival curves for different values of nodes
. local j 0
. foreach n of num 0 1 2 3 5 10 25 {
  2.          local nn = exp(-0.24 * `n´)
  3.          local ++j
  4.          predict s`j´, survival at(enodes_1 `nn´ `at´)
  5. }
. // Plot
. quietly bysort _t: drop if _n > 1
. line s1 s2 s3 s4 s5 s6 s7 _t, sort xtitle("Years from surgery")
> ytitle("S(t)") lpattern(l ..) legend(off)
> ylabel(0(0.2)1, angle(h) format(%4.1f))
> text(.55 10 "0 nodes", place(w)) text(.42 10 "1 node", place(w))
> text(.32 10 "2 nodes", place(w)) text(.25 10 "3 nodes", place(w))
> text(.18 10 "5 nodes", place(w)) text(.13 10 "10 nodes", place(w))
> text(.05 10 "25 nodes", place(w))
```

In this and the previous example, most of the work involves setting up the local macro `‘at’`, which holds the adjustment values of the covariates.

6.5.4 Survival probabilities in groups

Commonly, we use the prognostic index, $\mathbf{x}\widehat{\beta}$, of a model as a summary (on the appropriate scale) for each individual of the information from the prognostic variables. Often we categorize this index into groups and calculate Kaplan–Meier survival curves to display the group-specific prognosis. With fully parametric models, we can also compute the model-based mean survival curve for each prognostic group, which, of necessity, is a smooth function of t (as opposed to the Kaplan–Meier curves, which are more or less jagged step functions).

We stress that the correct method of calculating a mean survival curve for a group differs from calculating survival at the given value of the corresponding covariate (that is, a dummy variable for the group). To get a mean curve, we evaluate the survival curve for each individual at a fixed set of time points and average these values at each time point. The covariate patterns of the individuals in a given group may vary, giving rise to differing survival curves that we average at each chosen time point. See section 9.3 for more description of average survival curves.

An example for the model for the Rotterdam breast cancer data is shown in figure 6.6. Here we created five prognostic groups by categorizing the prognostic index at its 10th, 25th, 75th, and 90th centiles.

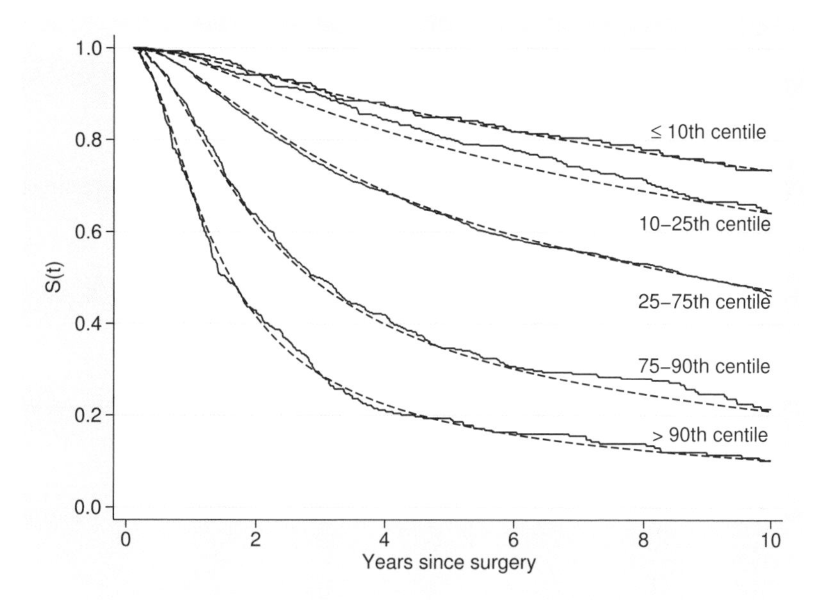

Figure 6.6. Rotterdam breast cancer data. Kaplan–Meier curves (jagged lines) and mean survival curves (dashed lines) in five prognostic groups. See text for further details.

The graph gives the general impression that the spread of prognoses for these patients is wide, as we also see in figure 6.2. The 10-year relapse-free survival probabilities range from 10%–73%.

The observed (Kaplan–Meier) and predicted mean survival curves generally agree very well. A minor exception is the second prognostic group, where the mean curve is slightly too low. The generally close agreement may be seen as crude confirmation of a good model fit.

The code to generate figure 6.6 is as follows:

```
. // Fit fractional polynomial model and predict prognostic index
. quietly xi: stpm2 age enodes_1 pr_1 i.size grade chemo hormon,
> scale(odds) df(2)
. predict xb, xbnobaseline
. // Form 5 prognostic groups using cut-points at 10, 25, 75 and 90 centiles
. centile xb, centile(10 25 75 90)
```

Variable	Obs	Percentile	Centile	— Binom. Interp. — [95% Conf.	Interval]
xb	2982	10	-2.778469	-2.81326	-2.740219
		25	-2.404464	-2.431199	-2.375563
		75	-1.073324	-1.173073	-.9961672
		90	-.1782056	-.242149	-.1187118

```
. generate cutpoints = .
(2982 missing values generated)
. forvalues j = 1 / 4 {
  2.        quietly replace cutpoints = r(c_`j´) in `j´
  3. }
. // Create grouping variable, xbc5, with 5 levels
. xtile xbc5 = xb, cutpoints(cutpoints)
. // Compute mean survival and Kaplan-Meier curves in each group
. forvalues j = 1 / 5 {
  2.        predict s`j´ if xbc5 == `j´, meansurv
  3.        sts gen km`j´ = s if xbc5 == `j´
  4. }
. // Plot
. line s1 s2 s3 s4 s5 km1 km2 km3 km4 km5 _t,
> sort connect(l l l l l J J J J J) lpattern(- - - - - l l l l l)
> xtitle("Years since surgery") ytitle("S(t)") yscale(r(0 1))
> ylabel(0(0.2)1, angle(h) format(%4.1f)) legend(off)
> text(.82 10 "{&le} 10th centile", place(w))
> text(.62 10 "10-25th centile", place(w))
> text(.45 10 "25-75th centile", place(w))
> text(.31 10 "75-90th centile", place(w))
> text(.16 10 "> 90th centile", place(w))
```

Note the `meansurv` option of `predict` for `stpm2`, to evaluate the mean survival curve over all individuals in a (prognostic) group. We emphasize that the mean survival curve is not the same as

- the Kaplan–Meier estimate for the group in question;
- the survival curve predicted at the mean covariate pattern of the group; or
- the survival curve predicted at the mean prognostic index for the group.

6.5.5 Plotting adjusted survival curves

Because of confounding, we often want to plot survival curves adjusted for one or more influential covariates. For a binary covariate, we would like to do this in the spirit of the Kaplan–Meier survival curve—that is, not to assume proportionality (of the hazards, for example) between the two levels, but still to adjust for confounding.

With RP models extended to allow for time-dependent effects, we can do such a plot—see section 7.10. Also see section 9.3 for details of calculation of adjusted survival curves.

6.5.6 Plotting differences between survival curves

We usually depict the results of randomized controlled trials with a time-to-event outcome by a Kaplan–Meier survival curve for each treatment group. Because of randomization and the ensuing approximate balance of prognostic factors across treatment groups, adjusting a comparison between treatment groups (for example, the hazard ratio [HR]) for other covariates rarely makes much difference to the estimated treatment effect. In observational studies, however, things can be very different.

In the Rotterdam breast cancer dataset, 339 patients received hormonal treatment. With the PO(2) model, the odds ratio (95% CI) for the effect of `hormon`, unadjusted for other variables, is 1.33 [1.08, 1.63]. Adjusted for the variables in the prognostic model of section 6.4.2, the odds ratio for `hormon` is 0.51 [0.41, 0.65]. Adjustment for prognostic factors has completely reversed the treatment effect, apparently from significantly harmful to significantly beneficial.

The reason for the reversal is that patients believed to be at higher risk of recurrence (that is, a worse prognosis) are more likely to receive hormonal treatment. For example, only node-positive patients (that is, with `nodes` > 0) received hormonal therapy, and as we have seen in figure 6.5, they have a relatively poor prognosis. In epidemiological language, `hormon` and prognosis are confounded (sometimes known in the treatment context as "confounding by indication").

To get a better estimate of the effect of `hormon`, we adjust for other prognostic factors. To gain a direct impression of the influence of a factor on a standardized scale, we plot the difference in adjusted survival curves between levels of the factor of interest, with 95% pointwise CIs. The upper panels of figure 6.7 show the difference in survival curves for the prognostic factor `grade`.

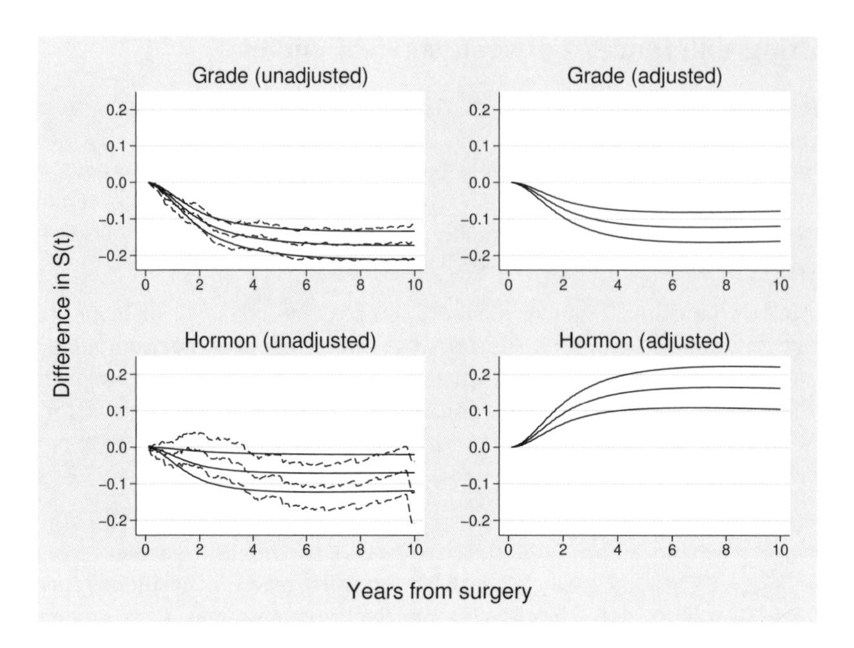

Figure 6.7. Rotterdam breast cancer data. Difference in survival curves with pointwise 95% CIs for two predictors: the prognostic factor **grade** and the treatment variable **hormon**. Unadjusted means univariate, adjusted means adjusted for the other variables in the prognostic model. Smooth lines, PO(2) models; jagged lines, from Kaplan–Meier estimates (univariate only).

We have centered the curves on median or modal values of the other prognostic factors in the model, as we described in section 6.5.3. Because the variable `grade` does not represent a treatment and is not susceptible to physician intervention, we would not expect as much confounding as for `hormon`.

The unadjusted and adjusted odds ratios for grade 3 versus grade 2 (there are no grade 1 tumors reported) are 2.00 $[1.71, 2.35]$ and 1.63 $[1.38, 1.93]$, respectively—a moderate difference. In contrast, the lower panels of figure 6.7 show the dramatic effect of adjustment on the direction of the estimated effect of `hormon`. The adjusted difference suggests an absolute relapse-free survival advantage of hormonal treatment of as much as 0.16 over a long period of time. The code for figure 6.7 is as follows:

```
. // Adjust to medians of continuous covariates
. local at _Isize_2 1 _Isize_3 0 chemo 0
. foreach var of varlist age pr_1 enodes_1 {
  2.         quietly centile `var', centile(50)
  3.         local at `at' `var' `=r(c_1)'
  4. }
```

```
. // Predict unadjusted survival for hormon and grade
. quietly stpm2 hormon, df(2) scale(odds)
. predict sunh, sdiff1(hormon 1) sdiff2(hormon 0) ci
. quietly stpm2 grade, df(2) scale(odds)
. predict sung, sdiff1(grade 3) sdiff2(grade 2) ci
. // Fit model for hormon and grade, adjusted for other variables
. quietly xi: stpm2 age enodes_1 pr_1 i.size grade chemo hormon,
> scale(odds) df(2)
. // Predict adjusted survival for hormon at grade 3 and grade at hormon 0
. predict sh, sdiff1(hormon 1 `at´ grade 3) sdiff2(hormon 0 `at´ grade 3) ci
. predict sg, sdiff1(hormon 0 `at´ grade 3) sdiff2(hormon 0 `at´ grade 2) ci
. // Get (unadjusted) differences in Kaplan-Meier curves
. stsurvdiff hormon, generate(kmh)
. stsurvdiff grade, generate(kmg)
. // Plot results
. generate tt = round(_t, 0.05)
. quietly bysort tt : drop if _n > 1
. global stuff xtitle("") ytitle("") sort legend(off)
> lpattern(l l l - ..) ylabel(, angle(h) format(%4.1f))
. line sung sung_* kmg kmg_lci kmg_uci tt, $stuff
> title("Grade (unadjusted)") name(g1, replace)
. line sg sg_* tt, $stuff title("Grade (adjusted)") name(g2, replace)
. line sunh sunh_* kmh kmh_lci kmh_uci tt, $stuff
> title("Hormon (unadjusted)") name(g3, replace)
. line sh sh_* tt, $stuff title("Hormon (adjusted)") name(g4, replace)
. graph combine g1 g2 g3 g4, ycommon xcommon b2title("Years from surgery")
> l1title("Difference in S(t)")
```

To more closely match the spirit of the difference in Kaplan–Meier plots, we generally recommend plotting time-dependent estimates of the effect of the factor of interest. We did not do this in figure 6.7, and we can see that the unadjusted curve for `hormon` does not match the Kaplan–Meier difference very accurately. Adding a time-dependent effect of `hormon` to the model improves the match between the Kaplan–Meier and unadjusted curves, but does not much affect the adjusted curve (not shown). There is no such problem for `grade`.

6.5.7 Centiles of the survival distribution

Something of potential interest that is not often done is to assess the distribution of survival times given covariate values or the prognostic index. We quite often estimate median survival time, typically in prognostic groups using the Kaplan–Meier method. With RP models, we can estimate any centiles of the survival distribution. As we will see, these estimates may involve extrapolation beyond the observed range of survival times. We should treat such estimates with due caution. They merely reflect the *unobserved* upper tail area of the distribution we have chosen to use to represent the data. We should not necessarily believe survival times beyond the observed maximum follow-up time. Also see section 6.9 for a different way to visualize survival distributions.

Following use of stpm2, the postestimation command `predict` *varname*, `centile()` `at()` computes arbitrary centiles of the survival distribution, conditional on covariate values. A useful way to do this is to condition on values of the prognostic index. Figure 6.8 shows the 10th, 50th, and 90th centiles of the relapse-free survival distribution for the Rotterdam breast cancer data, computed between the 5th and 95th centiles of the distribution of $\mathbf{x}\widehat{\boldsymbol{\beta}}$.

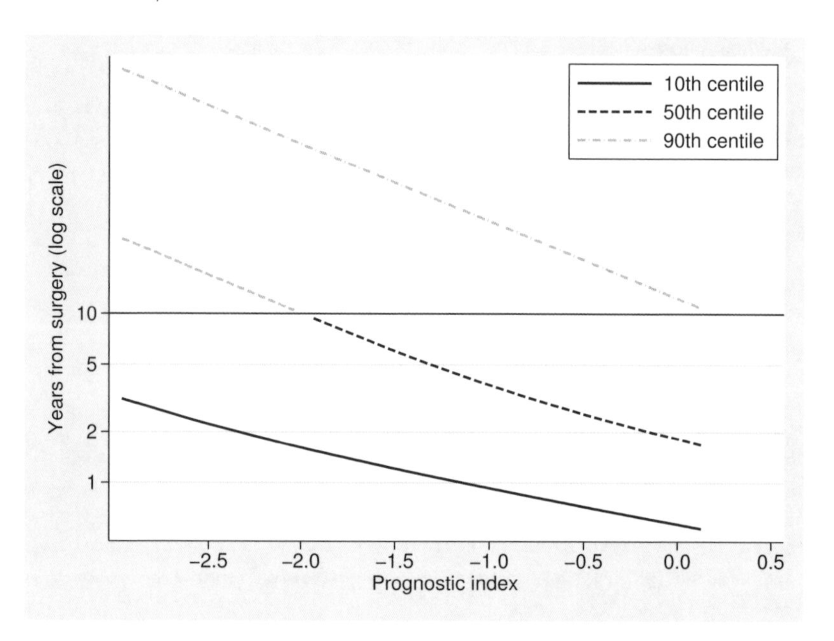

Figure 6.8. Rotterdam breast cancer data. Tenth, 50th, and 90th centiles of survival time according to the PO(2) model. The x axis gives values of the prognostic index $\mathbf{x}\widehat{\boldsymbol{\beta}}$ between the 5th and 95th centile. The horizontal line shows the limit of the observed follow-up time (10 years).

The horizontal line at $t = 10$ years shows the limit of observed times, and predictions above that are extrapolations that we have grayed out. Even the median survival time is an extrapolation when $\mathbf{x}\widehat{\boldsymbol{\beta}} < -2.0$ (the 47th centile of $\mathbf{x}\widehat{\boldsymbol{\beta}}$). The 90th centile is always an extrapolation.

The plot shows how enormously variable is the distribution of relapse-free survival time, given $\mathbf{x}\widehat{\boldsymbol{\beta}}$. At the median risk ($\mathbf{x}\widehat{\boldsymbol{\beta}} = -1.36$) the 10th, 50th, and 90th relapse-free survival-time centiles are 1.6, 9.4, and 94.3 years, respectively. In other words, 80% of patients at average risk of recurrence will wait between 1.6 and 94.3 (!) years after surgery until they experience an event. This shows why we should be cautious when extrapolating.

The code to create figure 6.8 is as follows:

```
. // Fit MFP model and predict prognostic index
. quietly xi: stpm2 age enodes_1 pr_1 i.size grade chemo hormon,
> scale(odds) df(2)
. predict xb, xbnobaseline
. quietly stpm2 xb, scale(odds) df(2)
. // Predict 3 centiles of survival time at different centiles of prog. index
. foreach thing in C10 C50 C90 xbval {
  2.         quietly gen `thing´ = .
  3. }
. local i 0
. forvalues j = 5 (5) 95 {
  2.         quietly centile xb, centile(`j´)
  3.         local xb_cent = r(c_1)
  4.         local ++i
  5.         quietly replace xbval = `xb_cent´ in `i´
  6.         forvalues k = 10 (40) 90 {
  7.                 predict c`k´, centile(`k´) at(xb `xb_cent´)
  8.                 quietly summarize c`k´
  9.                 quietly replace C`k´ = r(mean) in `i´
 10.                 drop c`k´
 11.         }
 12. }
. // Distinguish predicted median above observed follow-up time (10 years)
. generate C50a = C50 if C50 > 10
(2973 missing values generated)
. replace C50 = . if C50 > 10
(9 real changes made, 9 to missing)
. line C10 C50 C90 C50a xbval, sort lpattern(l - -. -) lwidth(medthick ..)
> ylabel(1 2 5 10, angle(h)) yscale(log) yline(10)
> ytitle("Years from surgery (log scale)")
> xtitle("Prognostic index") xlabel(-2.5 (0.5) 0.5, format(%4.1f))
> lcolor(gs2 gs2 gs12 gs12) legend(order(1 2 3) label(1 "10th centile")
> label(2 "50th centile") label(3 "90th centile") ring(0) pos(1) col(1))
```

We evaluated `C10`, `C50`, and `C90` (the predicted 10th, 50th, and 90th centile of survival time at a given value of $\mathbf{x}\widehat{\boldsymbol{\beta}}$) over all observations. Because these centiles are constant over observations, use of the mean is for convenience.

6.6 Goodness of fit

We may use martingale-like residuals from RP models, analogous to those from a Cox model, to assess goodness of fit of the linear predictor and of models for individual continuous covariates. The martingale-like residual, r_i, for the ith individual is

$$r_i = \delta_i - \widehat{H}_i\left(t_i\right)$$

where δ_i is the censoring indicator and $\widehat{H}_i\left(t_i\right)$ is the estimated cumulative hazard at the individual's failure or censoring time, t_i. After running `stpm2`, we compute the r_i using `predict` *varname*, `martingale`. The cumulative hazard function is available for any RP model, not just for a PH model. If the model is correct, then $E(r_i|x_i) = 0$ for any x in the model, and $E\left(r_i|\mathbf{x}_i\widehat{\beta}\right) = 0$.

Like ordinary residuals, martingale-like residuals are noisy. We can best glean diagnostic information by graphical methods. We recommend a smoothed scatterplot of the r_i against an x with pointwise CIs (see Royston and Sauerbrei [2008, 15]). Lack of fit should manifest as a systematic pattern of departure of the smooth line from the horizontal line $y = 0$. We should exercise caution when interpreting the plot. A pointwise CI is not a global CI; the value 0 may be excluded for some small range of x values, even when there is no serious lack of fit.

6.6.1 Example

Figure 6.9 shows smoothed martingale residuals with a 95% pointwise CI for the predictors `nodes` and `pr`.

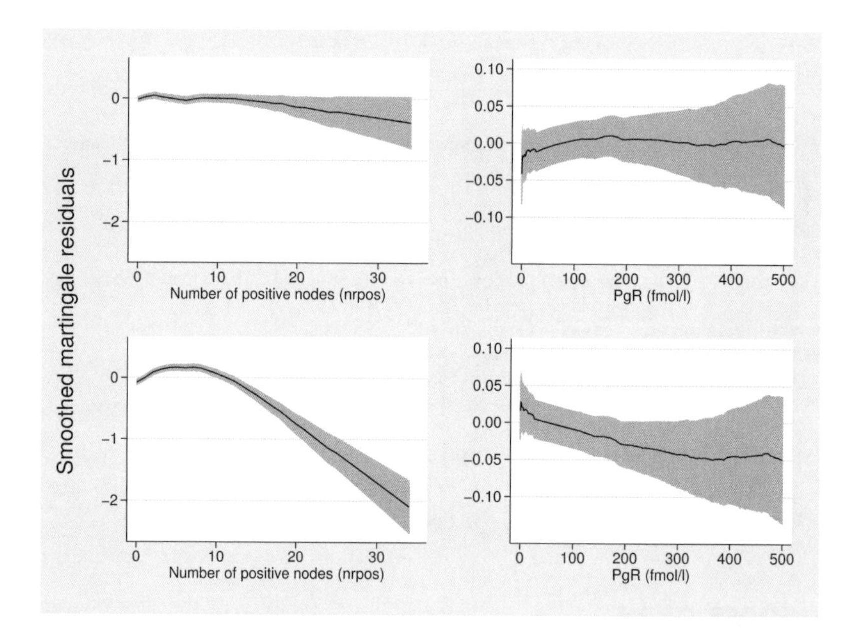

Figure 6.9. Rotterdam breast cancer data. Plots of smoothed martingale residuals against `nodes` (left panels) and `pr` (right panels). The upper panels are for a model including exponentially transformed `nodes` and log transformed `pr`, whereas the lower panels are for a misspecified model including linear `nodes` and `pr`.

The two upper panels are for the model we described in section 6.4.2. We see no sign of serious lack of fit. The lower panels are for a PO(2) model in which we modeled both `nodes` and `pr` as linear terms. The nonlinearity of `nodes` is obvious. The lack of fit for pr is subtle, but we see a suspicion of curvature in the plot. Clearly, the nonlinearity of nodes is much greater than of pr—note the different vertical scales we used for the two variables. The code for figure 6.9 is as follows:

```
. // Fit MFP model and predict residuals
. quietly xi: stpm2 age enodes_1 pr_1 i.size grade chemo hormon,
> scale(odds) df(2)
. predict mgale, martingale
. // Fit linear multivariable model and predict residuals
. quietly xi: stpm2 age nodes pr i.size grade chemo hormon, scale(odds) df(2)
. predict mgale2, martingale
. // Plot smoothed residuals
. global stuff nopts ci ytitle("") lineopts(lpattern(1)) title("")
. global yla1 ylabel(-2(1)0, angle(h)) yscale(r(-2.5 0.5))
> xlabel(0(10)30) xscale(r(0 35))
. global yla2 ylabel(-0.1(0.05).1, angle(h) format(%5.2f)) yscale(r(-0.15,0.1))
. running mgale nodes, $stuff $yla1 name(g1, replace)
. running mgale pr if pr <= 500, $stuff $yla2 name(g2, replace) span(1)
. running mgale2 nodes, $stuff $yla1 name(g3, replace)
. running mgale2 pr if pr <= 500, $stuff $yla2 name(g4, replace) span(1)
. graph combine g1 g2 g3 g4, l1title("Smoothed martingale residuals")
```

6.7 Discrimination and explained variation

The discrimination of a model reflects how well it can distinguish between patient outcomes. For example, a model that predicts a survival probability at 2 years that varies between 10% and 90% discriminates better than one whose $S(t)$ varies only between 30% and 60%. Rather than focusing on one or two time points, it is more natural for us to consider variability on the scale of the model. For the Cox model, for example, variations in the log relative hazard (that is, the prognostic index) are on the natural scale. This leads us to the idea that discrimination is a measure of spread (for example, standard deviation) of the outcome on the model's natural scale. It is also closely related to the notion of explained variation.

For the linear regression model $y \sim N\left(\mathbf{x}\beta, \sigma^2\right)$ with covariate vector $\mathbf{x}$ and parameter vector $\boldsymbol{\beta}$, the concept of explained variation or index of determination is familiar to data analysts. We may write the explained variation statistic R^2 less familiarly than usual as

$$R^2 = \frac{\mathrm{var}\left(\mathbf{x}\beta\right)}{\sigma^2 + \mathrm{var}\left(\mathbf{x}\beta\right)}$$

where we take the variance, $\mathrm{var}(\mathbf{x}\beta)$, over the distribution of $\mathbf{x}\beta$ between individuals. Following on from the considerations in our first paragraph above, several authors have proposed versions of explained variation statistics for use with (possibly censored) survival data. However, the measures have not necessarily been extensions of the linear regression R^2.

The motivation of Royston and Sauerbrei's (2004) D statistic is as a measure of discrimination—that is, of variation in outcome among patients on the appropriate scale, as just discussed. For a Cox model, for example, D is a function of the variance of the log relative hazard among patients. In the Cox model, a simple but numerically approximate interpretation of D is as the log HR between two groups created by dichotomizing $\mathbf{x}\widehat{\boldsymbol{\beta}}$ at its median. A similar interpretation applies to PH models on the log cumulative-hazard scale, whereas for PO models the equivalent is the log odds-of-failure ratio scale, and for probit models it is the difference between the groups on the scale of the probit of the failure probability.

We compute D by ordering the estimated prognostic index, $\mathbf{x}\widehat{\boldsymbol{\beta}}$, calculating the expected normal order statistics (rankits) corresponding to these values, scaling the rankits by dividing by a factor $\kappa = \sqrt{8/\pi} \simeq 1.60$, and performing an auxiliary regression on the scaled rankits. The scaling of the rankits by κ ensures that D has the character of a log HR between equal-sized prognostic groups—see section 3.2.2 of Royston and Sauerbrei (2004) for further details. The estimated regression coefficient on the scaled rankits is D. For D to be useful, the prognostic index must be approximately normally distributed, something the central limit theorem tends to fulfill, because $\mathbf{x}\widehat{\boldsymbol{\beta}}$ is a sum of random variables. In practice, D appears quite robust to departures from normality.

Royston and Sauerbrei's (2004) R^2_D is a monotonic transformation of the D measure, defined by

$$R^2_D = \frac{D^2/\kappa^2}{\sigma^2 + D^2/\kappa^2}$$

where

$$\sigma^2 = \begin{cases} \pi^2/6 & \text{(Weibull model; Cox model; PH models)} \\ \pi^2/3 & \text{(loglogistic model; PO models)} \\ 1 & \text{(lognormal model; models with a probit link)} \end{cases}$$

We can interpret D^2/κ^2 as an estimate of the variance of $\mathbf{x}\boldsymbol{\beta}$ across individuals, and R^2_D as a measure of explained variation on the natural scale of the model. The covariates in an RP model operate on a standardized scale whose scale parameter is σ^2. The values of σ^2 for the three classes of model are appropriate for the standard extreme value, logistic, and normal distributions; these correspond, respectively, to the cumulative hazards, cumulative odds, and probit scales. The σ^2 here is analogous to the residual variance of the linear regression model.

By construction, the statistics D and R^2_D are sensitive only to the *ranks* of $\mathbf{x}\widehat{\boldsymbol{\beta}}$. A subtle change in the model that alters $\mathbf{x}\widehat{\boldsymbol{\beta}}$ but leaves the rank order of its values unchanged does not affect D or R^2_D. The main advantage of this property is robustness to outliers; the disadvantage is that the auxiliary model on the rankits may not fit the data perfectly, resulting in underestimation (albeit typically minor) of the discrimination and explained variation.

The current version of the ado-file `str2d` (Royston 2006) recognizes RP models and so can be used directly. See Royston and Sauerbrei (2004) and Royston (2006) for further discussion and examples.

In the real datasets we have worked with, R_D^2 for prognostic models varies quite widely, from 0 to about 60%. Theoretically, R_D^2 can reach 100%, but we have never seen such an extreme case. In primary cancers, values up to about 40% are common; in advanced cancers, rather lower than that. We may see larger values of R_D^2 in diseases in which much is known about mechanisms or pathways leading to death; an example is bilirubin in primary cirrhosis of the liver. The "feel" of R_D^2 in a survival model is similar to that in a linear regression model. For example, a value of 30% can be regarded as rather low, because it means that considerable variation in the outcome is still unexplained by the model.

6.7.1 Example

For the PO(2) model for the Rotterdam breast cancer data, we give D and R_D^2 in the first row of table 6.2.

Table 6.2. Rotterdam breast cancer data. Effect of removing variables from the PO(2) model on discrimination (D) and explained variation (R_D^2). See text for further details.

Variable removed	Single		Cumulative		Cumulative (least first)		
	D	R_D^2	D	R_D^2	D	R_D^2	order
–	1.57	0.228	1.57	0.228	1.57	0.228	–
`nodes`	0.98	0.104	0.98	0.104	0.00	0.000	7
`size` (2 dummies)	1.51	0.214	0.60	0.041	1.31	0.170	6
`grade`	1.50	0.212	0.44	0.022	1.42	0.194	3
`pr`	1.53	0.218	0.18	0.004	1.53	0.218	1
`chemo`	1.50	0.212	0.17	0.003	1.35	0.178	5
`hormon`	1.55	0.223	0.09	0.001	1.51	0.213	2
`age`	1.51	0.214	–	–	1.36	0.180	4

The explained variation is modest (22.8%). Much of the variation among the survival curves in breast cancer is unaccounted for by standard prognostic factors.

str2d is simple to use. Code to compute D and R^2_D for the PO(2) model is as follows:

```
. xi: str2d stpm2 enodes_1 i.size grade pr_1 chemo hormon age, scale(odds) df(2)
i.size            _Isize_1-3          (naturally coded; _Isize_1 omitted)
[warning: not a proportional hazards model]
R^2 (explained variation - D method): Flexible parametric model with scale odds
```

Obs	Events	R^2	Std. err.	95% conf. interval		D	SE
2982	1477	0.228188	0.014652	0.199622	0.256961	1.574	0.065

We can gauge the importance of each variable in the model by examining the effect on D and R^2_D of removing the variable from the model. We show the results in the subsequent rows of table 6.2. The second and third columns show what happens when just one of the prognostic variables is removed. In the fourth and fifth columns, we remove variables cumulatively, with the most important first. In the sixth and seventh columns, we also remove variables cumulatively, but with the least important first. The column labeled "order" indicates which variable we removed first, second, and so on. For example, for the row labeled hormon, the model in columns two and three excludes only hormon, whereas that in columns four and five of the same row comprises only age. For the same row in columns six and seven, we have removed hormon and pr, leaving nodes, size, grade, chemo and age.

Removing variables other than nodes singly from the model has little effect on D and R^2_D, reducing the latter by 0.014 at most. Removing nodes reduces D and R^2_D by about one half (by 0.59 and 0.124, respectively). We see that nodes is easily the most important prognostic factor. On its own, nodes gives $D = 1.31$ and $R^2_D = 0.170$, which are the values following removal of the six lesser predictors as exhibited in the row labeled size. Adding the other variables contributes a further 15% (adding 0.26 to D and 0.058 to R^2_D). Removing nodes and the second most important factor, size, reduces D and R^2_D to a paltry 0.60 and 0.041, respectively.

The last three columns suggest that a model with almost as good performance as the original excludes (FP-transformed) pr and hormon. Removing further variables damages D and R^2_D more noticeably.

6.7.2 Harrell's C index of concordance

An alternative measure of discrimination is Harrell's C index, defined as the proportion of all usable subject pairs in which the predictions and outcomes are concordant (that is, in the same direction). It is available using estat concordance after fitting a Cox model. Because the C index is generic, we can use it after fitting an RP model without time-dependent effects. To implement the C index, we have produced an ado-file called stcstat2, a minor modification of the "factory" Stata routine stcstat that is used by estat concordance.

Although the C index is quite often used in practice, we are in general not too keen on it, for the following reasons. Its interpretation is not entirely clear, both substantively and with respect to the metric: for example, do we regard a value of 0.7 as large? Also, the C index increases with the amount of censoring, and the bias can be substantial if censoring is heavy. Gönen and Heller (2005) have proposed an improved version of the statistic for PH models that is insensitive to censoring. Gönen and Heller's (2005) statistic is available in Stata 12 through the `gheller` option of `estat concordance`.

6.8 Out-of-sample prediction: Concept and applications

One of the most powerful and useful features of Stata estimation commands is their ability to do out-of-sample prediction—that is, they can predict outcomes at covariate values or patterns that are not necessarily in the estimation sample. Our implementation of RP models in `stpm2` supports such prediction.

In survival analysis, there are at least two situations in which out-of-sample prediction is useful:

- interpolating or extrapolating the baseline or other survival functions at time points not represented in the estimation sample
- predicting survival probabilities or other quantities of interest from a model on a derivation sample onto individuals in an evaluation sample (that is, external validation)

Interpolation is helpful, for example, when we wish to plot a survival function for an individual, a group, or a covariate pattern as a smooth curve at a suitable choice of time points within the range of the observed follow-up time. We need extrapolation when we want to project a modeled survival function into the future. We usually require extrapolation in economic evaluation of a health care intervention, where we project costs over the hypothetical lifetime of the patient. For such extrapolation to be useful, it should be supported by quantitative evidence of long-term survival probabilities, perhaps in the framework of relative survival modeling.

Successful external validation is usually regarded as the gold standard of potential usefulness of a proposed prognostic model (Altman and Royston 2000)—or at least, as a necessary first step. Here we do not attempt to address the many issues that arise when considering what external validation of a prognostic model means or the details of how we should do it. We aim to show how the mechanics of out-of-sample prediction on an independent sample work with `stpm2`, to demonstrate in principle that validating an RP model is feasible, reasonably simple, and attractive.

6.8.1 Extrapolation of survival functions: Basic technique

In section 6.4.2, we developed a PO(2) model for the Rotterdam breast cancer data. Suppose that we wish to see what the model tells us about the baseline survival curve between the maximum follow-up time (10 years) and 30 years after surgery.

Here we choose to define baseline as meaning loosely "at average risk of an event". By subtracting the mean prognostic index, we compute the baseline survival curve at the average of the prognostic index across all patients in the dataset. We may do this by

1. fitting the PO model of interest;
2. predicting the prognostic index;
3. centering the prognostic index by subtracting its mean;
4. refitting the PO model with centered prognostic index as the only non–time-related covariate; and
5. predicting the baseline survival curve.

Stata code to carry out these steps is as follows:

```
xi: stpm2 age enodes_1 pr_1 i.size grade chemo hormon, scale(odds) df(2)
predict xb, xbnobaseline
summarize xb
replace xb = xb - r(mean)
stpm2 xb, scale(odds) df(2)
predict s0, survival zeros
```

The problem with this approach for extrapolation is that we predict baseline survival at all observed times, but not at times between 10 and 30 years after surgery (the extrapolation we seek). To remedy the defect, we can use the `timevar()` option of `predict`. We first create a variable containing the times at which we want to predict (suppose that these are at 1-year intervals from 0 to 30 years) and then use `predict` again:

```
range timev 0 30 31
predict s0, survival zeros timevar(timev)
replace s0 = 1 if timev == 0
```

Predicting survival at `timev` = 0 produces missing `s0`, so we replace the missing value with the correct value, `s0` = 1. The resulting curve is shown in figure 6.10.

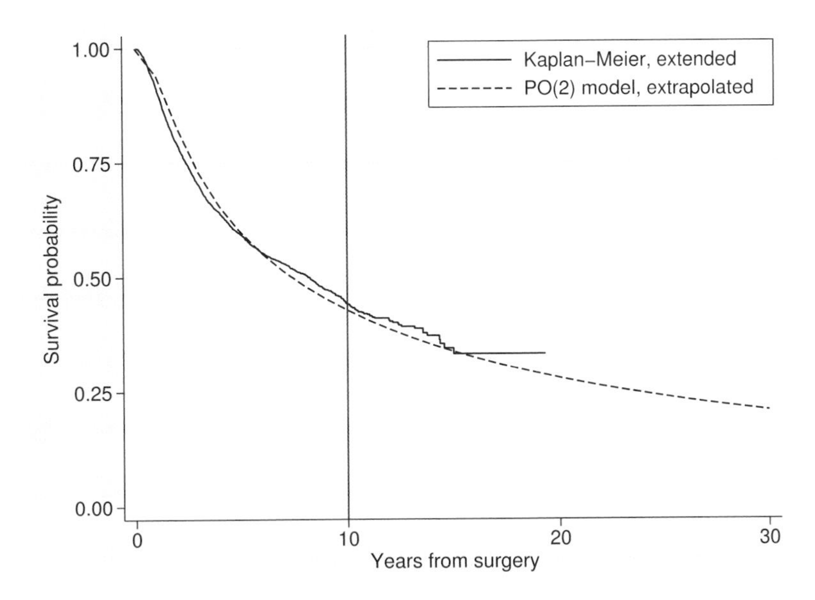

Figure 6.10. Rotterdam breast cancer data. Irregular solid line: Kaplan–Meier estimate of survival function for recurrence-free interval, all patients, extended follow-up. Dashed line: baseline survival curve from PO(2) prognostic model, extrapolated to 30 years. The vertical line shows the extent of follow-up time used when fitting the PO(2) model.

The smooth curve we see after 10 years is a transformation of the cumulative log odds of an event. The latter is a linear function of $\ln t$ beyond the right-hand boundary knot, a consequence of modeling with a restricted cubic spline function.

The Kaplan–Meier curve shown in figure 6.10 was obtained by using the Rotterdam data with 231 months of follow-up—that is, before it was truncated at 10 years (see section 3.2). We see that the extrapolation actually does quite well in the decade between 10 and 20 years; beyond that, of course, its performance cannot be judged.

6.8.2 Extrapolation of survival functions: Further investigations

We have seen that the PO(2) baseline distribution extrapolates reasonably well to 20 years and at least plausibly to 30 years. We may ask what happens if we vary other parameters—for example, the type of model (PH, POs, probit) and the d.f. To investigate this issue in a simple way, we model only the survival function—no covariates.

Figure 6.11 shows what happens when we extrapolate survival estimates from PH, POs, and probit models—each with 1, 2, 3, or 4 d.f.

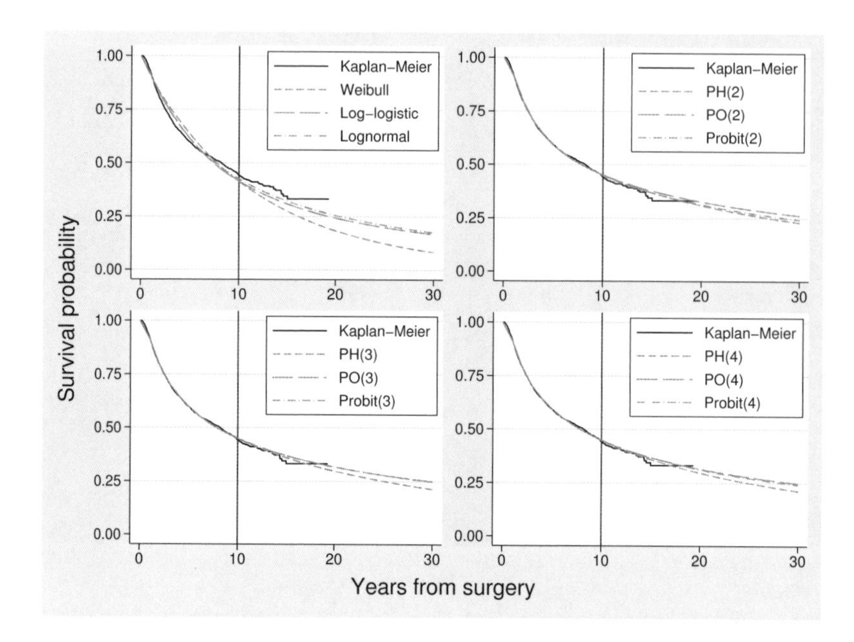

Figure 6.11. Rotterdam breast cancer data. Extrapolation of survival curves to 30 years. The irregular solid line is the Kaplan–Meier estimate for a recurrence-free interval with extended follow-up for all patients. The other curves show fitted and extrapolated survival functions from various standard parametric and RP models, as indicated in the legends.

The 1 d.f. models (Weibull, loglogistic, and lognormal) fit the data up to 10 years less well and do a worse job of prediction than the RP models with more than 1 d.f. The Weibull is the worst fit and the worst extrapolator. There is very little to choose among the RP models; they all predict survival quite well out to 20 years.

We also explored the effect of changing the right-hand boundary knot in the RP models. Because (on the appropriate scale) the predicted curves are linear in $\ln t$ to the right of the this knot, we might anticipate some effect of varying its value on the accuracy of the extrapolation. In fact, the predicted survival curves hardly changed when the position of the right-hand boundary knot was altered (data not shown).

Reducing the follow-up time to five years considerably lowered the accuracy of extrapolated survival from the 1 d.f. models, but little affected that from the RP models. Of the three RP model classes, the PH class provided the worst extrapolation. When we reduced follow-up to two years, however, all the models badly underestimated the survival curve beyond two years (data not shown).

While the results of these experiments are interesting, they do not prove anything about how well different models might extrapolate in different types of dataset. Much more experience is needed even to answer basic questions, such as "does a model that fits the observed data well extrapolate future survival better than a poorly fitting model?" The answer in the Rotterdam data seems to be yes, but we cannot meaningfully generalize the finding to other cases.

6.8.3 Validation of prognostic models: Basics

The basic principle of external validation is to create a model on a derivation or "training" dataset and evaluate its predictions on an independent validation or "test" dataset. The approach we describe here requires a single dataset containing individual patient data for all the relevant time-related and prognostic variables, and a binary variable that marks the derivation and validation datasets.

The beauty of fully specified parametric models, such as Poisson or RP models, is that out-of-sample prediction incorporates not only covariate effects but also the baseline survival distribution from the derivation dataset. With a partially specified model, such as the Cox model, we can predict only covariate effects, because we do not estimate the baseline hazard function or the baseline survival distribution.

As mentioned above, we give here only a flavor of what validation of an RP prognostic model might look like. In reality, we would need a more comprehensive and focused evaluation. See further comments in section 6.8.4.

To mimic external validation of the PO(2) model for the Rotterdam breast cancer dataset, we proceed as follows:

1. Split the dataset at random into equal, nonoverlapping subsamples, each of size 1,491 patients.
2. Create a variable called `half` with values of 1 and 2 indicating the subsamples (first and second halves of the data, respectively).
3. Fit the PO(2) model from section 6.4.2 to the first half.
4. Predict the prognostic index for all patients.
5. Create (for example) four prognostic groups for all patients, using cutpoints at (for example) the 15th, 50th, and 85th centiles of the prognostic index in the first half. These centiles approximately equal the "Cox cutpoints" (Cox 1957), which minimize the loss of information when discretizing a normally distributed continuous variable into a given number of groups.
6. Use `predict` with the `meansurv` option to predict the survival curve expected in each prognostic group in the second half.
7. Compute Kaplan–Meier survival curves in the four prognostic groups in the second half.
8. Compare predicted and Kaplan–Meier curves in the second half graphically.

We could also compare survival estimates predicted on the first and second halves from the model fit on the first half. The resulting curves (not shown) are closely similar in each prognostic group.

We show the results of the validation exercise in figure 6.12.

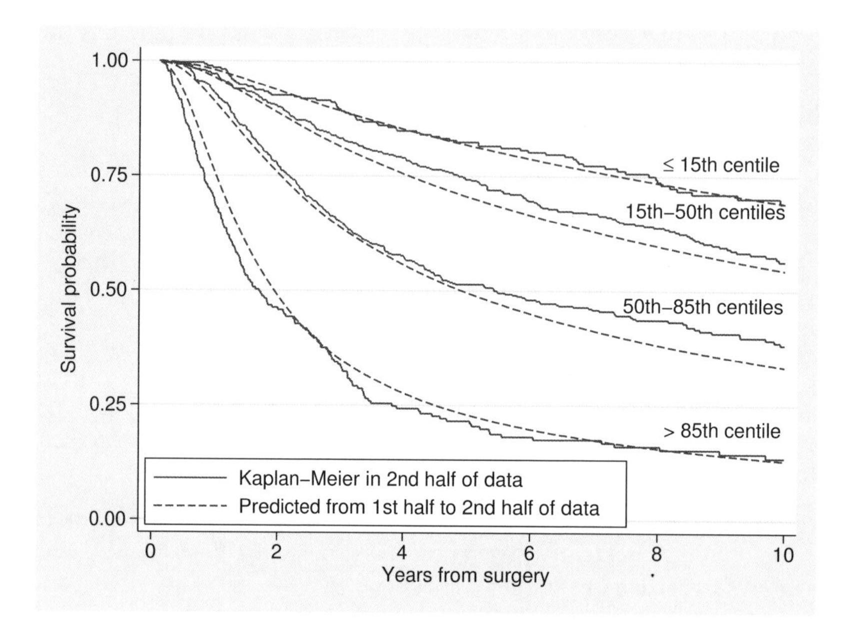

Figure 6.12. Rotterdam breast cancer data. Conceptual validation of an RP prognostic model. Solid lines: Kaplan–Meier survival curves in four prognostic groups in the second half of the data. Dashed lines: Mean survival functions in the same prognostic groups predicted in the second half by the model fit to the first half of the data.

The predicted survival curves (dashed lines) agree well with the nonparametric (Kaplan–Meier) estimates. Subjectively speaking, therefore, the model appears to validate well. Seeing much less separation between the Kaplan–Meier curves than between the predicted curves, and possibly even crossing survival curves, would be evidence that the model validated poorly.

Of course, we are not surprised by the good result, because we derived the model on the entire dataset and estimated the parameters on one half of the data, chosen at random. Nevertheless, it illustrates the general principle of validation: estimate something of interest on one dataset, predict onto another dataset, and evaluate the quality of the resulting estimate in the second dataset.

The Stata code generating the results shown in figure 6.12 is as follows:

```
. use rott2, clear
(Rotterdam breast cancer data, truncated at 10 years)
. // Create random 50:50 split of data
. set seed 111
. generate u = runiform()
. sort u
. generate byte half = cond(_n <= _N/2, 1, 2)
. // Fit MFP model to first half of data
. xi: stpm2 age enodes_1 pr_1 i.size grade chemo hormon if half == 1,
> scale(odds) df(2) all nolog
i.size            _Isize_1-3          (naturally coded; _Isize_1 omitted)
Log likelihood = -1706.3722                     Number of obs   =       1491

             |      Coef.   Std. Err.      z    P>|z|     [95% Conf. Interval]
-------------+----------------------------------------------------------------
xb           |
         age |  -.0192587   .0043575    -4.42   0.000    -.0277993   -.0107182
    enodes_1 |  -2.344021   .1739341   -13.48   0.000    -2.684926   -2.003117
        pr_1 |  -.0869466   .0230022    -3.78   0.000    -.1320302   -.0418631
    _Isize_2 |     .39374   .1095401     3.59   0.000     .1790455    .6084346
    _Isize_3 |   .6286078   .1833346     3.43   0.001     .2692786     .987937
       grade |   .4745347   .1216084     3.90   0.000     .2361866    .7128829
       chemo |  -.6636309   .1428891    -4.64   0.000    -.9436884   -.3835734
      hormon |  -.6678157   .1790259    -3.73   0.000      -1.0187   -.3169313
       _rcs1 |   1.305107    .041038    31.80   0.000     1.224673     1.38554
       _rcs2 |   .2192363   .0292782     7.49   0.000     .1618521    .2766206
       _cons |   .8942928   .4730848     1.89   0.059    -.0329363    1.821522
------------------------------------------------------------------------------

. // Predict prognostic index (PI) for all patients
. predict xb, xbnobaseline
. // Compute centiles of PI on first half and
. // create group indicators from saved cutpoints
. centile xb if half == 1, centile(15 50 85)
                                                       -- Binom. Interp. --
    Variable |     Obs  Percentile    Centile        [95% Conf. Interval]
-------------+-------------------------------------------------------------
          xb |    1491         15    -2.540645       -2.590883   -2.478303
             |                 50    -1.874788       -1.934024   -1.815976
             |                 85    -.4997558       -.6496682   -.3887834
. generate byte g1 = (xb <= r(c_1))
. generate byte g2 = (xb > r(c_1)) & (xb <= r(c_2))
. generate byte g3 = (xb > r(c_2)) & (xb <= r(c_3))
. generate byte g4 = (xb > r(c_3))
. // Predict mean survival curve in each group, at observed times.
. // Also predict corresponding Kaplan-Meier curves.
. forvalues j = 1 / 4 {
  2.         predict smean`j´ if (half == 2) & (g`j´ == 1), meansurv
  3.         sts gen km`j´ = s if (half == 2) & (g`j´ == 1)
  4. }
```

```
. line km1 km2 km3 km4 smean1 smean2 smean3 smean4 _t if half==2,
> sort c(J J J J l l l l) lpattern(l l l l - - - -) lcolor(gs4 ..)
> legend(order(1 5) label(1 "Kaplan-Meier in 2nd half of data")
> label(5 "Predicted from 1st half to 2nd half of data")
> ring(0) pos(7) col(1))
> xtitle("Years from surgery") ytitle("Survival probability")
> ysca(r(0 1)) yla(0(0.25)1, angle(horizontal) format(%4.2f))
> text(.78 10 "{&le} 15th centile", place(w))
> text(.66 10 "15th-50th centiles", place(w))
> text(.47 10 "50th-85th centiles", place(w))
> text(.20 10 "> 85th centile", place(w))
```

6.8.4 Validation of prognostic models: Further comments

As far as we know, graphs resembling figure 6.12 and its underlying methodology are not found in the literature. The following paradigm is more typical:

1. Construct a Cox model on a derivation sample and produce a prognostic index with cutpoints defining prognostic groups. Publish the model, including the estimates of β so that a prognostic index and corresponding groups can be created without needing the raw derivation data.
2. In a validation sample, construct the prognostic groups via the prognostic index.
3. Plot the Kaplan–Meier curves for the prognostic groups in the validation sample.

An example is figure 2 of van Houwelingen (2000), which depicts the discrimination of the International Prognostic Index for non-Hodgkin's lymphoma in an independent Dutch sample.

The main difference between the above procedure and that outlined in section 6.8.3 is that in the latter we predict mean survival curves out-of-sample from the derivation sample to the validation sample, whereas in the former, we use the prognostic index only to define prognostic groups and to estimate survival functions nonparametrically in each sample. The relative merits of the two approaches are an open issue, but we should realize that they are distinctively different. For example, our approach requires individual patient data, or failing that, a full description of all parameter values of the RP model fit to the derivation data. A comprehensive discussion of the topic is beyond the scope of our book. For a closely related proposal for external validation and updating of an RP model, see Royston, Parmar, and Altman (2010).

Finally, the approach to predicting survival functions we have discussed so far relates mainly to the calibration of a model. As we discuss in section 6.7, the other important property of a model is its *discrimination* according to suitable measures. For example, in the "toy" validation of the PO(2) model we presented for the Rotterdam data, the measure R^2_D, the percentage of variation explained by the model on the log odds scale, is 21.9% (SE 2.0) and 23.9% (SE 2.1) in the first and second half of the data, respectively. The corresponding values of Harrell's C index of concordance are 0.688 and 0.697. Thus model discrimination in the second half appears to be slightly better than in the first half—purely by chance, of course.

6.9 Visualization of survival times

A problem with censored survival data is how we can visualize the observed survival times. Because of censoring, standard visualization tools, such as scatterplots, are not helpful. To improve visualization, Royston, Parmar, and Altman (2008) proposed imputation of the censored observations followed by the use of scatterplots and other tools. The imputation has two components. First, we require a prognostic model with which to describe the distribution of survival time given the covariates (prognostic factors). Second, we make a random draw from the conditional distribution of survival time given covariates and survival up to the time of censoring. Because in a parametric framework "everything is known", the calculations are quite straightforward. We have written an ado-file called `stsurvimpute` that uses `stpm2` to do the imputations.

Scatterplots of (log) survival time against the prognostic index, possibly with prognostic-group cutpoints shown, can be particularly revealing, as we demonstrate shortly. The main message from such plots is that the separation or discrimination between prognostic groups afforded by the model is much less than the corresponding Kaplan–Meier survival curves suggest. The plots help point us to a more realistic assessment of the prognostic ability of the model.

6.9.1 Example

With the PO(2) prognostic model described in section 6.4.2, we use `stsurvimpute` to impute the 1,505 censored survival times in the Rotterdam breast cancer data. Figure 6.13 is a scatterplot of the log survival-time for all patients against the prognostic index, with its 10th, 25th, 75th, and 90th centiles marked.

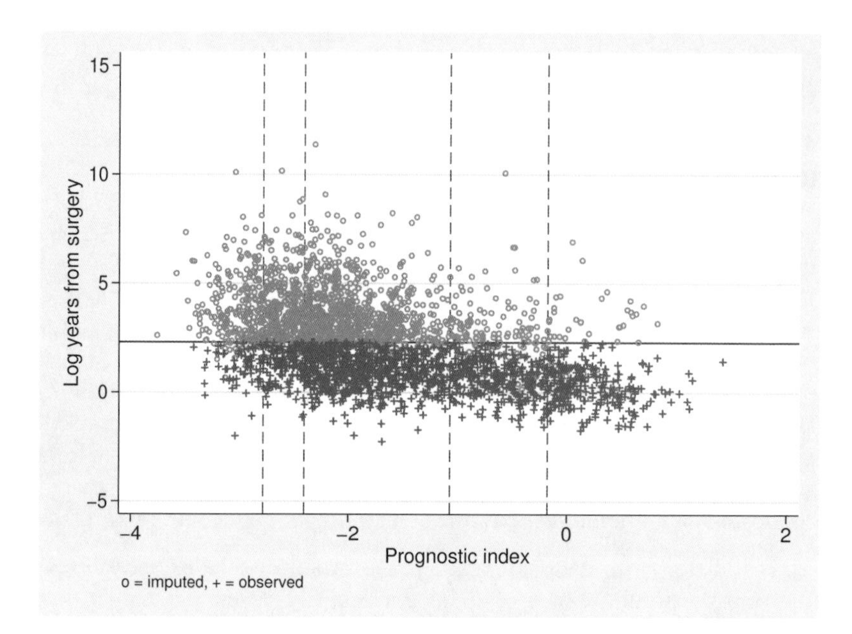

Figure 6.13. Rotterdam breast cancer data. Visualization of data by imputation under a PO(2) model. Scatterplot of log years since surgery (dark gray, observed = +; pale gray, imputed = o) against the prognostic index from the PO(2) model. Horizontal line shows the limit of follow-up (10 years, log transformed). Vertical dashed lines are cutpoints at the 10th, 25th, 75th, and 90th centiles of the distribution of the prognostic index.

The relationship is approximately linear. The top half of the scatterplot is massively dominated by imputed censored observations (marked as "o" symbols). Note the large variance of the log times at any given value of the prognostic index: prediction of survival times at the individual level is very imprecise. Also the distributions of survival times between neighboring prognostic groups exhibit considerable overlap. Of course, prognosis is not constant within a group—regression on the prognostic index remains.

The code for figure 6.13 exemplifies use of `stsurvimpute` and is as follows:

```
. // Fit MFP model and predict prognostic index (excluding the spline terms)
. quietly xi: stpm2 age enodes_1 pr_1 i.size grade chemo hormon,
> scale(odds) df(2)

. predict xb, xbnobaseline

. // Impute censored times to event under PCO(2) model
. stsurvimpute xb, seed(111) gen(timp) scale(odds) df(2)
-> fitting: stpm2 xb, df(2) scale(odds)

1505 censored observations imputed from 1477 event times

. // Refit model to prognostic index and estimate survival probabilities
. quietly stpm2 xb, scale(odds) df(2)

. local obs +
```

```
. local imp o
. label define d 0 "`imp´" 1 "`obs´"
. label values _d d
. // Get cutpoints on predicted survival time for plotting
. quietly centile xb, centile(10 25 75 90)
. forvalues j = 1 / 4 {
  2.         local cut`j´ = r(c_`j´)
  3. }
. generate lnt = ln(timp)
. quietly regress lnt xb
. predict lntf
(option xb assumed; fitted values)
. local logten = ln(10)
. generate lnt0 = lnt if _d == 0
(1477 missing values generated)
. generate lnt1 = lnt if _d == 1
(1505 missing values generated)
. scatter lnt0 lnt1 xb, ms(oh +) mcolor(gs9 gs6) msize(*.75 ..)
> yline(`logten´) ylabel(, angle(horizontal))
> xline(`cut1´ `cut2´ `cut3´ `cut4´, lpattern(dash) lwidth(thin))
> xtitle("Prognostic index") ytitle("Log years from surgery")
> note("`imp´ = imputed, `obs´ = observed") legend(off)
```

As we did in section 6.5.7, we must express a word of caution here. The data marked "o" in figure 6.13 are *extrapolated into the future*, based on the RP model we fit the observed distribution of survival times. The most extreme survival time in the dataset is 10 years—which is only at the 55th centile of the observed and imputed distribution. We do not observe a large part of the upper tail of the relapse-free survival distribution. The imputed values give us almost an "artist's impression" of what the survival distribution could look like if the model were correct. The model may fit the observed data well, but that does not make it correct! A different model (for example, an RP probit(2) model) would have different upper-tail behavior. As Royston, Parmar, and Altman (2008) point out, we should use imputed data only for visualizing what complete survival times might look like under the model—not for any kind of formal inference.

A related graphical use of imputation of survival times is shown in figure 6.14, a smoothed scatterplot of log survival-time against `nodes`.

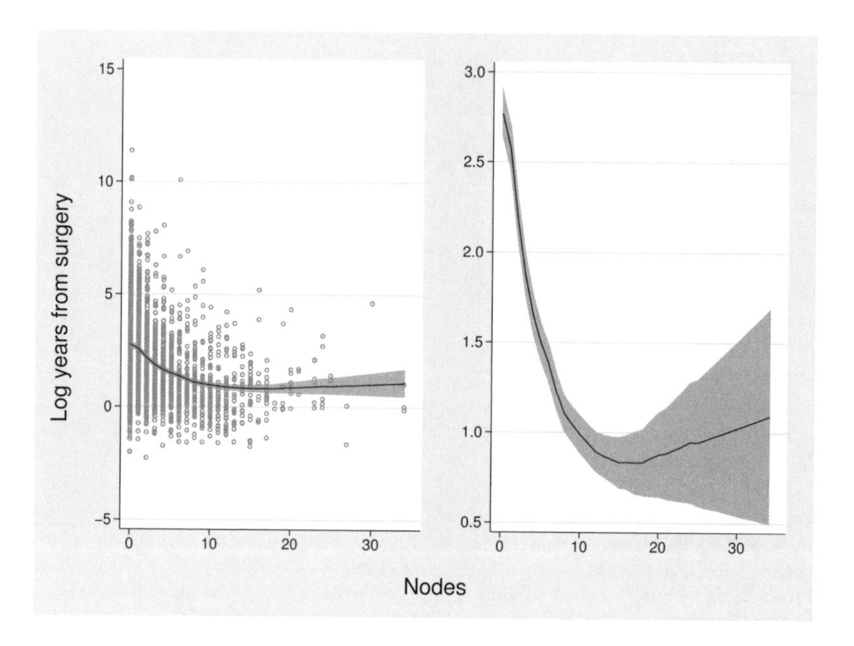

Figure 6.14. Rotterdam breast cancer data. Smoothed scatterplot of observed and imputed log relapse-free survival time against `nodes`, the number of positive lymph nodes. The right panel focuses on the regression relationship, omitting the scatterplot of the raw data. Note the different scales of the two graphs.

Figure 6.14 nicely shows the strong relationship between `nodes` and time to relapse. Beyond about 15 nodes, the prognosis (mean log time to event) does not seem to change much. Such a type of relationship is reflected by the preliminary negative exponential transformation applied to `nodes` before FP modeling. See also figure 6.5.

6.10 Discussion

In this chapter, we have touched on several aspects of prognostic modeling and how we perform it using RP models. We have not attempted to deal with the many generic issues that affect prognostic modeling. These include assessing the instability of model selection (which we may address using bootstrap resampling), model validation (a topic in its own right, of which we have only scratched the surface), investigating interactions between covariates, use of other systems of flexible models for nonlinearity in the covariates (for example, regression splines), coping with missing covariate observations, and robustification of FP functions to reduce the effect of influential observations. None of these issues presents additional difficulty in the context of RP models. Apart from model validation and missing data, all the issues are discussed in various places in Royston and Sauerbrei (2008).

We finish with a speculative point. Of essentially all the datasets we have analyzed from a prognostic-factors angle, the best model was a PO model. In no case did a PH model fit better, suggesting that PH models are suboptimal in most cases. We suspect that the PO assumption is a better bet a priori than PH. The reason for this may be (as we indicated earlier) that the PO scaling automatically causes the HR between different levels of a covariate to converge to 1 as t tends to infinity. We feel that PO is biologically more plausible than PH, because we cannot reasonably expect the baseline (historical) value of a covariate to have a persistent effect on the hazard "for all time". However, we need experience with a wider range of datasets to test our speculation further.

7 Time-dependent effects

Summary

1. When the relative effect of a covariate varies over follow-up time, then we no longer have proportional hazards (PH) on the log hazard scale. In other words, the effect of the covariate is time-dependent (TD).
2. One way of fitting a model with nonproportional hazards is to fit the model on an alternative scale. For example, with proportional odds (PO) models, the hazard rates are forced to converge as follow-up time increases.
3. Because both the Poisson and Royston–Parmar (RP) models include the effect of time as covariates in the linear predictor, TD effects can be included by fitting interactions between the covariate of interest and the covariates defining the effect of time.
4. TD effects can be estimated in a piecewise fashion by categorization of time scale or in continuous time with splines.
5. Complex TD effects can be estimated using spline functions.
6. With splines, the number of parameters needed to model the TD effects is usually fewer than the number of parameters needed to model the baseline.
7. TD effects are also useful for modeling on other time scales (for example, age).

7.1 Introduction

This chapter extends the models we have described previously to cases in which the effect of a covariate cannot be summarized by a single number and is thus considered to be a function of follow-up time. For example, in a PH model, a covariate effect is usually expressed as a single hazard ratio (HR), whereas in a nonproportional hazards model, the relative effect of a covariate varies over follow-up time. When the effect of a covariate depends upon follow-up time, it is known as a TD effect.

A proportional effect on one scale usually leads to a nonproportional effect on another scale. For example, both PO (Bennett 1983) and accelerated failure-time models (Patel, Kay, and Rowell 2006) have been advocated in situations where the hazards are nonproportional. The disadvantage of such approaches is that the interpretation of the covariate effects differs from what most practitioners are used to—that is, a (log) HR.

The PH assumption implies that the relative effect of a covariate is the same at all points of the time scale. Sometimes this may not be a sensible assumption. For example, if the effect of a treatment is only expected to work in the short term and its impact is likely to diminish over time, we would expect the HR to converge to 1 as follow-up time increases.

7.2 Definitions

It is important to give some definitions because some of the following terms have been used interchangeably in the literature. We adopt the following definitions in our book.

Time-fixed covariate: A covariate whose value is measured once, at $t = 0$. This is also known as a baseline covariate. So far in our book, we have only considered covariates that are time-fixed.

Time-varying covariate: A covariate whose value is measured at $t = 0$ and at least once at $t > 0$. For example, a subject may start on treatment A, but switch to treatment B after six months, or they may have a biomarker measured several times during follow-up.

Time-fixed effect: A covariate whose regression coefficient (in whatever scaling the model uses) is constant over time. An HR from a PH model is a time-fixed effect, as is an odds ratio from a PO model. A time-fixed effect can apply to a time-fixed or time-varying covariate.

Time-dependent (TD) effect: A covariate whose regression coefficient (in whatever scaling the model uses) changes over time. A TD effect can apply to a time-fixed or time-varying covariate.

Up to this point, we have only considered time-fixed effects. This chapter is concerned with extending models to incorporate TD effects for covariates measured at baseline that is, for time-fixed covariates. First, in section 7.3 we review how TD effects can be estimated with a Cox model. In section 7.4, we show how TD HRs can be estimated by assuming proportional effects on various other scales. Section 7.5 shows how TD effects can be estimated using Poisson models, and section 7.6 shows how they can be estimated using RP models. Section 7.7 shows how continuous covariates can be simultaneously nonlinear and TD. Section 7.8 describes how TD effects can be used when considering age as the time scale, and section 7.9 demonstrates how to model more than one time scale. Section 7.10 shows how the prognostic models described in the previous chapter can be extended to include TD effects. Section 7.11 discusses issues raised in the chapter.

7.3 What do we mean by a TD effect?

The usual way to report an effect of a covariate in survival analysis is an HR. In a PH model, we assume that the HR—that is, the relative increase or decrease in the hazard rate—is the same throughout the follow-up period. This may not always be a sensible assumption because the relative increase or decrease in the hazard rate may depend on the elapsed time from follow-up.

We first show how TD effects can be estimated within the Cox modeling framework. We use the England and Wales breast cancer dataset described in section 3.3. Specifically, we look at a subset that consists of 24,889 women aged under 50 years of age diagnosed with breast cancer in England and Wales between 1986 and the end of 1990, with follow-up to the end of 1995. The event is death from any cause, although given their age, most women who die will die of their cancer. We explore differences in survival by deprivation group as measured by the Carstairs index (Coleman et al. 1999). There are five deprivation groups, ranging from the most to the least deprived quantile in the population. Follow-up is restricted to five years after diagnosis. For simplicity, we initially compare only the most and least deprived groups in the population, leading to 6,755 women in the least deprived group and 2,944 women in the most deprived group. The larger number in the least deprived group reflects the higher incidence of breast cancer in young women in this group. A Kaplan–Meier curve by deprivation group, obtained using `sts graph`, can be seen in figure 7.1. There is a clear difference in survival between the two groups. The proportion of women who survive five years or more is 72.6% in the least deprived group and 66.3% in the most deprived group.

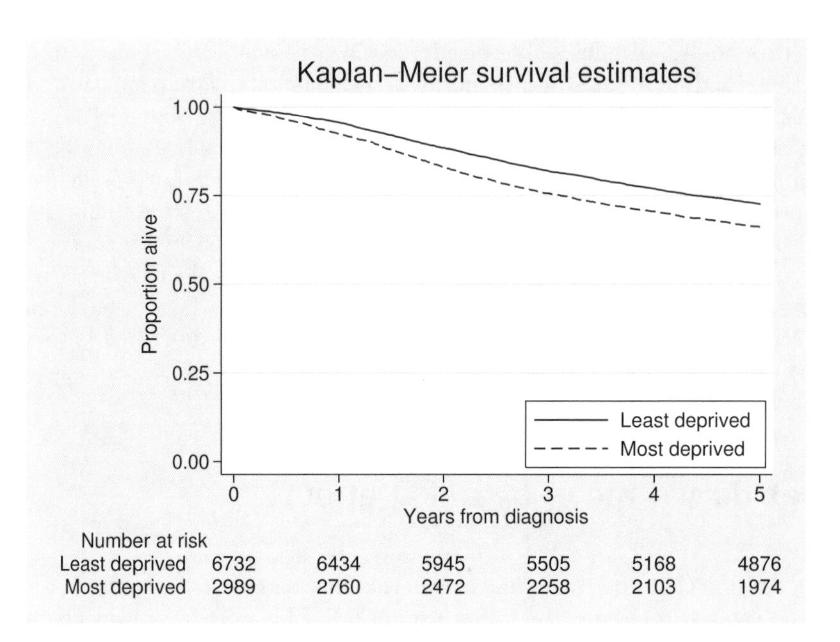

Figure 7.1. England and Wales breast cancer data. Kaplan–Meier estimates of the survival function for women aged ≤ 50 years diagnosed with breast cancer, by deprivation group.

A Cox PH model can be fit as follows:

```
. use ew_breast_ch7
(England and Wales Breast Cancer: Age<=50: least and most deprived)
. stset survtime, failure(dead==1) exit(time 5) id(ident)

                id:  ident
     failure event:  dead == 1
obs. time interval:  (survtime[_n-1], survtime]
 exit on or before:  time 5

------------------------------------------------------------------------------
      9721  total obs.
         0  exclusions
------------------------------------------------------------------------------
      9721  obs. remaining, representing
      9721  subjects
      2847  failures in single failure-per-subject data
  40919.28  total analysis time at risk, at risk from t =         0
                             earliest observed entry t =         0
                                  last observed exit t =         5
```

```
. stcox dep5, nolog noshow
Cox regression -- Breslow method for ties
No. of subjects =         9721                    Number of obs   =       9721
No. of failures =         2847
Time at risk    =    40919.284
                                                  LR chi2(1)      =      45.88
Log likelihood  =   -25649.634                    Prob > chi2     =     0.0000

          _t   Haz. Ratio   Std. Err.      z    P>|z|     [95% Conf. Interval]

        dep5     1.309158    .0513214    6.87   0.000     1.212337    1.413711
```

We see that the mortality rate in the most deprived group is about 31% higher than that in the least deprived group. Because we have fit a PH model, we are assuming that there is an 31% increase in the mortality rate after one day, one week, one month, one year and five years and at all time points in between. The underlying mortality (hazard) rate can of course vary over this period; it is only the ratio of the hazard rates that is assumed constant. However, the hazard rate is not directly estimated in the Cox model.

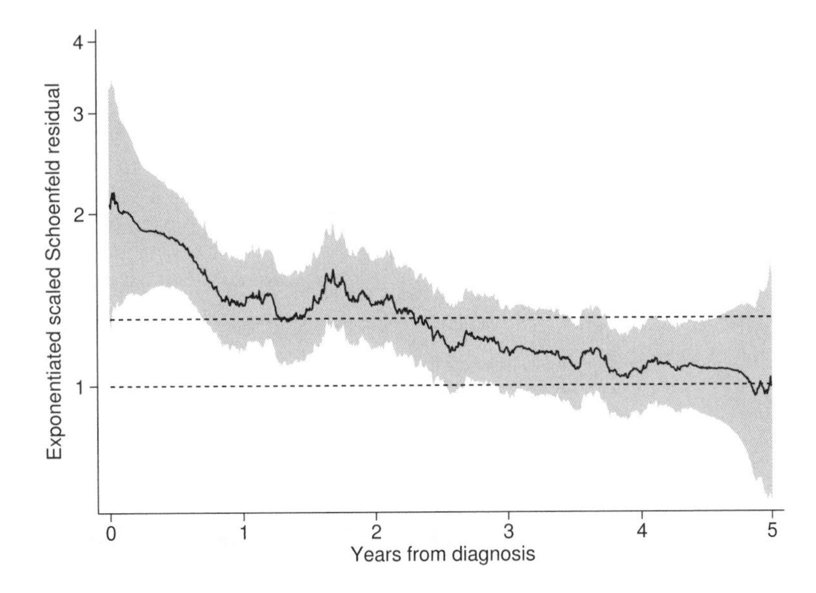

Figure 7.2. England and Wales breast cancer data. Smoothed Schoenfeld residuals for deprivation group.

The scaled Schoenfeld residuals for dep5 can be obtained after fitting a Cox model using

```
. predict sca1, scaledsch
```

This enables us to investigate the PH assumption graphically. If the PH assumption is reasonable, then the scaled Schoenfeld residuals should have an average value approximately equal to the log HR and there should be no trend with time (Grambsch and Therneau 1994). These plots are available using `estat phtest`, but we prefer to use symmetric nearest-neighbor smoothing of the Schoenfeld residuals against time using the `running` command and then transform to the HR scale. The code below produces the plot shown in figure 7.2:

```
running sca1 _t if _d == 1, gen(smooth_sca) gense(smooth_sca_se) nodraw
gen smooth_esca = exp(smooth_sca)
gen smooth_esca_lci = exp(smooth_sca - 1.96*smooth_sca_se)
gen smooth_esca_uci = exp(smooth_sca + 1.96*smooth_sca_se)
local beta = exp(_b[dep5])
twoway (rarea smooth_esca_lci smooth_esca_uci _t, pstyle(ci) sort) ///
       (line smooth_esca _t, sort clpattern(solid))                ///
       (function y = 1, lpattern(shortdash) range(_t))             ///
       (function y = `beta´, lpattern(shortdash) range(_t)),       ///
       legend(off)                                                 ///
       ytitle("Exponentiated scaled Schoenfeld residual")          ///
       xtitle("Years from diagnosis")                              ///
       ylabel(,angle(h)) yscale(log) scheme(sj)
```

After doing the smoothing, we have exponentiated the estimates. The smoother is important because it is usually impossible to judge the average value as a function of time, especially in models including a number of covariates. Reference lines have been added to the plot at 1 (null effect) and at the estimated value of the HR for dep5. We see a trend in the running line smoother, with the effect of deprivation group reducing as follow-up time increases. The formal test of a nonzero slope is obtained using `estat phtest` and the output is shown below:

```
. estat phtest, log
      Test of proportional-hazards assumption
      Time:  Log(t)
```

	chi2	df	Prob>chi2
global test	16.54	1	0.0000

The resulting p-value is < 0.001, indicating that the relationship is unlikely to be due to chance. The test can be sensitive to the choice of time scaling (here we have used log time), but given that the p-value is so small, changing the time scale in this case is unlikely to make much difference. The test assumes a linear relationship between the scaled Schoenfeld residuals and (log) time, and thus any departure from a linear trend may give an inappropriate p-value.

Thus there is strong evidence that the hazard rates in the two groups are not proportional, and just reporting the HR of 1.31 does not fully describe the underlying effect. We explore two different ways of modeling TD effects using the Cox model—namely, splitting the time scale to obtain piecewise HRs and making the log HR a linear function of log time.

If we split the time scale, a separate HR can be estimated within each time interval defined by the split times. As a simple example, we can use `stsplit` to split the time scale at one and two years and estimate three HRs, one for the effect of deprivation group before one year, one for one to two years, and one for after two years. This is done by the code below:

```
. stsplit sptime, at(1 2)
(17611 observations (episodes) created)
. stcox i1.dep5#ibn.sptime, nolog noshow
Cox regression -- Breslow method for ties
No. of subjects =         9721                 Number of obs    =      27332
No. of failures =         2847
Time at risk    =    40919.284
                                               LR chi2(3)       =      64.67
Log likelihood  =   -25640.241                 Prob > chi2      =     0.0000

          _t   Haz. Ratio   Std. Err.      z    P>|z|     [95% Conf. Interval]

 dep5#sptime
         1 0     1.760192    .1549884    6.42   0.000     1.481187    2.091751
         1 1     1.398539    .1043885    4.49   0.000     1.208203    1.618859
         1 2     1.136001    .0619193    2.34   0.019     1.020899     1.26408
```

`stsplit` creates a new variable, `sptime`, that defines the time categories. To estimate a separate parameter for each interval, we use factor-variable notation to include in the model an interaction between `sptime` and `dep5`. The output from `stcox` shows that we have now estimated three HRs for the effect of deprivation group. The HR up to one year is 1.76, for one to two years it is 1.40, and for after two years it is 1.14, clearly showing a reduction in the HR as follow-up time increases. This is what we should expect, given the trend seen in the scaled Schoenfeld residuals in figure 7.2 (although it could be argued that the step function is oversimplified). The difference in $-2\ln L$ between the PH model and the model using three time intervals for the HR is 18.31 with 2 degrees of freedom (d.f.), giving strong evidence of nonproportionality.

There are always issues with piecewise models in the selection of the cutoffs. In chapter 4, we saw this when using piecewise Poisson models for the baseline hazard. However, given that we are usually more interested in HRs, the choice of cutoffs becomes more crucial. If the decision is made after examining the data, any p-values become irrelevant because they will be conditional on having seen some difference in the data. If too many intervals are selected, a separate parameter is needed for each interval, potentially leading to unstable estimates and a reduction in power for the detection of nonproportionality.

An alternative approach with stcox is to allow the log HR to vary as a continuous function of time. This is implemented in Stata with the tvc() option. We are effectively introducing an interaction between the covariate of interest and time, or more usually, log time. As a reminder, the PH model for the effect of dep5 can be written,

$$h(t) = h_0(t)\exp(\beta_1 \texttt{dep5})$$

In this model, only the baseline hazard, $h_0(t)$, varies over time, but the effect of the covariate, dep5, is constant over time. Thus β_1 estimates the log HR for dep5. The model is extended by adding a time-by-covariate interaction for dep5, as follows:

$$h(t) = h_0(t)\exp\{\beta_1 \texttt{dep5} + \beta_2 \texttt{dep5} \times \ln(t)\}$$

We now have two parameters that summarize the effect of dep5. The log HR is a linear function of $\ln(t)$ and can be written

$$\ln(\text{HR}) = \beta_1 + \beta_2 \ln(t)$$

If $\beta_2 = 0$, then the model reduces to a PH model. A formal test of PH can be performed by assessing whether $\beta_2 = 0$. We do not have to use $\ln(t)$, but can use untransformed time or some other transformation of time. However, given the usual skewed distribution of survival times, using $\ln(t)$ is a common approach.

To fit this model in Stata, we must apply stjoin to convert the split data back to single-record data. We first have to drop sptime because it varies within individuals. Having done this, we fit a model in which the effect of dep5 is TD.

```
. drop sptime
. stjoin
(17611 obs. eliminated)
. stcox dep5, tvc(dep5) texp(ln(_t)) nohr nolog noshow

Cox regression -- Breslow method for ties

No. of subjects =         9721                 Number of obs    =       9721
No. of failures =         2847
Time at risk    =    40919.284
                                               LR chi2(2)       =      61.95
Log likelihood  =   -25641.601                 Prob > chi2      =     0.0000

------------------------------------------------------------------------------
          _t |      Coef.   Std. Err.      z    P>|z|     [95% Conf. Interval]
-------------+----------------------------------------------------------------
main         |
        dep5 |   .3560444   .0446557     7.97   0.000     .2685208    .4435681
-------------+----------------------------------------------------------------
tvc          |
        dep5 |  -.1608519   .0401304    -4.01   0.000     -.239506   -.0821977
------------------------------------------------------------------------------
Note: variables in tvc equation interacted with ln(_t)
```

The tvc() option of stcox specifies any covariates that are to have TD effects estimated. The texp(ln(_t)) option means that the log HR is estimated as a function of $\ln(t)$. Thus the log HR for dep5 is $\beta_1 + \beta_2 \ln(t)$.

There are now two estimated parameters for the effect of `dep5`, one is the intercept, β_1 (equation `[main]`), and the other the gradient, β_2 (equation `[tvc]`), and thus the HR can be calculated as $\exp\{0.356 - 0.161 \ln(t)\}$. Using `predictnl`, this function can be estimated with a 95% confidence interval (CI).

```
. range temptime 0.03 5 200
(9521 missing values generated)
. predictnl lhr = [main][dep5] + [tvc][dep5]*ln(temptime), ci(lhr_lci lhr_uci)
(9521 missing values generated)
note: Confidence intervals calculated using Z critical values
. generate hr = exp(lhr)
(9521 missing values generated)
. generate hr_lci = exp(lhr_lci)
(9521 missing values generated)
. generate hr_uci = exp(lhr_uci)
(9521 missing values generated)
```

Because we do not need to plot all 9749 observations, we first create a time variable with 200 observations over the same range as `_t`. The resulting function with a 95% CI can be seen in figure 7.3. We see that the reduction in the HR for deprivation group 5 is greatest early on in the time scale. Also shown on the plot are the piecewise estimates of the HR obtained from splitting the time scale. While there is general agreement that the HR is higher earlier on the time scale, we see that the piecewise estimates may not be capturing the effect within the first year where there appears to be a fairly rapid reduction in the HR.

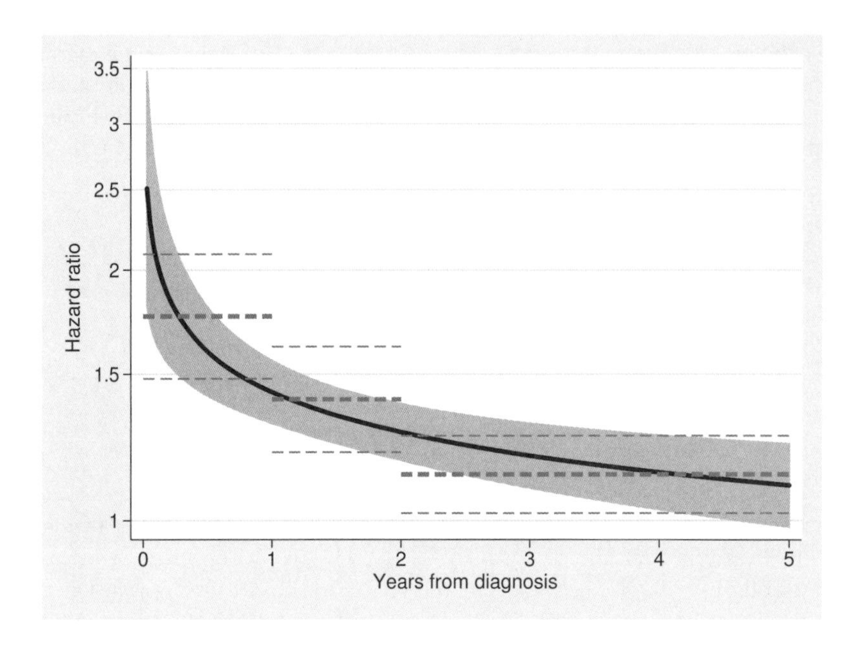

Figure 7.3. England and Wales breast cancer data. TD HR for deprivation group from a Cox model with the `tvc()` option.

There are some limitations in what we can do with a Cox model when modeling TD effects. Firstly, of course we are not directly estimating the baseline hazard function, and thus we have not estimated what the HR is relative to. This is one of the main reasons why we advocate parametric models. Secondly, the shape of the log HR seen in figure 7.3 is the shape we expect to see with a log function. Therefore, what we observe may be due to the fact that we have not fit a more flexible function. With the `tvc()` option in `stcox`, we cannot use more than one term—for example, we cannot use a quadratic function or splines. If, for example, the TD function had a turning point, we would never see it using a simple transformation of time, such as $\ln(t)$.

7.4 Proportional on which scale?

If the effect of a covariate is assumed to be proportional over time on one scale, then generally this implies nonproportionality on another scale. In chapter 5, models on the log cumulative hazard and log cumulative odds scales were compared, and in some cases a better fitting model was found when fitting on the log cumulative odds scale because the hazard rates were not proportional. When fitting a model on the log cumulative odds scale, the relative difference in the hazard rates between any two groups decreases over time; that is, the HR converges to 1 as follow-up time increases (Bennett 1983). Given this is what we have observed in the breast cancer data, it is worthwhile assessing if a model on the log cumulative odds scale adequately captures the declining HR.

The following output shows the estimates from an RP PO model with **dep5** as a covariate and 5 d.f. (2 boundary knots and 4 interior knots) for the baseline distribution.

```
. use ew_breast_ch7, clear
(England and Wales Breast Cancer: Age<=50: least and most deprived)
. stset survtime, failure(dead==1) exit(time 5) id(ident)
  (output omitted)
. stpm2 dep5, scale(odds) df(5) eform nolog
Log likelihood = -8758.2476                    Number of obs   =       9721
```

	exp(b)	Std. Err.	z	P>|z|	[95% Conf.	Interval]
xb						
dep5	1.397421	.0647891	7.22	0.000	1.276036	1.530354
_rcs1	2.226502	.0347686	51.26	0.000	2.159389	2.295701
_rcs2	.9555388	.0111276	-3.91	0.000	.9339761	.9775993
_rcs3	1.047527	.0069646	6.98	0.000	1.033965	1.061267
_rcs4	1.007728	.0035753	2.17	0.030	1.000745	1.01476
_rcs5	.9994118	.001829	-0.32	0.748	.9958334	1.003003
_cons	.2627584	.0071077	-49.41	0.000	.2491903	.2770652

The most deprived group has an increased odds of dying of 39% compared with the least deprived group. Because this is a PO model, we assume that the relative increase in odds is the same throughout the time scale. However, because the cumulative odds are proportional, the hazard rates are nonproportional and, as stated above, the relative difference in any two hazard rates decreases over follow-up time.

Also included in the output under the **exp(b)** heading is an estimate of **exp(_[_cons])**, the exponentiated constant. Its inclusion is a new feature of Stata 12. While for standard models such as logistic and Poisson such an estimate would be interpreted as the baseline odds or the baseline incidence rate, respectively, this estimate has no practical interpretation in **stpm2** models. Instead, **_cons** merely serves as a scaling parameter that affects the vertical positioning of the flexible baseline hazard.

The HR can be obtained from this model using

```
. range temptime 0.03 5 200
(9521 missing values generated)
. predict hr_po, hrnumerator(dep5 1) timevar(temptime) ci
```

Note the use of the **hrnumerator()** option, which defines the covariate pattern for the numerator of the HR. There is an associated **hrdenominator()** option for the denominator of the HR. All covariate values not specified using the **hrdenominator()** option are set to zero by default, which is exactly what we want here and so there is no need to use this option. The **ci** option requests that CIs be calculated. The standard errors (SEs) are estimated on the log HR scale using the delta method. The resulting function is shown in figure 7.4, which shows the effect of the deprivation group reducing (slightly) over time. As we stated above, when fitting a PO model, the HR always approaches the null (that is, 1) as follow-up time increases. However, the shape of this curve is very different from that observed with the Cox model in figure 7.3 and different from the general pattern seen in the piecewise estimates. These differences are because neither PH nor proportional cumulative odds is a reasonable assumption for the data.

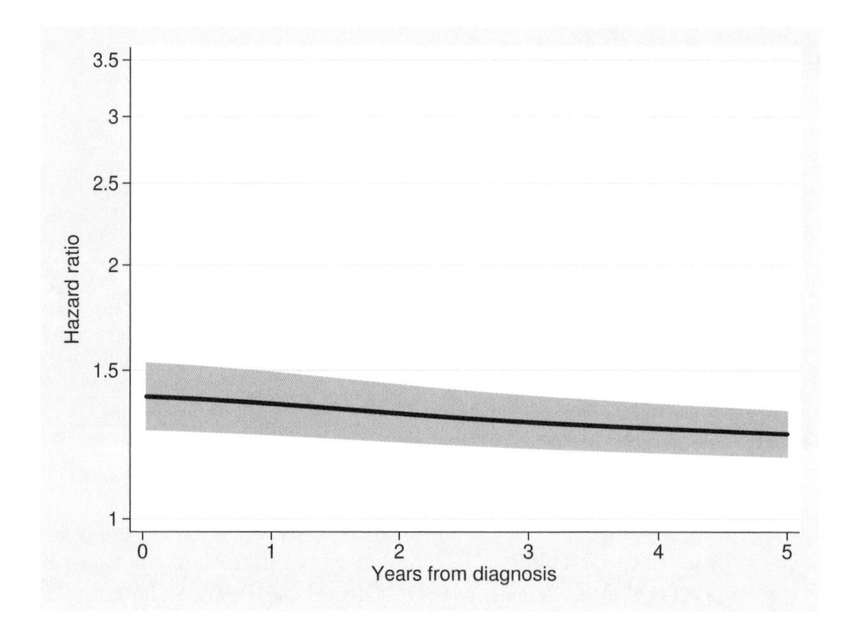

Figure 7.4. England and Wales breast cancer data. HR for deprivation group from a proportional cumulative odds model.

In section 5.6, we showed that a parameter, θ, could be estimated for the Aranda-Ordaz link function for the survival distribution in RP models, and that the PO and PH model were special cases of this more general link function. Such a model is fit below using the scale(theta) option of stpm2.

```
. stpm2 dep5, scale(theta) df(5) nolog
Log likelihood = -8755.3404                     Number of obs   =      9721

------------------------------------------------------------------------------
             |      Coef.   Std. Err.      z    P>|z|     [95% Conf. Interval]
-------------+----------------------------------------------------------------
xb           |
        dep5 |   .5279887   .1017753     5.19   0.000     .3285127    .7274646
       _rcs1 |   .9679653   .0816226    11.86   0.000     .8079879    1.127943
       _rcs2 |   -.120458   .0381569    -3.16   0.002    -.1952441   -.0456719
       _rcs3 |    .019412   .0156699     1.24   0.215    -.0113004    .0501244
       _rcs4 |   .0080387   .0044589     1.80   0.071    -.0007005    .0167779
       _rcs5 |  -.0025147   .0027277    -0.92   0.357    -.0078608    .0028314
       _cons |  -.8849205   .2210825    -4.00   0.000    -1.318234   -.4516068
-------------+----------------------------------------------------------------
ln_theta     |
       _cons |   1.404777   .3338622     4.21   0.000     .7504195    2.059135
------------------------------------------------------------------------------
```

The estimate of θ is $\exp(1.40) = 4.06$, which is a long way from a PH ($\theta = 0$) or a PO ($\theta = 1$) model. We can use the `predict` command to obtain the TD HR.

```
. predict hr_theta, hrnum(dep5 1) timevar(temptime) ci
```

The estimated HR as a function of time is shown in figure 7.5. The SE of the log HR used in calculation of the 95% CI again employs the delta method. There is a greater decrease in the HR as a function of time than was seen for the PO model, but the fitted function is noticeably different from that seen for the Cox model in figure 7.3. So which model, if any, is correct? We believe that to answer this question, it is better to allow the effect of a covariate to be TD on the scale you are modeling on. In section 7.5, we show how this is done for Poisson models, and in section 7.6 for RP models.

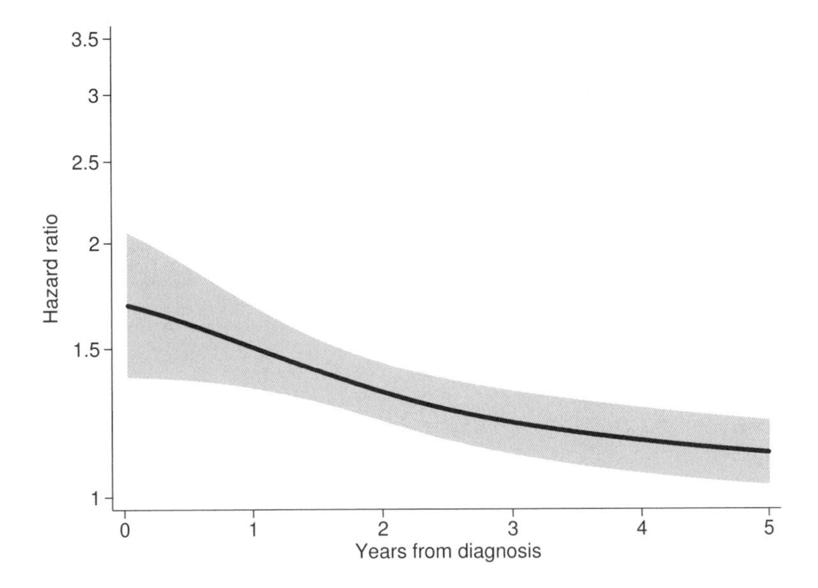

Figure 7.5. England and Wales breast cancer data. Estimated HR with 95% CI from an RP model where θ is estimated.

7.5 Poisson models with TD effects

In the Poisson models described in chapter 4, we included follow-up time in the model with a number of covariates, either as a step function with a dummy covariate for each interval or with a large number of intervals and estimating a smooth function using restricted cubic splines or fractional polynomials (FPs). The Poisson models in chapter 4 were all PH models in that they assumed that the effect of a covariate of interest was constant at all levels of other covariates and, in particular, at all levels of the covariates used to describe the effect of time. If we believe that the hazard rates are nonproportional, we are saying that the effect of the covariate of interest differs at different levels of the covariates we use to describe the effect of time. In other words, there is an interaction between our covariate of interest and time. In this section, we describe how we can easily extend piecewise models and models incorporating restricted cubic splines for the effect of time to include TD effects—that is, nonproportional hazards. We simply add interaction terms to the models.

7.5.1 Piecewise models

Recall that with the piecewise Poisson approach, we can write a PH model as

$$
\begin{aligned}
d_{ij} &\sim \text{Poisson}(\mu_{ij}) \\
\ln(\mu_{ij}) &= \ln(y_{ij}) + \alpha_j + \beta x_i
\end{aligned}
$$

where subscript i denotes the subject and subscript j denotes the time interval. For simplicity, we assume that there is only one binary covariate, x_i. The effect of this covariate, β, is assumed to be the same for all time intervals. The log baseline hazard is estimated in each time interval by the α_j parameters. The model can be extended to nonproportional hazards, where the effect of covariate x_i is time dependent, by adding a subscript j to β and thus estimating a separate (log) HR for each interval:

$$
\begin{aligned}
d_{ij} &\sim \text{Poisson}(\mu_{ij}) \\
\ln(\mu_{ij}) &= \ln(y_{ij}) + \alpha_j + \beta_j x_i
\end{aligned}
$$

The model can be fit by simply adding interactions between the covariate of interest and the dummy variables we are using to define the time scale. To fit a Poisson model to the England and Wales breast cancer data, we first need to set up the data in the appropriate format:

```
. use ew_breast_ch7, clear
(England and Wales Breast Cancer: Age<=50: least and most deprived)
. stset survtime, failure(dead==1) exit(time 5) id(ident)
  (output omitted)
. stsplit split_time, every(1)
(32644 observations (episodes) created)
. generate risktime = _t - _t0
. collapse (min) start=_t0 (max) end=_t (count) n=_d (sum) risktime _d,
> by(split_time dep5)
```

We have used the every(1) option in stsplit, which means that intervals are one year in length. We collapse the data because this speeds up model fitting. We can now fit a PH model.

```
. glm _d ibn.split_time dep5, family(poisson) lnoffset(risktime) nocons nolog
> eform noheader

------------------------------------------------------------------------------
             |                 OIM
          _d |        IRR   Std. Err.      z    P>|z|     [95% Conf. Interval]
-------------+----------------------------------------------------------------
  split_time |
          0  |   .0506709   .0023264   -64.96   0.000     .0463103    .0554421
          1  |   .0798247   .0030896   -65.31   0.000     .0739931    .0861158
          2  |   .0736876   .0030646   -62.71   0.000     .0679193    .0799458
          3  |   .0594125   .0028141   -59.61   0.000     .0541453    .0651921
          4  |   .0545722   .0027673   -57.35   0.000     .0494092    .0602748
             |
        dep5 |   1.308883   .0513104     6.87   0.000     1.212082    1.413413
ln(risktime) |          1  (exposure)
------------------------------------------------------------------------------

. estimates store poiss_ph
```

We use factor variables for the baseline hazard in section 4.3.1. The estimated HR for dep5 is 1.31, which is the same as that obtained from the Cox model. This is despite the poor way we have modeled the effect of time, which is assumed to be constant within each yearly interval. We define smaller intervals later in this section, but for now we continue with these large intervals to explain how the model can be extended to fit a TD effect for a deprivation group.

We need to define an interaction between our deprivation group covariate, dep5, and five dummy covariates defining the time scale. We use the factor-variable notation introduced in Stata 11 to do this.

```
. glm _d ibn.split_time ibn.split_time#dep5, family(poisson) lnoffset(risktime)
> nocons nolog eform noheader

------------------------------------------------------------------------------
             |                 OIM
          _d |        IRR   Std. Err.      z    P>|z|     [95% Conf. Interval]
-------------+----------------------------------------------------------------
  split_time |
          0  |   .0450445   .0026137   -53.43   0.000     .0402022      .05047
          1  |   .0779281   .0035495   -56.03   0.000     .0712727    .0852051
          2  |   .0762258   .0036506   -53.75   0.000     .0693963    .0837273
          3  |   .0625992   .0034253   -50.64   0.000     .0562332    .0696858
          4  |   .0580232   .0034014   -48.56   0.000     .0517254    .0650879
             |
 split_time# |
        dep5 |
        0 1  |   1.758491   .1548368     6.41   0.000      1.47976    2.089726
        1 1  |   1.398081   .1043533     4.49   0.000     1.207809    1.618327
        2 1  |   1.184562   .0990255     2.03   0.043     1.005541    1.395453
        3 1  |   1.117276   .1093159     1.13   0.257     .9223111    1.353453
        4 1  |   1.084407   .1150133     0.76   0.445     .8808726     1.33497
ln(risktime) |          1  (exposure)
------------------------------------------------------------------------------

. estimates store poiss_tvc
```

There are now five HRs, one for each of the intervals. The HR is highest in the first interval and then decreases with increasing follow-up time. A likelihood-ratio test comparing the PH model with the TD model is shown below:

```
. lrtest poiss_ph poiss_tvc
Likelihood-ratio test                                 LR chi2(4)  =     19.17
(Assumption: poiss_ph nested in poiss_tvc)            Prob > chi2 =    0.0007
```

This output gives strong evidence that the effect of deprivation group varies over time.

One of the problems with the approach we have adopted here is that the number of parameters used to model the TD effect depends on the number of intervals used to model the baseline hazard rate. This is illustrated in figure 7.6, which shows the estimated HRs within each interval for intervals of length one month, one quarter of a year, one half a year, and one year. There are two main features of the graphs to note: First, there is more noise (that is, random variation) as the number of intervals increases. Second, the CIs become wider as the intervals become narrower. Both these features are to be expected; as the intervals become narrower, the number of events within each interval drops, and thus the uncertainty associated with any interval-specific estimate increases. In these models, we are making no assumptions about a relationship between the intervals. In fact, because there is only one covariate in the model, we would obtain identical estimates if we fit a separate model to each of the intervals.

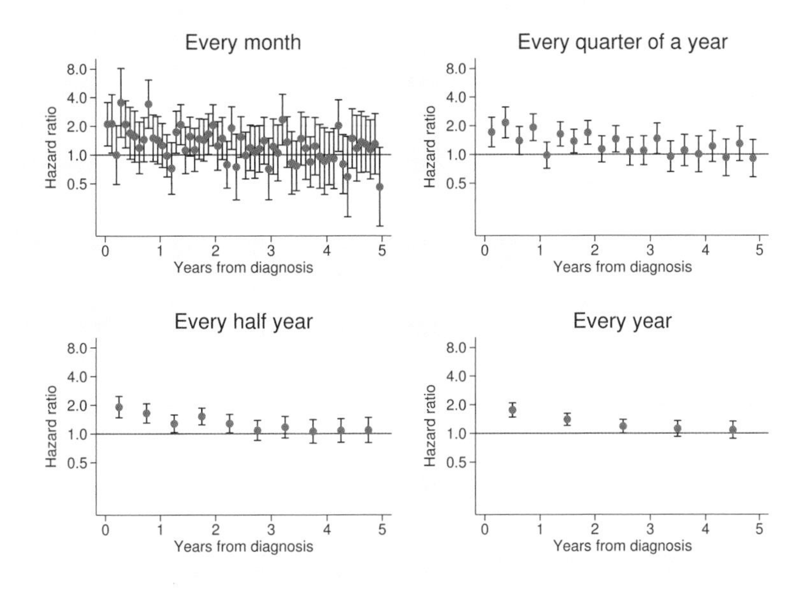

Figure 7.6. England and Wales breast cancer data. Panels show TD HRs from piecewise Poisson models with different split times every month, every quarter year, every half year, and every year.

We want to increase the number of intervals so that we are not making such strong assumptions about the baseline hazard. However, we do not want too many parameters because this makes the TD HRs too noisy. In our view, the best way to do this is to move away from step functions toward either Poisson models with restricted cubic splines or RP models, as described in section 7.6. However, if we prefer to stay with step functions, we do not have to have the same number of parameters for the TD effect as there are for the baseline hazard. One solution is to decide on intervals where we would expect the TD effect to be approximately constant. For example, we could estimate one HR for the first year of follow-up, one for the second year, and one more for years three through five, as we did for the Cox model in section 7.3. We do this below for the model with split times every month:

```
. use ew_breast_ch7, clear
(England and Wales Breast Cancer: Age<=50: least and most deprived)
. stset survtime, failure(dead==1) exit(time 5) id(ident)
  (output omitted)
. stsplit split_time, every(`=1/12´)
(482752 observations (episodes) created)
. gen risktime = _t - _t0
. collapse (min) start=_t0 (max) end=_t (count) n=_d (sum) risktime _d,
> by(dep5 split_time)
```

```
. egen interval = group(split_time)
. recode start (min/1 = 1) (1/2 = 2) (2/max=3), gen(td_int)
(120 differences between start and td_int)
. glm _d ibn.interval i.td_int#i1.dep5, family(poisson) lnoffset(risktime)
> nolog nocons noheader eform
```

_d	IRR	OIM Std. Err.	z	P>|z|	[95% Conf.	Interval]
interval						
1	.0562382	.0078218	-20.69	0.000	.0428197	.0738618
(output omitted)						
60	.0537985	.009555	-16.45	0.000	.0379831	.076199
td_int#dep5						
1 1	1.760397	.1550064	6.42	0.000	1.48136	2.091995
2 1	1.39865	.1043968	4.49	0.000	1.208299	1.618989
3 1	1.136014	.06192	2.34	0.019	1.020911	1.264095
ln(risktime)	1	(exposure)				

Three HRs have been created: one for zero to one year, one for one to two years, and one for three to five years. All are significant at the 5% level, but the magnitude of the HR decreases over follow-up time. They are almost identical to the HRs from the Cox model with piecewise HRs in section 7.3. The major disadvantage of such an approach is that these intervals are completely arbitrary. For the p-values to have any relevance, the intervals must be chosen prior to seeing the data. Although there is a clear TD effect for this dataset, in other datasets the effect may be less obvious. Any test of significance depends strongly on the number of intervals chosen for the TD effect, which is not desirable.

7.5.2 Using restricted cubic splines

In chapter 4, we described how a step function for the baseline hazard function was not the only option in Poisson models. We pointed out that we could fit a continuous function by defining narrow intervals and using either restricted cubic splines or FPs. The extension to TD effects follows the same principle as the piecewise models described above, in that interactions are formed between the covariates used to describe the effect of time and the covariates of interest. We first need to define narrow time intervals, which we choose here to be of length one week.

```
. use ew_breast_ch7, clear
(England and Wales Breast Cancer: Age<=50: least and most deprived)
. stset survtime, failure(dead==1) exit(time 5) id(ident)
  (output omitted)
. stsplit sp_time, every(`=1/52.18')
(2127598 observations (episodes) created)
. generate risktime = _t - _t0
. collapse (min) start=_t0 (max) end=_t (count) n=_d (sum) risktime _d,
> by(dep5 sp_time)
```

A PH model is first fit using 3 d.f. for the restricted cubic spline function used to estimate the baseline hazard function. The restricted cubic spline function is generated with log time. We showed in chapter 4 that this led to a better fit for the Rotterdam breast cancer data, and it is the same for the England and Wales breast cancer dataset used here.

```
. generate midtime = (start + end)
. generate lntime = ln(midtime)
. rcsgen lntime, df(3) gen(rcs) fw(_d) orthog
Variables rcs1 to rcs3 were created
. glm _d rcs* dep5, family(poisson) lnoffset(risktime) nolog eform
Generalized linear models                         No. of obs      =        522
Optimization     : ML                             Residual df     =        517
                                                  Scale parameter =          1
Deviance         =  589.4507401                   (1/df) Deviance =   1.140137
Pearson          =  565.6616566                   (1/df) Pearson  =   1.094123
Variance function: V(u) = u                       [Poisson]
Link function    : g(u) = ln(u)                   [Log]
                                                  AIC             =   4.513367
Log likelihood   = -1172.988905                   BIC             =  -2645.763

------------------------------------------------------------------------------
             |                 OIM
          _d |        IRR   Std. Err.      z    P>|z|     [95% Conf. Interval]
-------------+----------------------------------------------------------------
        rcs1 |   1.033444   .0203234     1.67   0.094     .9943687    1.074055
        rcs2 |   1.066464   .0202456     3.39   0.001     1.027513    1.106892
        rcs3 |   1.174232   .0229925     8.20   0.000     1.130021    1.220172
        dep5 |   1.309601   .0513388     6.88   0.000     1.212747    1.414189
       _cons |    .062716   .0014843  -117.01   0.000     .0598733    .0656937
ln(risktime) |          1  (exposure)
------------------------------------------------------------------------------
. estimates store pois_rcs_ph
```

The HR in the PH model is 1.31, which (as should come as no surprise) is the same as in the Cox model and the piecewise models in the previous section. To extend the model to TD effects, we use factor-variable notation:

```
. glm _d i.dep5##c.rcs*, family(poisson) lnoffset(risktime) nolog
Generalized linear models                         No. of obs      =        522
Optimization     : ML                             Residual df     =        514
                                                  Scale parameter =          1
Deviance         =  571.3748157                   (1/df) Deviance =   1.111624
Pearson          =  549.7399366                   (1/df) Pearson  =   1.069533
Variance function: V(u) = u                       [Poisson]
Link function    : g(u) = ln(u)                   [Log]
                                                  AIC             =   4.490233
Log likelihood   = -1163.950943                   BIC             =  -2645.066

------------------------------------------------------------------------------
             |                 OIM
          _d |      Coef.   Std. Err.      z    P>|z|     [95% Conf. Interval]
-------------+----------------------------------------------------------------
      1.dep5 |   .2460437   .0407188     6.04   0.000     .1662363     .325851
        rcs1 |   .0974977   .0258872     3.77   0.000     .0467597    .1482358
        rcs2 |   .0568394   .0252797     2.25   0.025     .0072921    .1063867
        rcs3 |   .1486538    .024408     6.09   0.000      .100815    .1964926
             |
 dep5#c.rcs1 |
          1  |  -.1711919   .0407214    -4.20   0.000    -.2510044   -.0913795
             |
 dep5#c.rcs2 |
          1  |   .0377089   .0392366     0.96   0.337    -.0391935    .1146113
             |
 dep5#c.rcs3 |
          1  |   .0389086   .0413411     0.94   0.347    -.0421186    .1199357
             |
       _cons |   -2.76561   .0237546  -116.42   0.000    -2.812168   -2.719052
ln(risktime) |          1  (exposure)
------------------------------------------------------------------------------

. estimates store rcs_tvc_df3
```

The parameters associated with the restricted cubic spline terms are impossible to interpret individually, but we can predict both the hazard rate and the TD HR as follows:

```
. predict log_hazard, xb nooffset
. generate hazard = 1000*exp(log_hazard)
. predictnl log_hr = _b[1.dep5] + _b[1.dep5#c.rcs1]*rcs1 +
> _b[1.dep5#c.rcs2]*rcs2 + _b[1.dep5#c.rcs3]*rcs3,
> ci(log_hr_lci log_hr_uci)
note: Confidence intervals calculated using Z critical values
. generate hr = exp(log_hr)
. generate hr_lci = exp(log_hr_lci)
. generate hr_uci = exp(log_hr_uci)
```

The plot of the hazard functions (on the log scale) is shown in figure 7.7. The estimated hazard functions for the PH model using restricted cubic splines are also shown on the plot. There is a larger difference between the mortality rates in the two groups early on in the time since diagnosis. The distance between the two lines from the TD model narrows as follow-up time increases. For the PH model, the distance between the two lines is forced to be constant (on the log scale, as presented) over follow-up time.

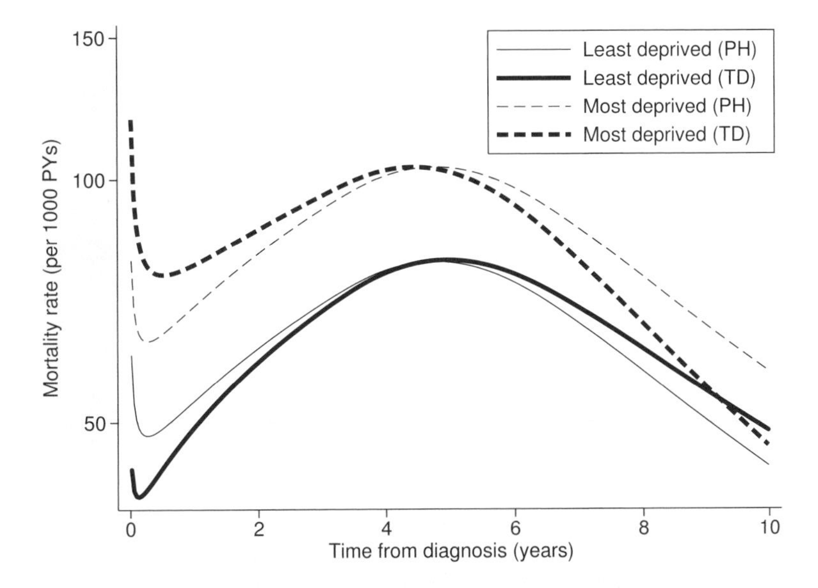

Figure 7.7. England and Wales breast cancer data. Estimated mortality rates from a Poisson model incorporating restricted cubic splines. PYs stands for person-years.

The estimated TD HR with 95% CI is plotted in figure 7.8.

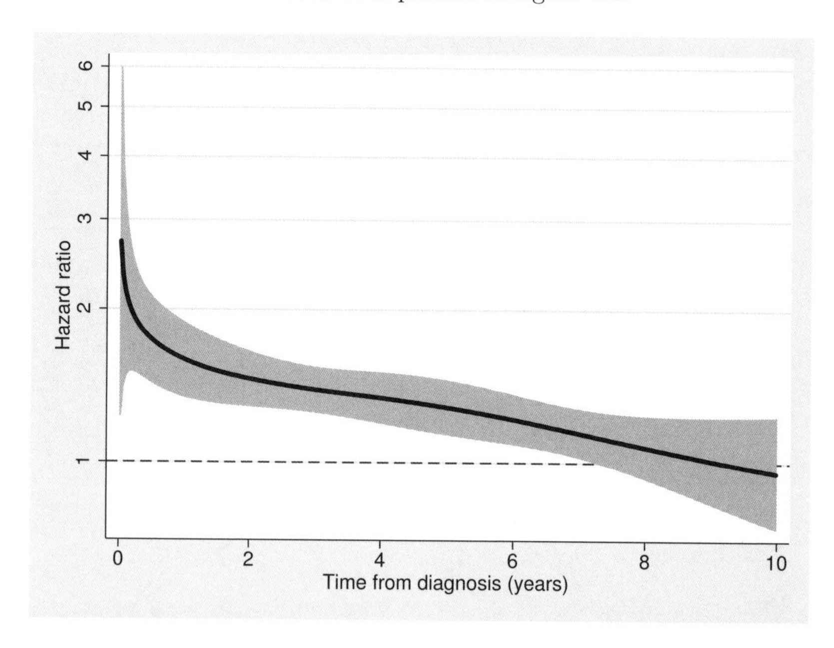

Figure 7.8. England and Wales breast cancer data. Estimated TD HR for the most deprived compared with the least deprived group from a Poisson model incorporating restricted cubic splines.

The HR is seen to be a decreasing function of time, which is to be expected after seeing the estimates of the hazard functions in figure 7.7. One criticism of this model could be that the TD effect is overparameterized because the difference between the two (log) hazard rates is assumed to have the same complexity as the baseline hazard rate; that is, the same number of spline variables are used. It is possible that the difference between the (log) hazard rates can be summarized using fewer parameters. In the code below, we fit a model where the TD effect is assumed to be a linear function of log(time) and a second model where 2 d.f. are used for the spline variables. We can use the Akaike information criterion (AIC) or Bayes information criterion (BIC) to compare such models. This is shown below:

```
. qui glm _d rcs1-rcs3 i1.dep5##c.lntime, family(poisson) lnoffset(risktime)
. estimates store lntime
. rcsgen lntime, df(2) gen(rcs_df2_) fw(_d) orthog
Variables rcs_df2_1 to rcs_df2_2 were created
. quietly glm _d rcs1-rcs3 i.dep i1.dep#c.(rcs_df2_*), family(poisson)
> lnoffset(risktime)
. estimates store rcs_tvc_df2
. summarize _d, meanonly
```

```
. estimates stats lntime rcs_tvc_df2 rcs_tvc_df3, n(`r(sum)´)
```

Model	Obs	ll(null)	ll(model)	df	AIC	BIC
lntime	2847	.	-1164.736	6	2341.472	2377.196
rcs_tvc_df2	2847	.	-1164.353	7	2342.706	2384.384
rcs_tvc_df3	2847	.	-1163.951	8	2343.902	2391.534

Note: N=2847 used in calculating BIC

The model with just 1 d.f., in which the TD effect is a function of log time, has the lowest AIC and BIC. A plot of this function with the corresponding estimate from the model with a full interaction is shown in figure 7.9. As it happens, the two estimated TD effects convey a similar message. However, the spline model is much more general than the simple log function and could represent more complex TD effects if they were present.

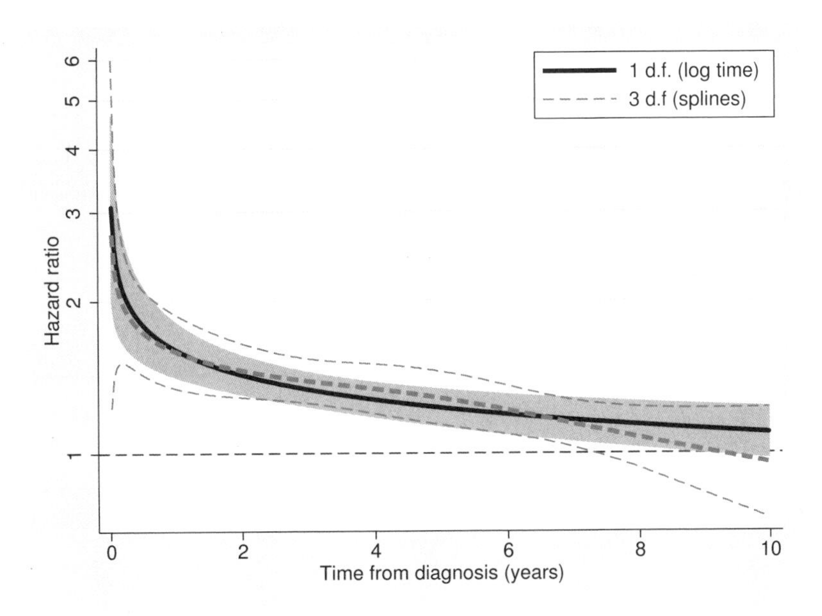

Figure 7.9. England and Wales breast cancer data. Estimated TD HR for the most deprived compared with the least deprived group from a Poisson model incorporating restricted cubic splines where the TD effect is a linear function of ln(time).

7.6 RP models with TD effects

In this section, we demonstrate how the RP models discussed in chapter 5 can be extended to model TD effects. We first show how to estimate piecewise HRs and some limitations of this approach. We then discuss continuous TD effects. In general, we favor the latter approach.

7.6.1 Piecewise HRs

In section 7.3, we showed that by using **stsplit** to split the time scale, we can estimate different HRs in predefined time intervals with a Cox model. Using the same process, we can also fit RP models with piecewise constant HRs. We can do this with stpm2 because it allows for delayed entry; each failure time does not necessarily have to start at time $t = 0$.

We first fit a PH model with 5 d.f. for the baseline, which is shown in the output below:

```
. use ew_breast_ch7, clear
(England and Wales Breast Cancer: Age<=50: least and most deprived)
. stset survtime, failure(dead==1) exit(time 5) id(ident)
  (output omitted)
. stpm2 dep5, scale(hazard) df(5) eform nolog
Log likelihood = -8760.4204                    Number of obs    =      9721
```

	exp(b)	Std. Err.	z	P>|z|	[95% Conf. Interval]	
xb						
dep5	1.309129	.0513202	6.87	0.000	1.21231	1.413679
_rcs1	2.121704	.0325627	49.01	0.000	2.058832	2.186495
_rcs2	.9759501	.0112833	-2.11	0.035	.9540839	.9983175
_rcs3	1.054759	.0067851	8.29	0.000	1.041544	1.068142
_rcs4	1.00741	.003317	2.24	0.025	1.000929	1.013932
_rcs5	.9998765	.00163	-0.08	0.940	.9966868	1.003076
_cons	.2306123	.0054703	-61.85	0.000	.2201362	.241587

The estimated HR of 1.31 is identical to that obtained from the Cox model in section 7.3. As we stated in chapter 5, we have yet to find an example where the estimated HR from a PH RP model differs markedly from the estimated HR from a Cox PH model. We now split the time scale into the same three intervals as before (that is, zero to one year, one to two years, and after two years) and use an RP model on the log cumulative hazard scale to estimate a separate HR for each interval.

```
. stsplit split_time, at(1 2)
(17611 observations (episodes) created)
. qui tab split_time, gen(int)
. forvalues i = 1/3 {
  2.        gen dep5int`i´ = dep5*int`i´
  3. }
```

```
. stpm2 dep5int1-dep5int3, scale(hazard) df(5) eform nolog
note: delayed entry models are being fitted
Log likelihood =   -8751.94                     Number of obs   =      27332

------------------------------------------------------------------------------
             |     exp(b)   Std. Err.      z    P>|z|     [95% Conf. Interval]
-------------+----------------------------------------------------------------
xb           |
    dep5int1 |   1.641424   .1346268     6.04   0.000     1.397677     1.92768
    dep5int2 |   1.472792   .1033083     5.52   0.000     1.283613    1.689851
    dep5int3 |   1.133265   .0611072     2.32   0.020     1.019609    1.259591
       _rcs1 |   2.214027   .0391198    44.98   0.000     2.138666    2.292044
       _rcs2 |   .9783114   .0091116    -2.35   0.019     .9606151    .9963337
       _rcs3 |   1.065473   .0099565     6.79   0.000     1.046136    1.085167
       _rcs4 |   1.006942   .0023338     2.98   0.003     1.002378    1.011526
       _rcs5 |   1.000054   .0012291     0.04   0.965     .9976475    1.002465
       _cons |   .1118691   .0035897   -68.26   0.000     .1050502    .1191306
------------------------------------------------------------------------------

. range temptime 0 5 200
(27132 missing values generated)
. predict h_stpm2, hazard zeros timevar(temptime)
. estimates store stpm2
```

We have had to create our own dummy variables because, at the time of writing, `stpm2` did not allow factor variables. The HRs for the first two intervals are different from those we observed for the Cox model (1.76 versus 1.64 for zero to one year and 1.40 versus 1.47 for one to two years). Furthermore, the SEs are slightly lower for the RP model. This is the first time there has been any more than a negligible difference between the Cox model and an RP model. So why has this happened? The reason for the difference is that when we split the time scale for the Cox model and estimate an HR within each interval, this is equivalent to fitting three separate models, one for each interval. In the RP model, we are still estimating a smooth baseline hazard function, and thus there is some sharing of information across intervals. If we fit a separate RP model to each interval, then we restore the similarity of estimates between the two approaches. This is shown in the output below:

```
. qui stcox dep5int1-dep5int3
. estimates store cox
. range timevar1 0 1 200
(27132 missing values generated)
. range timevar2 1 2 200
(27132 missing values generated)
. range timevar3 2 5 200
(27132 missing values generated)
. forvalues i = 1/3 {
  2.          qui stpm2 dep5int`i´ if int`i´ == 1, df(5) scale(hazard)
  3.          estimates store stpm2_int`i´
  4.          predict h_int`i´ if int`i´ == 1, hazard zeros timevar(timevar`i´)
  5. }
```

```
. estimates table cox stpm2 stpm2_int1 stpm2_int2 stpm2_int3,
> equations(1) eform se(%6.4f) b(%6.4f) modelwidth(10)
> drop(dxb: xb0: _rcs1 _rcs2 _rcs3 _rcs4 _rcs5 _cons)
```

Variable	cox	stpm2	stpm2_int1	stpm2_int2	stpm2_int3
dep5int1	1.7602	1.6414	1.7603		
	0.1550	0.1346	0.1550		
dep5int2	1.3985	1.4728		1.3986	
	0.1044	0.1033		0.1044	
dep5int3	1.1360	1.1333			1.1360
	0.0619	0.0611			0.0619

legend: b/se

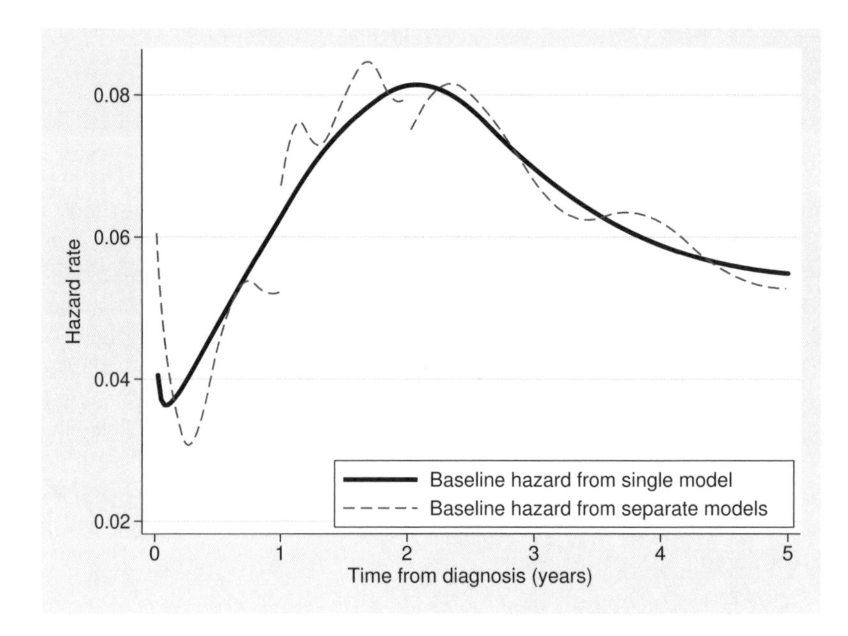

Figure 7.10. England and Wales breast cancer data. Estimated baseline hazard from an RP model with three piecewise HRs and from three separate models.

The estimates from the three separate RP models (**stpm2_int1**, **stpm2_int2**, and **stpm2_int3**) are virtually identical to those estimates from the Cox model. So do we really want to fit separate models to each interval? Generally, we would say no, and if we believe the underlying hazard rate to be smooth, then we should model it as such and use it to our advantage. Figure 7.10 shows the estimated baseline hazard function from the initial RP model together with those from the three separate RP models. To get the same estimates as we could get from a Cox model, we have to fit a discontinuous function that is clearly overfitted and has local turning points. We find the continuous function biologically much more plausible. However, if there are piecewise HRs, then although the baseline hazard is a smooth function, hazard functions for other covariate patterns will not be. This can be seen by plotting the predicted hazard function for each of the two deprivation groups, as is shown in figure 7.11. Although the baseline hazard (that is, for the least deprived group) is smooth and biologically plausible, the hazard rate for the most deprived group has jumps at the split point for the time intervals. Such jumps make no biological sense, so we generally prefer modeling TD HRs as smooth, continuous functions.

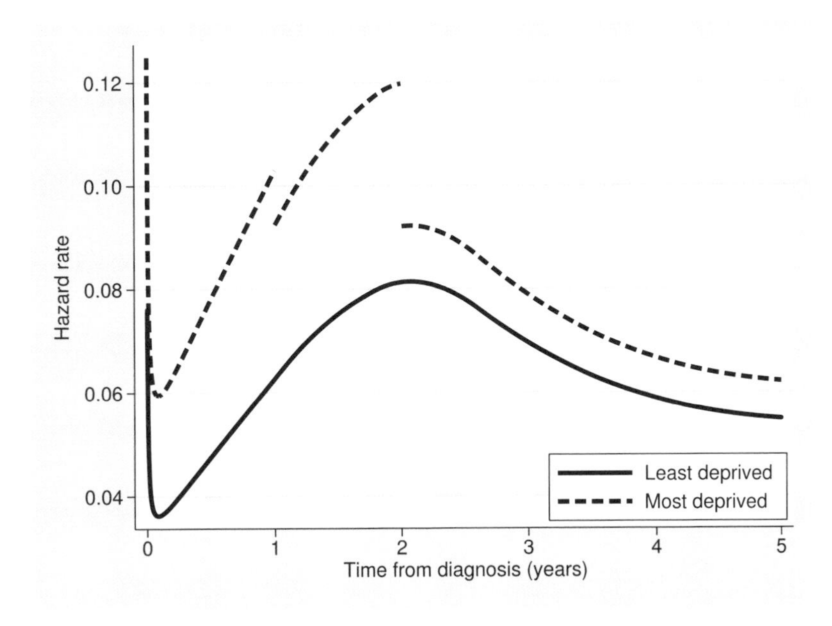

Figure 7.11. England and Wales breast cancer data. Estimated hazard rate from an RP model with piecewise HRs.

7.6.2 Continuous TD effects

When we used RP models in chapter 5, we assumed that the effects of covariates were constant over time. For example, in a model on the log cumulative-hazards scale, a PH model can be written as

$$\ln H(t|x) = \eta = s\left\{\ln(t)|\gamma, \mathbf{k}_0\right\} + \mathbf{x}\boldsymbol{\beta} \tag{7.1}$$

There is an assumption that the effect of each covariate does not depend on time. Royston and Parmar (2002) discussed that TD effects could be fit by including interactions between a covariate and the spline variables in $s\left\{\ln(t)|\gamma, \mathbf{k}_0\right\}$. In `stpm`, the first implementation of these models in Stata, the same number and location of knots were used for modeling a TD effect as for the baseline hazard. In situations where the shape of the baseline hazard was complex—requiring, for example, 6 knots—any TD effects also needed to use the same 6 knots. This tended to overfit the TD effects. Here we describe a more general approach in which there can be a different number of knots (in potentially different locations) for TD effects than for the baseline hazard. In nearly all situations, the number of knots for TD effects is lower than for the baseline hazard.

If there are D TD effects, then (7.1) can be extended by defining $\mathbf{k}_j$ to denote the knots for the jth TD effect with associated parameters, $\boldsymbol{\delta}_j$. The log cumulative hazard for such a model is

$$\ln\{H(t|\mathbf{x})\} = s\{\ln(t)|\boldsymbol{\gamma}, \mathbf{k}_0\} + \sum_{j=1}^{D} s\{\ln(t)|\boldsymbol{\delta}_j, \mathbf{k}_j\}\mathbf{x}_j + \mathbf{x}\boldsymbol{\beta}$$

In the original RP approach, $\mathbf{k}_j = \mathbf{k}_0$ for any TD effects, while in the above approach, $\mathbf{k}_j$ can vary between different TD effects. This approach is implemented by calculating different sets of spline variables—one set for the baseline hazard rate and one set for each of the TD effects. The use of smaller numbers of d.f. for the TD effects creates a more parsimonious and generally smoother model.

The default knot locations for TD effects in `stpm2` are the same as for the log cumulative baseline hazard shown in table 5.2. TD effects are implemented in `stpm2` using the `tvc()` and `dftvc()` options. We initially use 3 d.f. for the TD effect of deprivation (`dep5`) in the England and Wales breast cancer data, but we investigate alternatives later. The code is shown below:

```
. use ew_breast_ch7, clear
(England and Wales Breast Cancer: Age<=50: least and most deprived)
. stset survtime, failure(dead==1) exit(time 5) id(ident)
  (output omitted)
. stpm2 dep5, scale(hazard) df(5) tvc(dep5) dftvc(3) nolog
Log likelihood = -8751.4069                    Number of obs    =        9721

xb
          dep5     .3002045   .0400425     7.50   0.000     .2217227    .3786864
         _rcs1     .7910191   .0208548    37.93   0.000     .7501444    .8318938
         _rcs2    -.0303248   .0163107    -1.86   0.063    -.0622932    .0016436
         _rcs3     .0533709   .0076104     7.01   0.000     .0384548     .068287
         _rcs4     .0074656     .00348     2.15   0.032      .000645    .0142862
         _rcs5    -.0001605   .0016233    -0.10   0.921     -.003342     .003021
   _rcs_dep51    -.0970783   .0306738    -3.16   0.002     -.157198   -.0369587
   _rcs_dep52     .0196883   .0230925     0.85   0.394    -.0255721    .0649487
   _rcs_dep53     .0012431   .0098042     0.13   0.899    -.0179728    .0204591
         _cons    -1.480394   .0240537   -61.55   0.000    -1.527538    -1.43325
```

There are now 10 parameters estimated. The terms `_rcs1` through `_rcs5` are the spline variables for the baseline log cumulative hazard. These appear through use of the `df(5)` option. The terms `_rcs_dep51` through `_rcs_dep53` are the three spline variables associated with the TD effect of `dep5`, and they are included because of the `tvc(dep5)` and `dftvc(3)` options. The likelihood-ratio test comparing this model with a nonproportional hazards model (that is, without the tvc(dep5) and dftvc(3) options) gives $\chi^2_3 = 17.35$ and $P = 0.0006$, again giving strong evidence of a nonproportional effect for dep5. Each individual parameter is difficult to interpret, but we can make use of the predict command to obtain informative predictions. First, we estimate the cumulative hazard to demonstrate how this is now a nonproportional cumulative hazards model.

```
. range temptime 0.003 5 200
(9521 missing values generated)
. predict ch_dep0, cumhaz timevar(temptime) at(dep5 0)
(9521 missing values generated)
. predict ch_dep1, cumhaz timevar(temptime) at(dep5 1)
(9521 missing values generated)
```

We have used the at() option to obtain predictions at specified values of covariates. The cumulative hazard functions are shown in figure 7.12. The cumulative hazards (on the log scale) in the two groups get closer together as follow-up time increases. In a PH model, there would be a constant difference between the two lines (on the log scale).

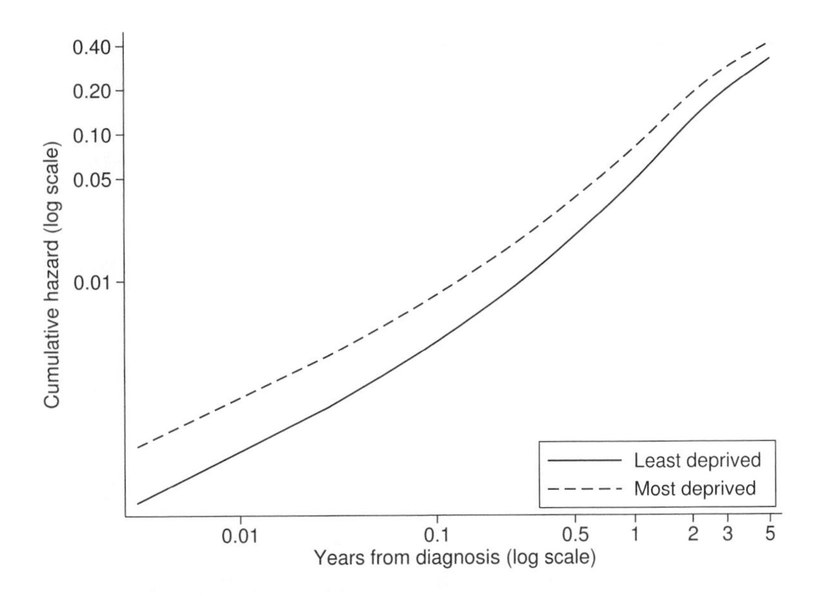

Figure 7.12. England and Wales breast cancer data. Estimated cumulative hazard from an RP model with a TD effect.

It is more useful to report hazard rates than cumulative hazards, and these hazard rates can be predicted in the same way as before:

```
. predict h_tvc_dep0, hazard timevar(temptime) at(dep5 0) per(1000)
. predict h_tvc_dep1, hazard timevar(temptime) at(dep5 1) per(1000)
```

The `per(1000)` option multiplies the predicted hazard rates by 1,000 to give the mortality rate per 1,000 person-years. The resulting hazard rates are plotted in figure 7.13, together with the estimated hazard rates from a PH model. Early on in the time scale, there is a greater difference between the hazard rate for the model with a TD effect compared with the PH model. Later on the difference is smaller, and in fact, the hazard rates for the two groups almost touch by five years of follow-up.

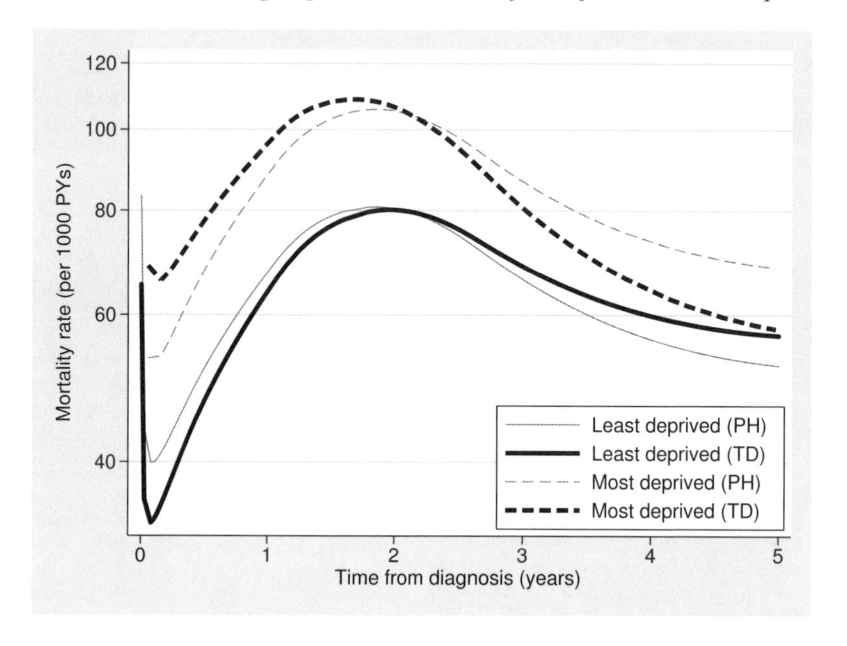

Figure 7.13. England and Wales breast cancer data. Estimated mortality rates from an RP model with TD effects. PYs stands for person-years.

As the time dependence is modeled on the log cumulative-hazard scale, it is a bit more complicated to obtain the SE (and thus the CI) for the HR. The log HR turns out to be a nonlinear function of the model parameters, and the delta method is used to obtain CIs. For a dichotomous covariate, x_1, the log HR at time t_0 can be written:

$$\ln(\text{HR}) = \ln\{s'(t_0|\gamma, \mathbf{k}_0) + s'(t_0|\boldsymbol{\delta}_1, \mathbf{k}_1)\} - \ln\{s'(t_0|\gamma, \boldsymbol{k}_0)\} + s(t_0|\boldsymbol{\delta}_1, \mathbf{k}_1) + \beta_1$$

The `predict` command performs these calculations by working out what formula needs to be given to `predictnl`. There is an issue when there is more than one factor with a TD effect because the TD effect of one covariate can depend on the value of another TD covariate. See section 7.6.3 for a discussion of this issue. The following code predicts the HR together with a 95% CI:

```
. predict hr, hrnum(dep5 1) hrdenom(dep5 0) timevar(temptime) ci
```

We have included the `hrdenominator()` (abbreviated `hrdenom()`) option for illustration, although actually it is not needed here because `predict` sets all covariate values to zero by default. Figure 7.14 shows the resulting HR with 95% CI. As we have seen with previous analyses and the Schoenfeld residuals in figure 7.2, the HR approaches 1 as follow-up time increases. Figure 7.14 is similar to figure 7.3, where a Cox model with a TD effect of $\ln(t)$ was fit for `dep5`.

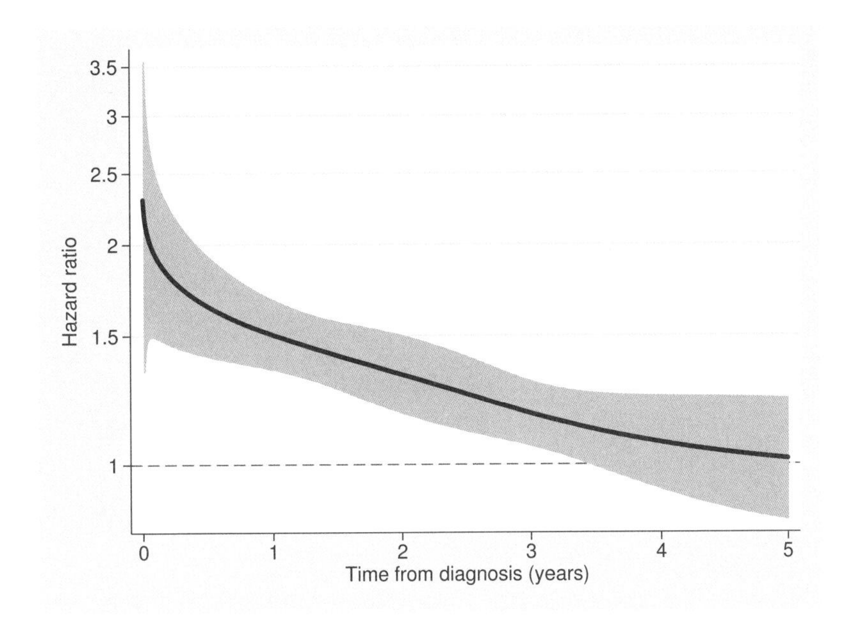

Figure 7.14. England and Wales breast cancer data. Estimated HR and 95% CI from an RP model with TD effect for deprivation group.

One of the advantages of the parametric approach is that various other functions of model parameters can be used to obtain useful predictions. If we are concerned with the impact of a covariate in a population, it is sensible to consider absolute levels of risk. If the underlying risk of the event is very low, then even a large HR has little impact in population terms. An alternative way to quantify the difference between two groups is to investigate the difference in hazard rates. To calculate a SE and hence a CI, the delta method is again used. The difference in hazard rates can be obtained using the `hdiff1()` and `hdiff2()` options of the `predict` command, which work in a similar way to `hrnumerator()` and `hrdenominator()`. This command is shown below:

```
. predict hdiff, hdiff1(dep5 1) hdiff2(dep5 0) timevar(temptime) ci per(1000)
```

The `per(1000)` option multiplies the predicted hazard rates by 1,000 to give the difference in the mortality rate per 1,000 person-years. The difference in hazard rates with a 95% CI is shown in figure 7.15. There is a large difference very early in the time scale, but for most of the first 1.5 years, the difference in hazard rates is fairly constant at just over 30 extra deaths per 1,000 person-years in the most deprived group compared with the least deprived group. The difference decreases to close to zero by four years, which is to be expected because an HR close to 1, as seen in figure 7.14, implies a hazard difference close to zero.

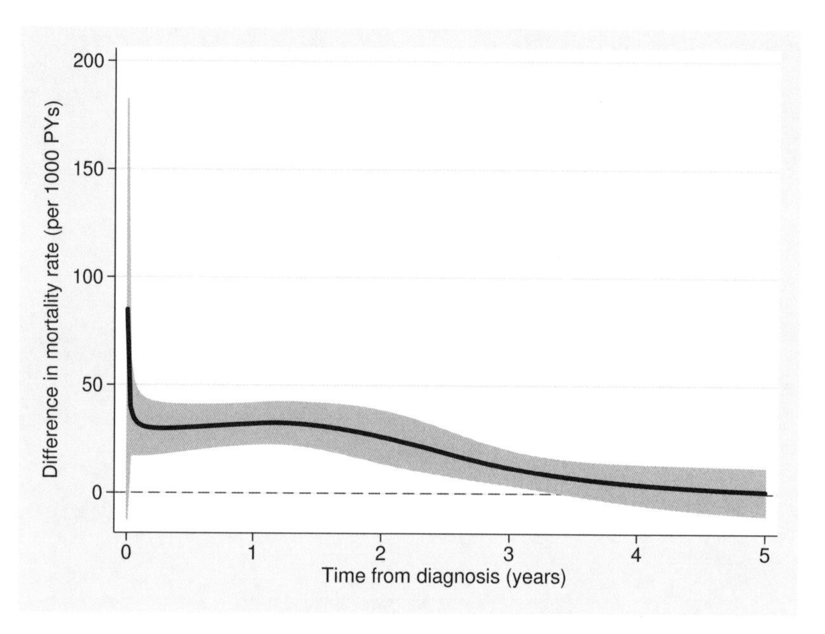

Figure 7.15. England and Wales breast cancer data. Estimated difference in mortality rates from an RP model with a TD effect for deprivation group. PYs stands for person-years.

An alternative measure to quantify differences between two groups is the difference in survival curves (Altman and Andersen 1999), which gives, as a function of follow-up time, the difference in the probability of being alive. Calculation of CIs again makes use of the delta method. Calculation of the survival difference is implemented using the `sdiff1()` and `sdiff2()` options of the `predict` command. First, the survival function in each group is estimated:

```
. predict s0, survival timevar(temptime) at(dep5 0)
. predict s1, survival timevar(temptime) at(dep5 1)
```

These estimates are plotted in figure 7.16 and show a similar pattern to the one previously observed for the Kaplan–Meier curves in figure 7.1.

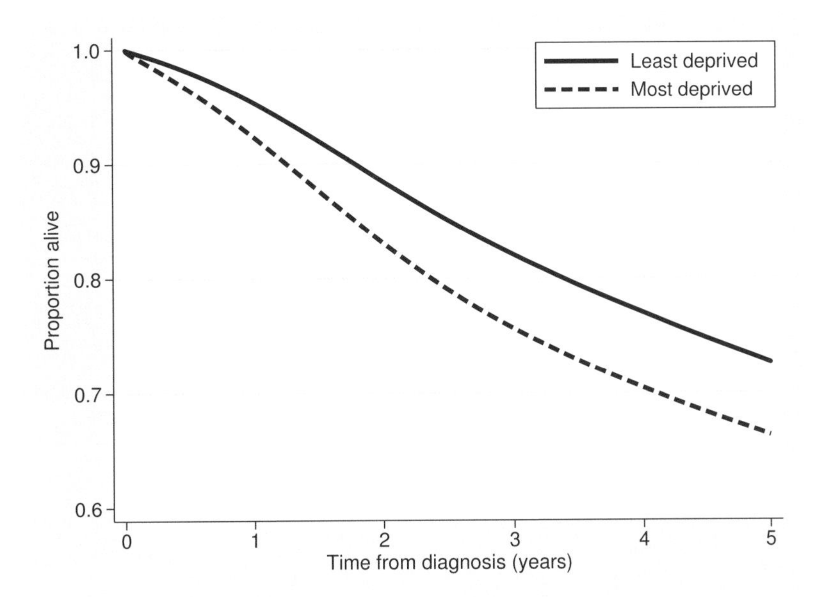

Figure 7.16. England and Wales breast cancer data. Estimated survival curves from an RP model with TD effect for deprivation group.

The difference in these two survival curves with a 95% CI is calculated as follows:

```
. predict sdiff, sdiff1(dep5 1) sdiff2(dep5 0) timevar(temptime) ci
```

The corresponding graph is shown in figure 7.17, which shows that the difference increases until just after two years postdiagnosis, where it appears to stabilize at an absolute difference of just over 6%.

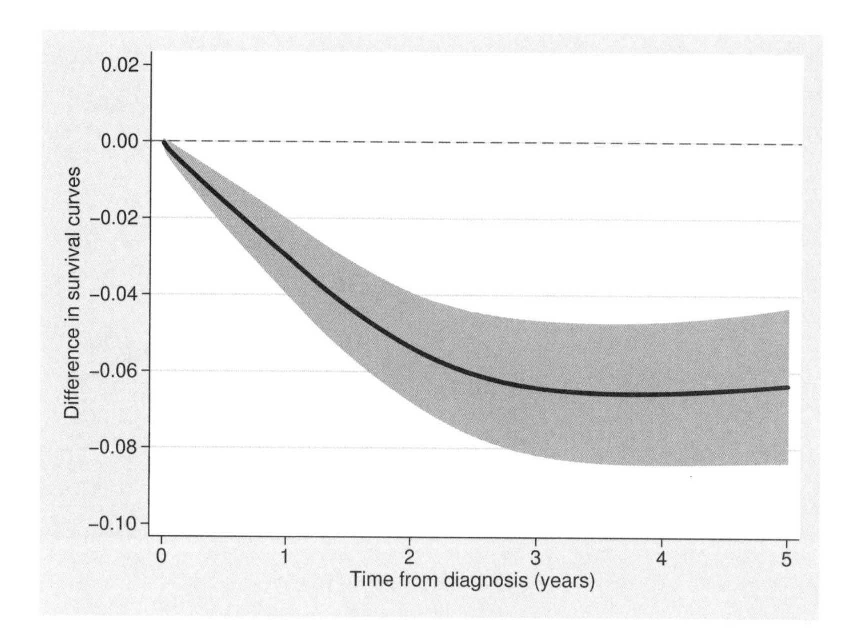

Figure 7.17. England and Wales breast cancer data. Estimated survival difference with 95% CI from an RP model with a TD effect for deprivation group.

In clinical trials, a popular message to communicate the result of trials is the number needed to treat (NNT). In studies with a time-to-event outcome, the NNT changes as a function of follow-up time and can be calculated as the reciprocal of the difference in survival curves (Altman and Andersen 1999). See section 9.2 for more discussion of estimating the NNT using RP models.

All the predictions above come from a model with 3 d.f. for the TD effect. We can use the AIC or BIC to compare the model with varying number of knots for the TD effect. We can do this in a loop as follows:

```
forvalues i = 1/5 {
     stpm2 dep5, scale(hazard) df(5) tvc(dep5) dftvc(`i´)
     estimates store df`i´
     predict hr`i´, hrnum(dep5 1) timevar(timevar) ci
}
```

The above code allows between 1 d.f. and 5 d.f. for the TD effect. The baseline has 5 d.f. Recall that 1 d.f. corresponds to the TD effect being a linear function of $\ln(t)$. The predicted HRs and the AIC and BIC for each model are shown in figure 7.18, exhibiting broadly similar estimates of the TD HR. There is some evidence of overfitting for 5 d.f., with local maxima and minima. The lowest AIC and BIC are for the model with 1 d.f.; that is, the TD effect on the log cumulative-hazard scale is a linear function of $\ln(t)$.

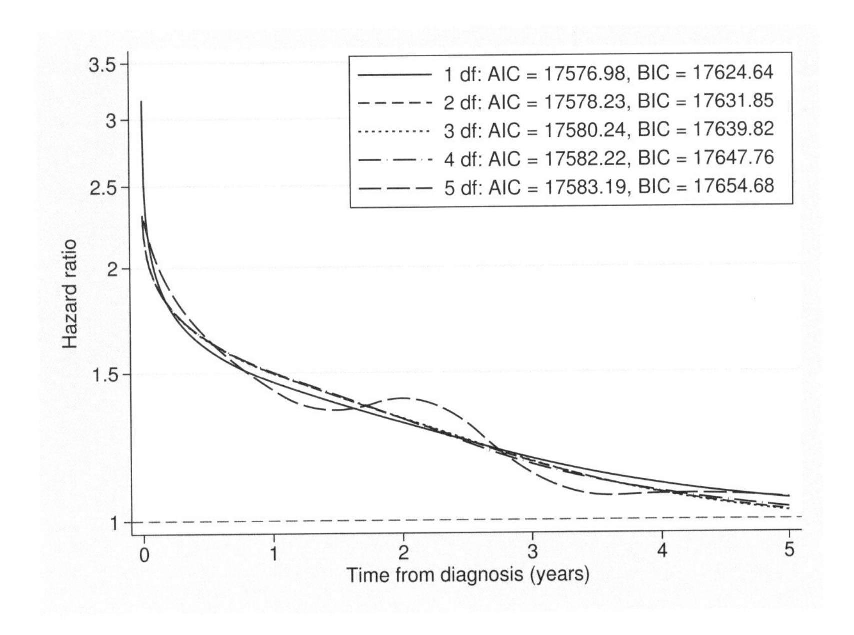

Figure 7.18. England and Wales breast cancer data. Comparison of TD HRs for models with 5 d.f. for baseline.

7.6.3 More than one TD effect

A disadvantage of modeling on the log cumulative-hazard scale compared with the more standard log-hazard scale is that when there are two variables with TD effects, the HR for the first variable can depend on the level of the second variable. We demonstrate this by adding year of diagnosis to the model as a binary covariate, `yr8990`, with 1 denoting 1989–1990 and 0 denoting 1986–1988. This is shown below:

```
. generate byte yr8990 = year(datediag)>=1989
. stpm2 dep5 yr8990, scale(hazard) df(5) nolog tvc(dep5 yr8990) dftvc(3)
Log likelihood = -8747.2862                     Number of obs   =       9721

------------------------------------------------------------------------------
             |      Coef.   Std. Err.      z    P>|z|     [95% Conf. Interval]
-------------+----------------------------------------------------------------
xb           |
        dep5 |   .3013247   .0400411     7.53   0.000     .2228455    .3798039
      yr8990 |   -.076046   .0391812    -1.94   0.052    -.1528397    .0007478
       _rcs1 |   .7649538   .0231769    33.00   0.000     .7195279    .8103797
       _rcs2 |  -.0331247   .0173594    -1.91   0.056    -.0671486    .0008992
       _rcs3 |   .0519867   .0082261     6.32   0.000     .0358638    .0681096
       _rcs4 |   .0075426   .0036779     2.05   0.040     .0003341    .0147511
       _rcs5 |  -.0001628   .0016217    -0.10   0.920    -.0033412    .0030156
  _rcs_dep51 |  -.0999033    .030603    -3.26   0.001     -.159884   -.0399225
  _rcs_dep52 |   .0193171   .0228974     0.84   0.399     -.025561    .0641951
  _rcs_dep53 |   .0015211   .0097798     0.16   0.876    -.0176469    .0206891
_rcs_yr89901 |   .0776693   .0333092     2.33   0.020     .0123845    .1429541
_rcs_yr89902 |   .0180702     .02703     0.67   0.504    -.0349077     .071048
_rcs_yr89903 |   .0007674   .0101983     0.08   0.940    -.0192208    .0207556
       _cons |  -1.450495   .0287376   -50.47   0.000     -1.50682    -1.39417
------------------------------------------------------------------------------

. predict hr_dep5_early, timevar(temptime)
> hrnum(dep5 1 yr8990 0) hrdenom(dep5 0 yr8990 0) ci
. predict hr_dep5_late, timevar(temptime)
> hrnum(dep5 1 yr8990 1) hrdenom(dep5 0 yr8990 1) ci
```

Both `dep5` and `yr8990` are considered TD because they are included in the `tvc()` option. Note the use of the `hrnum()` and `hrdenom()` options to obtain the HR for `dep5` at each of the two levels of `yr8990`. The predicted HRs are plotted in figure 7.19. The HR and its 95% CI, for deprivation group has been calculated at both levels of `yr8990`. Although there is close agreement between the two HRs, they are not identical, as they would be when modeling on the log-hazard scale. However, the estimates are very similar and the same substantive conclusions would be drawn.

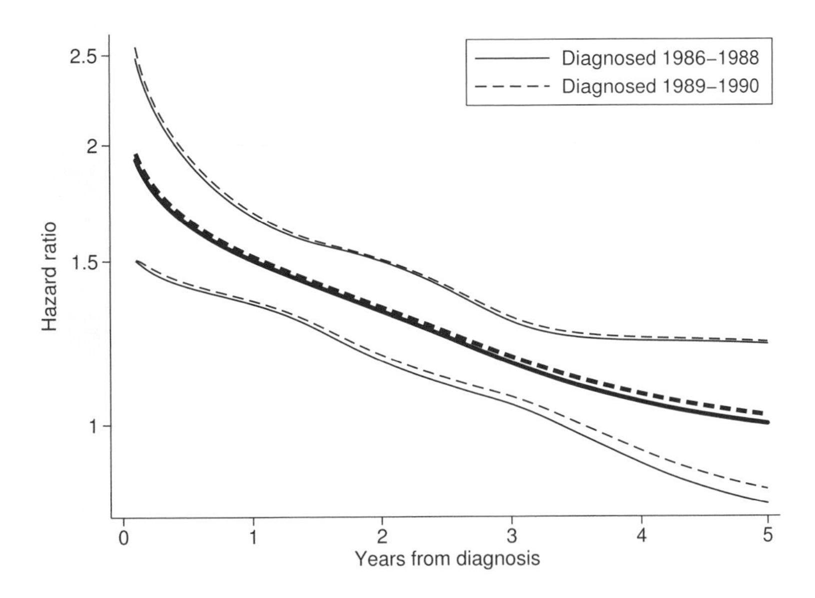

Figure 7.19. England and Wales breast cancer data. HR for deprivation group for those diagnosed in 1986–1988 and 1989–1990.

7.6.4 Stratification is the same as including TD effects

With Cox models, one way of dealing with nonproportional effects for categorical covariates that are not of direct interest is to stratify by them. In a stratified model, the baseline hazard function is assumed to be different at each level of the stratification factor. In such models, the covariate of interest is usually assumed to have PH within each of the strata. Such an approach is sometimes used in multicenter clinical trials where the shape of the baseline hazard may vary between centers, but the treatment effect is taken to be the same within each center. In addition, the treatment effect is assumed to be constant over time; that is, PH is assumed within each center (Harrell 2001).

There are nine recorded regions of England and Wales in the breast cancer data. A Cox model and an RP model for the effect of `dep5`, stratified by region, are fit in the output below:

```
. stcox dep5, strata(region) nolog noshow
Stratified Cox regr. -- Breslow method for ties
No. of subjects =         9721                  Number of obs   =       9721
No. of failures =         2847
Time at risk    =    40919.284
                                                LR chi2(1)      =      41.54
Log likelihood  =    -19509.71                  Prob > chi2     =     0.0000

          _t   Haz. Ratio   Std. Err.      z    P>|z|     [95% Conf. Interval]

        dep5     1.307217    .0537468     6.52   0.000     1.206008     1.41692

                                                             Stratified by region
. xi: stpm2 dep5 i.region, scale(hazard) df(5) nolog tvc(i.region)
> dftvc(5) eform
i.region          _Iregion_1-9        (naturally coded; _Iregion_1 omitted)
Log likelihood = -8722.411                     Number of obs   =       9721

                   exp(b)   Std. Err.      z    P>|z|     [95% Conf. Interval]

xb
        dep5     1.307149    .0537432     6.51   0.000     1.205947    1.416844
  (output omitted)
```

The estimates for dep5 are very similar. In the RP model, 5 d.f. are used for all the nine regions. It would be possible to use fewer d.f. for the TD effect, but doing so is unlikely to alter the estimates. Figure 7.20 shows the estimated baseline hazard rates for each region. With the exception of one region (Wales) these show broadly similar shapes. In the Cox model, the baseline hazards are not directly estimated.

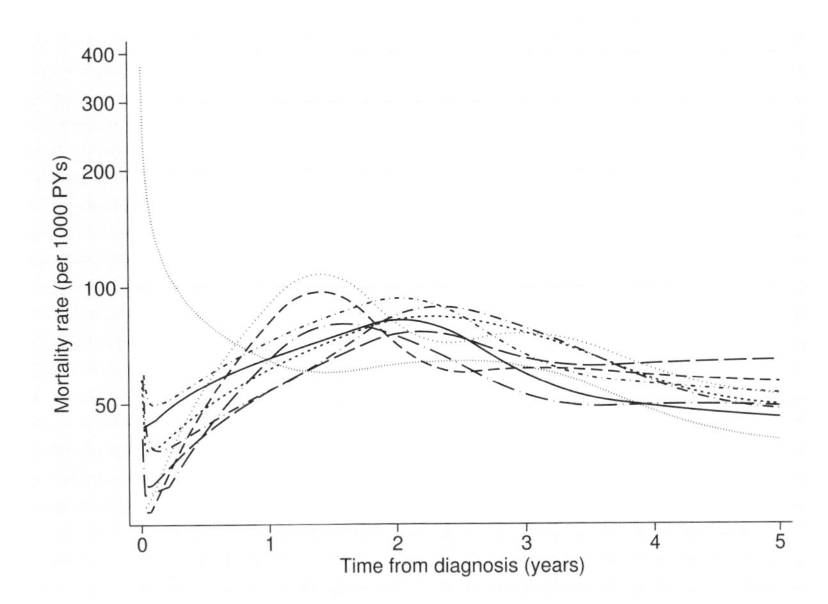

Figure 7.20. England and Wales breast cancer data. Baseline hazards for each region from model with TD effect for region—that is, a stratified model. PYs stands for person-years.

7.7 TD effects for continuous variables

There are many reasons to keep continuous covariates continuous, as opposed to converting them to categories (categorization). If the effect of a covariate is nonlinear, then various alternatives, such as splines or FPs, exist to model the nonlinear relationship. However, what if the potentially nonlinear effect of a covariate is itself TD? To illustrate the issues, we fit the effect of age to the breast cancer data. All 24,889 women aged under 50 are analyzed and the effect of deprivation group is ignored. To model the effect of age, we use restricted cubic splines with 5 knots (2 boundary and 3 interior), giving 4 d.f. The splines are generated below, followed by fitting a PH model:

```
. use ew_breast_alldep_ch7, clear
(England and Wales Breast Cancer: Age<=50: All deprivation groups)
. stset survtime, failure(dead==1) exit(time 5) id(ident)
                id:  ident
     failure event:  dead == 1
obs. time interval:  (survtime[_n-1], survtime]
 exit on or before:  time 5

      24889  total obs.
          0  exclusions

      24889  obs. remaining, representing
      24889  subjects
       7366  failures in single failure-per-subject data
     104639  total analysis time at risk, at risk from t =         0
                                  earliest observed entry t =         0
                                       last observed exit t =         5
. rcsgen agediag, df(4) gen(agercs) orthog
Variables agercs1 to agercs4 were created
. global ageknots `r(knots)'
. matrix R=r(R)
. stpm2 agercs1-agercs4, scale(hazard) df(5) nolog
Log likelihood = -22468.579                     Number of obs   =      24889

             |      Coef.   Std. Err.      z    P>|z|     [95% Conf. Interval]
-------------+----------------------------------------------------------------
xb           |
     agercs1 |  -.1019283   .0110129    -9.26   0.000    -.1235133   -.0803434
     agercs2 |  -.0492079   .0109589    -4.49   0.000     -.070687   -.0277288
     agercs3 |  -.0599475   .0113939    -5.26   0.000    -.0822793   -.0376158
     agercs4 |   .0072852    .011778     0.62   0.536    -.0157993    .0303697
       _rcs1 |   .7552168   .0095756    78.87   0.000     .7364489    .7739846
       _rcs2 |  -.0191509   .0075445    -2.54   0.011    -.0339379   -.0043639
       _rcs3 |   .0556031   .0041392    13.43   0.000     .0474905    .0637158
       _rcs4 |   .0053724   .0020786     2.58   0.010     .0012984    .0094463
       _rcs5 |   .0022085   .0010198     2.17   0.030     .0002098    .0042073
       _cons |  -1.376082   .0120139  -114.54   0.000    -1.399629   -1.352535
```

Notice that now we are modeling the effect of age with one spline function (in age) and the baseline log cumulative-hazard function with a different spline function (in log time). The knot locations created by `rcsgen` are stored in the return list macro, `r(knots)`, which is saved for future use. In addition, the **R** matrix is returned. The **R** matrix transforms the orthogonalized splines back to their untransformed form. It is needed for some predictions below. The PH model assumes that the effect of age is the same throughout the time scale, but it is difficult from simple investigation of the model parameters to know what the effect of age actually is. To quantify the effect of age, it is useful to define a reference age. Here age 45 is chosen as the reference and all other ages are compared with this reference. To obtain an HR as a function of age, we need to know the values of the spline variables at the reference age. The following code generates these values and uses them in the `predict` command to get the HR as a function of age, with age 45 as the reference.

```
. generate refage = 45 in 1
(24888 missing values generated)
. rcsgen refage in 1, knots($ageknots) gen(ragercs) rmatrix(R)
(24888 missing values generated)
Variables ragercs1 to ragercs4 were created
. local c1 = ragercs1[1]
. local c2 = ragercs2[1]
. local c3 = ragercs3[1]
. local c4 = ragercs4[1]
. predict hr, hrnumerator(agercs1 . agercs2 . agercs3 . agercs4 .)
> hrdenominator(agercs1 `c1´ agercs2 `c2´ agercs3 `c3´ agercs4 `c4´) ci
```

We first calculate the reference age in `refage` with only a single observation. We obtain the values of the spline variables at the reference age using the previously saved knots and R matrix. Doing so is important because the orthogonalization is data-dependent, but the values of the spline variables that correspond to the original calculation are needed. The values of the spline variables at the reference age are then stored in local macros `c1`–`c4`. The periods (.) in the `hrnumerator()` option indicate that we want the HR calculated at the values of the spline variables in the dataset. We want to compare each of these values with the reference, so we use the local macros `c1`–`c4` in the `hrdenominator()` option. A plot of this function is provided in figure 7.21. It shows an increase in risk for both younger and older women compared with those aged 45. However, because this is a PH model, the relative effect at each age compared with age 45 is assumed to be the same throughout follow-up. Note the zero variance of the curve at the reference age of 45.

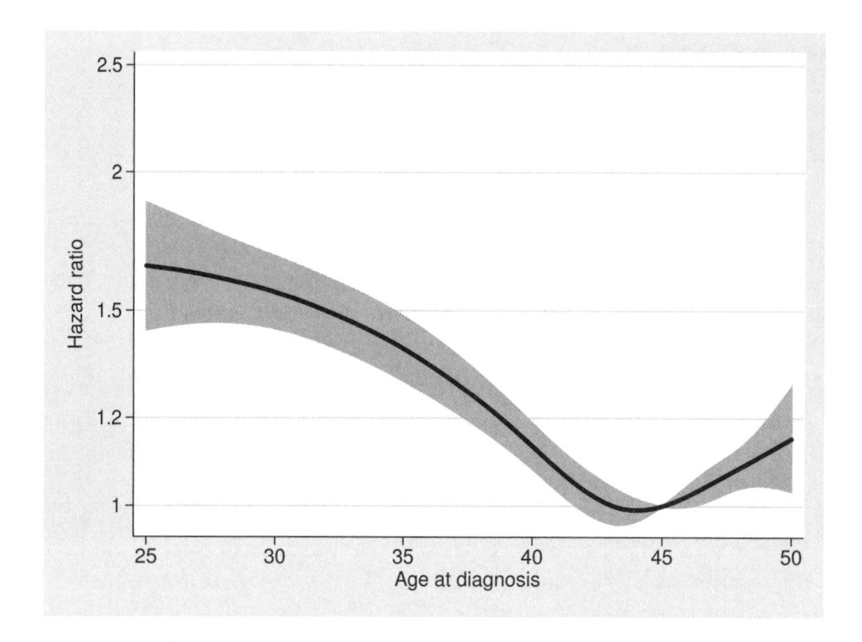

Figure 7.21. England and Wales breast cancer data. HR as a function of age with age 45 as the reference value from an RP model.

The model can be extended to a nonproportional hazards model by allowing the coefficients of the spline parameters to vary as a function of follow-up time. This can be done as before by using the `tvc()` and `dftvc()` options.

```
. stpm2 agercs1-agercs4, scale(hazard) df(5) nolog tvc(agercs1-agercs4) dftvc(4)
Log likelihood = -22445.963                     Number of obs   =      24889

------------------------------------------------------------------------------
             |      Coef.   Std. Err.      z    P>|z|     [95% Conf. Interval]
-------------+----------------------------------------------------------------
xb           |
     agercs1 |  -.0958559   .0112515    -8.52   0.000    -.1179085   -.0738033
     agercs2 |  -.0582562   .0111786    -5.21   0.000    -.0801658   -.0363465
     agercs3 |  -.0536617   .0116593    -4.60   0.000    -.0765135   -.0308099
     agercs4 |    .008645   .0120711     0.72   0.474     -.015014    .0323039
       _rcs1 |   .7577448   .0096917    78.18   0.000     .7387494    .7767403
       _rcs2 |  -.0174274   .0076327    -2.28   0.022    -.0323872   -.0024675
       _rcs3 |   .0549198   .0041716    13.17   0.000     .0467436    .0630959
       _rcs4 |   .0054832    .002083     2.63   0.008     .0014007    .0095658
       _rcs5 |   .0023477   .0010224     2.30   0.022     .0003439    .0043516
_rcs_ager~11 |  -.0166192   .0090008    -1.85   0.065    -.0342605    .0010222
_rcs_ager~12 |   .0059569   .0073908     0.81   0.420    -.0085287    .0204425
_rcs_ager~13 |  -.0123183    .003529    -3.49   0.000    -.0192349   -.0054017
_rcs_ager~14 |   .0018654   .0014735     1.27   0.206    -.0010225    .0047533
_rcs_ager~21 |   .0257508    .008268     3.11   0.002     .0095458    .0419557
_rcs_ager~22 |  -.0152562   .0065876    -2.32   0.021    -.0281676   -.0023449
_rcs_ager~23 |   .0065558   .0033904     1.93   0.053    -.0000894    .0132009
_rcs_ager~24 |  -.0000733   .0014854    -0.05   0.961    -.0029846    .0028379
_rcs_ager~31 |  -.0253429   .0089261    -2.84   0.005    -.0428377    -.007848
_rcs_ager~32 |  -.0062537   .0071319    -0.88   0.381     -.020232    .0077245
_rcs_ager~33 |  -.0067089   .0036454    -1.84   0.066    -.0138538     .000436
_rcs_ager~34 |   .0023423   .0015786     1.48   0.138    -.0007517    .0054363
_rcs_ager~41 |  -.0034147   .0093865    -0.36   0.716     -.021812    .0149826
_rcs_ager~42 |  -.0007353   .0074937    -0.10   0.922    -.0154226     .013952
_rcs_ager~43 |   .0021679   .0037778     0.57   0.566    -.0052365    .0095723
_rcs_ager~44 |   -.000946   .0015948    -0.59   0.553    -.0040717    .0021797
       _cons |  -1.376872   .0120255  -114.50   0.000    -1.400442   -1.353303
------------------------------------------------------------------------------
```

There are an additional $4 \times 3 = 12$ parameters when compared with the PH model. There are 3 restricted cubic-spline variables for follow-up time for each of the 4 spline variables for age. Individual parameters are almost impossible to interpret, and so we use the `predict` command again, together with looping over the ages of interest—that is, 25, 35, 40, and 50. Again we use age 45 as the reference age.

```
range temptime 0.003 5 200
foreach age in 25 35 40 50 {
     gen agetmp = `age´ in 1
     rcsgen agetmp in 1, knots($ageknots) gen(tmprcs) rmatrix(R)
     local b1 = tmprcs1[1]
     local b2 = tmprcs2[1]
     local b3 = tmprcs3[1]
     local b4 = tmprcs4[1]
     predict hr`age´,                                                        ///
          hrnumerator(agercs1 `b1´ agercs2 `b2´ agercs3 `b3´ agercs4 `b4´)   ///
          hrdenominator(agercs1 `c1´ agercs2 `c2´  agercs3 `c3´ agercs4 `c4´) ///
          timevar(temptime) ci
     predict s`age´,                                                         ///
          survival at(agercs1 `b1´ agercs2 `b2´ agercs3 `b3´ agercs4 `b4´)   ///
          timevar(temptime)
     drop agetmp tmprcs*
}
```

A plot of the four generated graphs can be seen in figure 7.22. The shape of the curves is broadly similar for women aged 35, 40, and 50, but for those aged 25 there is a noticeable difference with a higher initial HR.

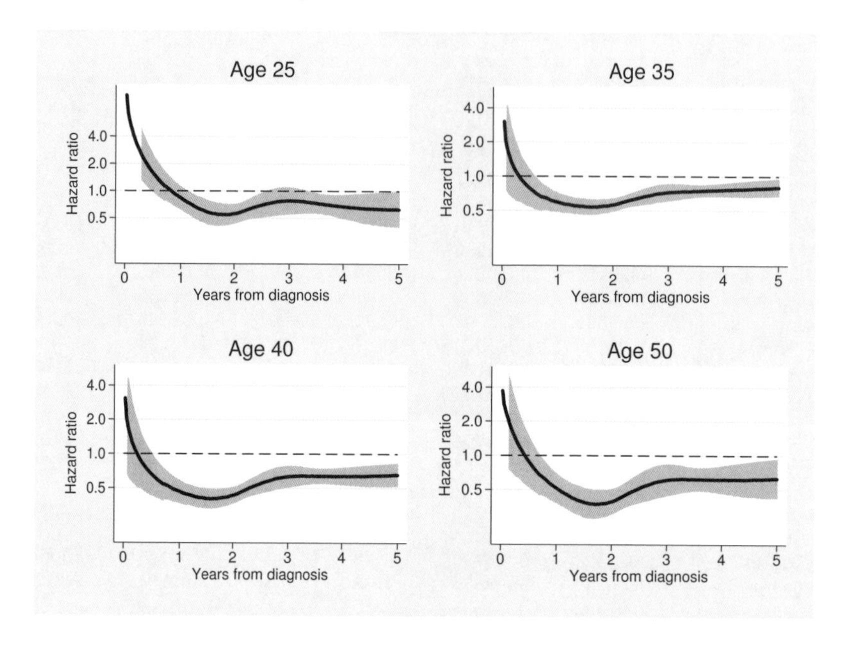

Figure 7.22. England and Wales breast cancer data. Estimated HRs from an RP model with age 45 as the reference age for four selected ages.

An alternative way to present the data is in tabular form, as shown in table 7.1, where the HRs for each of the selected ages are shown at years one through five. This is essentially a subset of the information presented in figure 7.22.

Table 7.1. Hazard ratios with 95% CI at years one through five for selected ages with age 45 as the reference

Year	Age 25	Age 35	Age 40	Age 50
1	1.95 [1.57, 2.41]	1.38 [1.24, 1.54]	1.09 [1.01, 1.18]	1.21 [1.02, 1.44]
2	1.59 [1.28, 1.98]	1.60 [1.44, 1.78]	1.23 [1.14, 1.33]	1.12 [0.94, 1.34]
3	1.41 [1.03, 1.93]	1.31 [1.14, 1.50]	1.14 [1.04, 1.25]	1.11 [0.89, 1.37]
4	1.26 [0.94, 1.69]	1.42 [1.26, 1.61]	1.19 [1.09, 1.30]	1.15 [0.94, 1.41]
5	1.17 [0.75, 1.84]	1.49 [1.23, 1.80]	1.22 [1.07, 1.39]	1.18 [0.87, 1.59]

One of the perceived advantages of categorizing continuous variables is that it makes it easier to present and interpret the results. We believe that if care is taken with the presentation, either in tabular or graphical form, more information can be communicated.

This section has concentrated on using restricted cubic splines to model nonlinearity. An alternative would be to use FPs.

7.8 Attained age as the time scale

In most standard survival analyses, the time scale starts at time $t = 0$. For example, we are often interested in time from diagnosis of disease or time from randomization in a clinical trial. If an adjustment for the effect of age at recruitment is needed, it is usually included in the model, either as a series of dummy variables to denote age categories or as a continuous (often linear) function of age at baseline. In epidemiological cohort studies, subjects are followed up prospectively after being recruited into the study. Age is usually a very important confounder because for many diseases it is so strongly associated with incidence. There is increasing popularity in using attained age as the main time scale in these types of study as a better way of controlling for age, as opposed to including age at baseline as a covariate. See Korn, Graubard, and Midthune (1997), Cheung, Gao, and Khoo (2003), and Thiébaut and Bénichou (2004) for more details about the advantages of using attained age as the main time scale.

7.8.1 The orchiectomy data

The dataset we use to illustrate age as the time scale is a large study of men diagnosed with prostate cancer in Sweden, which was briefly described in section 3.4. The study compares incidence of hip fracture in 17,731 men diagnosed with prostate cancer treated with bilateral orchiectomy (removal of the testicles) with 43,230 men with prostate cancer not treated with bilateral orchiectomy and 362,354 male controls randomly selected from the general population (Dickman et al. 2004a). The outcome of interest was fracture of the neck of the femur. The risk of fracture is likely to vary by age, and thus age is used as the main time scale. In section 7.9, we also consider multiple time scales where we simultaneously model attained age and time from diagnosis of prostate cancer.

7.8.2 Proportional hazards model

To incorporate attained age as the time scale, we apply stset to variables stored in date format. The following variables are recorded:

enddate	date of hip fracture or censoring
startdate	date of recruitment (6 months postdiagnosis)
datebirth	date of birth
id	identification number
fracture	event indicator
exp2	indicator for men with prostate cancer without orchiectomy
exp3	indicator for men with prostate cancer with orchiectomy

With this information, we can stset the data:

```
. stset enddate, failure(fracture = 1) enter(startdate) origin(birthdate)
> id(id) scale(365.24) exit(time birthdate+100*365.24)

                id:  id
     failure event:  fracture == 1
obs. time interval:  (enddate[_n-1], enddate]
 enter on or after:  time startdate
 exit on or before:  time birthdate+100*365.24
    t for analysis:  (time-origin)/365.24
            origin:  time birthdate

------------------------------------------------------------------------------
   423312  total obs.
       14  obs. begin on or after exit
------------------------------------------------------------------------------
   423298  obs. remaining, representing
   423298  subjects
    11002  failures in single failure-per-subject data
  2120262  total analysis time at risk, at risk from t =         0
                             earliest observed entry t =  38.53357
                                  last observed exit t =       100
```

In Stata, dates are recorded in days. The scale(365.24) option converts the days to years. The age at entry is determined by subtracting the origin date from the entry date (that is, startdate − datebirth), and the age at the event or censoring is determined by enddate − datebirth. Through use of the exit() option, the maximum age is truncated at 100 years because of the very small number of individuals older than 100. This truncation has had the effect of removing 14 observations from the analysis because these men were diagnosed when they were over 100 years of age, and so they cannot contribute to the time at risk. Two covariates, exp2 and exp3, denote the prostate cancer patients without and with a bilateral orchiectomy, respectively. Thus the population controls form the reference group. A PH model can be fit as follows:

```
. stpm2 exp2 exp3, df(5) scale(hazard) eform nolog
note: delayed entry models are being fitted
Log likelihood = -16476.437                     Number of obs   =     423298

------------------------------------------------------------------------------
             |     exp(b)   Std. Err.      z    P>|z|     [95% Conf. Interval]
-------------+----------------------------------------------------------------
xb           |
        exp2 |   1.366154   .0472293     9.02   0.000     1.276652    1.461929
        exp3 |   2.098076   .0880827    17.65   0.000     1.932349    2.278017
       _rcs1 |   2.343558   .1670524    11.95   0.000     2.037984     2.69495
       _rcs2 |    .882192   .0237304    -4.66   0.000     .8368861    .9299506
       _rcs3 |   1.027474   .0052656     5.29   0.000     1.017205    1.037846
       _rcs4 |   1.003319   .0027064     1.23   0.219     .9980288    1.008638
       _rcs5 |   1.003879    .001723     2.26   0.024     1.000508    1.007262
       _cons |   .0417206   .0032904   -40.28   0.000     .0357452    .0486948
------------------------------------------------------------------------------

. estimates store ph
```

Because we are modeling the incidence of hip fracture, we can interpret the covariate effects as (log) incidence-rate ratios (IRRs). The results of this model indicate that prostate cancer patients who are not treated with bilateral orchiectomy have an incidence rate of hip fracture 37% higher than the control group, while the incidence rate for those treated with bilateral orchiectomy is over twice that of the control group. We can predict the incidence rates using the following:

```
. summarize _t, meanonly
. range temptime `r(min)´ `r(max)´ 500
(422812 missing values generated)
. predict h1, h timevar(temptime) zeros per(1000)
. predict h2, h timevar(temptime) at(exp2 1 exp3 0) per(1000)
. predict h3, h timevar(temptime) at(exp2 0 exp3 1) per(1000)
```

Because there are over 400,000 observations in the dataset, a new variable with 500 observations, `temptime`, has been created with the same range as `_t`. The predicted hazard rates have been multiplied by 1,000 (using the `per(1000)` option) to give the age-specific incidence rates per 1,000 person-years. A plot of the hazard rates can be seen in figure 7.23. The large increase in incidence as age increases is clear. For the youngest men, the incidence of hip fracture is less than 1 event per 1,000 person-years, whereas for the oldest men it is almost 75 events per 1,000 person-years in prostate cancer patients treated with bilateral orchiectomy.

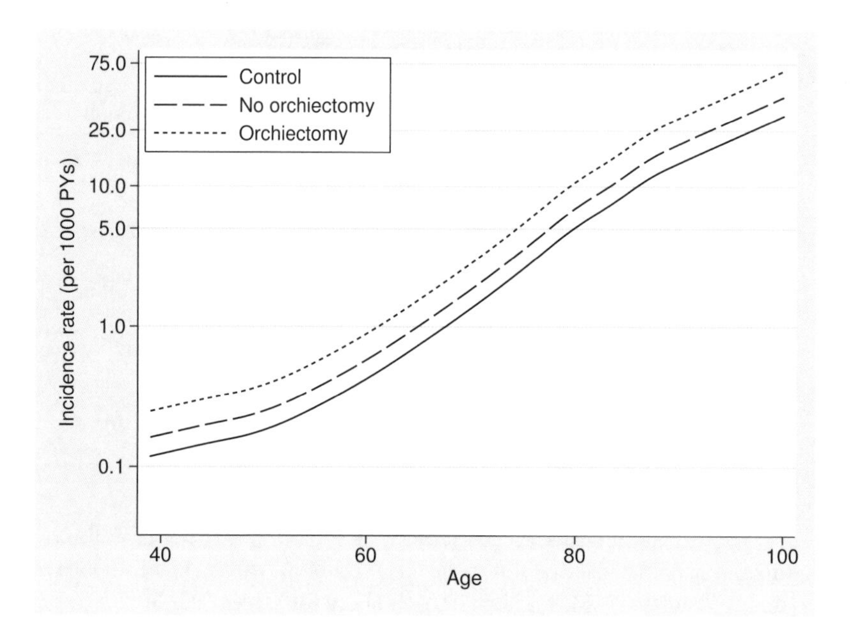

Figure 7.23. Orchiectomy data. Age-specific incidence rates for hip fracture for men diagnosed with prostate cancer in Sweden from a PH model. PYs stands for person-years.

7.8.3 TD model

The model in the previous section assumes that the relative increase in the incidence rate is the same for all ages—that is, the hazards are proportional. This may be too strict an assumption. We can fit a nonproportional hazards model in the same way as before—that is, by specifying the `tvc()` and `dftvc()` options:

```
. stpm2 exp2 exp3, df(5) scale(hazard) tvc(exp2 exp3) dftvc(3) nolog
note: delayed entry models are being fitted
Log likelihood = -16442.896                    Number of obs   =     423298

------------------------------------------------------------------------------
             |      Coef.   Std. Err.      z    P>|z|     [95% Conf. Interval]
-------------+----------------------------------------------------------------
xb           |
        exp2 |   .4309167   .1194747     3.61   0.000     .1967506    .6650827
        exp3 |   1.376789   .2482991     5.54   0.000      .890132    1.863447
       _rcs1 |   .7810457   .0407606    19.16   0.000     .7011565    .8609349
       _rcs2 |  -.1676213   .0083716   -20.02   0.000    -.1840294   -.1512133
       _rcs3 |   .0297331    .006193     4.80   0.000      .017595    .0418712
       _rcs4 |   .0063803   .0025485     2.50   0.012     .0013854    .0113753
       _rcs5 |   .0032496   .0016572     1.96   0.050     1.56e-06    .0064977
  _rcs_exp21 |  -.0519804   .0851685    -0.61   0.542    -.2189077    .1149469
  _rcs_exp22 |   .0580354   .0239236     2.43   0.015      .011146    .1049249
  _rcs_exp23 |  -.0218126   .0122625    -1.78   0.075    -.0458466    .0022215
  _rcs_exp31 |  -.3101977   .1212204    -2.56   0.010    -.5477854    -.07261
  _rcs_exp32 |   .0930658   .0229677     4.05   0.000     .0480499    .1380818
  _rcs_exp33 |    -.05176   .0108191    -4.78   0.000    -.0729651   -.0305548
       _cons |  -3.112282   .0552941   -56.29   0.000    -3.220656   -3.003907
------------------------------------------------------------------------------

. estimates store tvc
```

This model contains six extra parameters because 3 d.f. were used for each of the two TD effects. A likelihood-ratio test is shown below:

```
. lrtest ph tvc
Likelihood-ratio test                                 LR chi2(6)  =     67.08
(Assumption: ph nested in tvc)                        Prob > chi2 =    0.0000
```

The test gives a highly significant result. However, given the large sample size, even a small departure from PH is likely to be statistically significant. The parameters are difficult to interpret on their own, but we can see the effect of modeling the nonproportional effect by calculating and plotting the incidence rates. The result is shown in figure 7.24, which indicates a greater difference (on the log scale) between the groups at younger ages. We would therefore expect a larger IRR for younger ages. The TD IRR is calculated as follows:

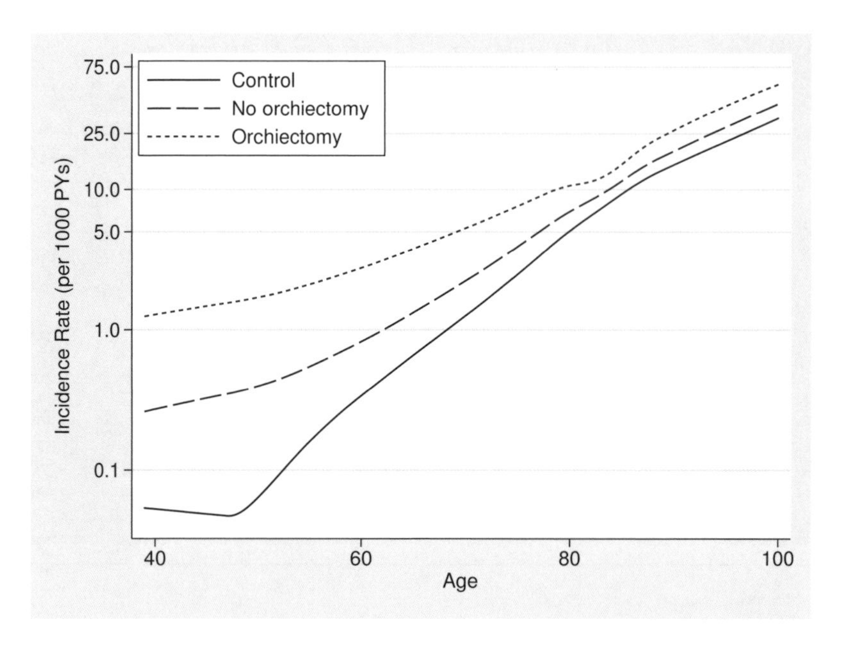

Figure 7.24. Orchiectomy data. Age-specific incidence rates for hip fracture for men diagnosed with prostate cancer in Sweden from a TD model. PYs stands for person-years.

```
. predict hr2, hrnum(exp2 1) ci timevar(temptime)
. predict hr3, hrnum(exp3 1) ci timevar(temptime)
```

The resulting estimates for the orchiectomy group are shown in figure 7.25. The age scale has been cut off at 50 because the width of the CIs distorts the figure if men aged less than 50 are included. There is over a 20-fold increase in risk for men aged 50. The IRR decreases with age until it stabilizes just below 85 years of age. However, even for those aged greater than 85, there is still almost a doubling of the IRR. The horizontal lines denote the estimates from a Poisson model with piecewise estimates of the baseline incidence and the IRR. The two approaches are in broad agreement, although the extremely high IRR in the youngest men is hidden in the categorized analysis.

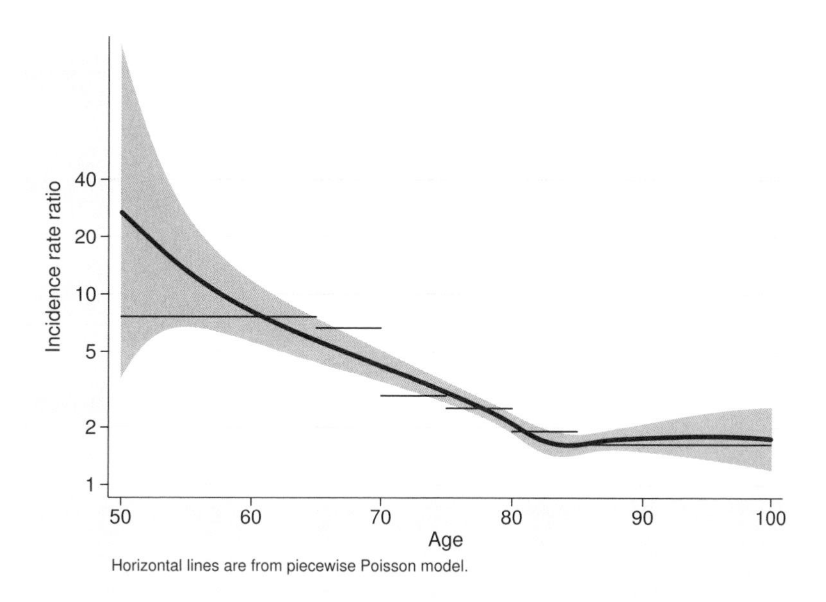

Figure 7.25. Orchiectomy data. Age-dependent IRR (orchiectomy group versus control) for hip fracture for men diagnosed with prostate cancer in Sweden from a TD model.

The underlying incidence rate is very dependent on age. As seen in figure 7.24, the incidence of hip fracture increases dramatically with age. The impact of the age-dependent IRR is difficult to fully understand without considering the absolute risks. The hazard differences can be considered by using the `hdiff1()` and `hdiff2()` options.

```
. predict hdiff2, hdiff1(exp2 1) ci timevar(temptime) per(1000)
. predict hdiff3, hdiff1(exp3 1) ci timevar(temptime) per(1000)
```

The hazard differences for the orchiectomy group are shown in figure 7.26. The `per(1000)` option has been used to obtain the difference in the incidence rate of hip fracture per 1,000 person-years. Although we saw in figure 7.25 that younger men have the largest relative increase in risk, this is actually less important in terms of the number of individuals affected. The difference in incidence rates at younger ages, where the relative increase is greatest, is lower than at older ages. This is due to the incidence rate being so low at younger ages.

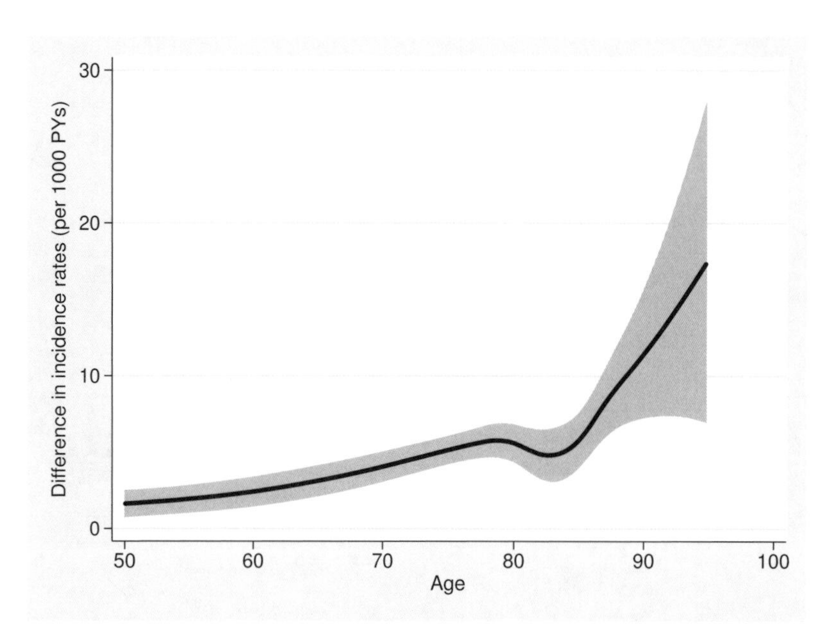

Figure 7.26. Orchiectomy data. Age-dependent incidence-rate differences (orchiectomy group − control) for hip fracture for men diagnosed with prostate cancer in Sweden from a TD model. PYs stands for person-years.

This example demonstrates an important aspect of the RP approach, namely the ease with which we can estimate absolute levels of risk as well as relative measures. One weakness of the Cox model is that it cannot directly estimate absolute measures of risk. As a result, researchers might neglect the potential impact of an HR on the population in terms of risk differences.

7.9 Multiple time scales

There are in fact two time scales of interest in the orchiectomy study. Not only is the age of the patient of interest, but also the time since orchiectomy. Multiple time scales are usually modeled using Poisson regression (Carstensen 2006). In `stpm2`, a second time scale can be modeled by applying `stsplit` and including dummy covariates for each time interval. Thus one time scale is modeled continuously and the other is modeled using categories, as shown in the output below, where follow-up time has been split into nine intervals.

```
. stsplit fu, at(1 2 3 4 5 7 10 15) after(startdate)
(1475689 observations (episodes) created)
. xi: stpm2 i.fu exp2 exp3, df(5) scale(hazard) nolog eform
i.fu              _Ifu_0-15           (naturally coded; _Ifu_0 omitted)
note: delayed entry models are being fitted
Log likelihood = -16475.755                     Number of obs   =    1898987
```

	exp(b)	Std. Err.	z	P>|z|	[95% Conf. Interval]	
xb						
_Ifu_1	1.023665	.0363249	0.66	0.510	.9548884	1.097394
_Ifu_2	1.00649	.0371512	0.18	0.861	.936247	1.082004
_Ifu_3	1.008599	.0387418	0.22	0.824	.9354543	1.087463
_Ifu_4	.9863619	.0398926	-0.34	0.734	.9111926	1.067732
_Ifu_5	.9995298	.0353706	-0.01	0.989	.9325541	1.071316
_Ifu_7	1.005216	.0361301	0.14	0.885	.9368388	1.078583
_Ifu_10	1.008974	.0407266	0.22	0.825	.9322268	1.092039
_Ifu_15	.967987	.0629761	-0.50	0.617	.8521015	1.099633
exp2	1.365013	.0473074	8.98	0.000	1.275372	1.460956
exp3	2.095076	.0883953	17.53	0.000	1.928795	2.275693
_rcs1	2.313684	.1901324	10.21	0.000	1.969494	2.718026
_rcs2	.8731451	.0237405	-4.99	0.000	.8278326	.9209378
_rcs3	1.023755	.0050971	4.72	0.000	1.013813	1.033794
_rcs4	1.002019	.0023897	0.85	0.398	.997346	1.006713
_rcs5	1.003068	.0013672	2.25	0.025	1.000392	1.005752
_cons	.0317691	.0032251	-33.98	0.000	.0260373	.0387628

This is a PH model. The `_rcs` terms model the baseline (log) cumulative hazard as a function of attained age. The `_Ifu_` terms are dummy variables for years since diagnosis, where the coefficients are HRs comparing all intervals with the reference (zero to one year). There appears to be little effect of follow-up, as was found in the original article (Dickman et al. 2004a). TD effects could be added for age by using the `tvc()` and `dftvc()` options. TD effects for years since diagnosis could be added by incorporating interactions between the exposure covariates (`exp2` and `exp3`) and the `_Ifu_` terms.

7.10 Prognostic models with TD effects

It is common to find that time-fixed covariates in prognostic models have TD effects. It seems intuitively reasonable that the prognostic importance of a quantity measured once at baseline ($t = 0$) should change with time. In most cases, the effect reduces over time. It is important to extend the development of a prognostic model, as described in chapter 6, to include a systematic assessment of TD effects. Including such effects in the model should improve the fit and hence the predictive accuracy of the model, and also give insight into the functional form of the prognostic influence of a variable over time. The latter is conveniently expressed as a plot of the estimated HR (with 95% pointwise CI) against time.

One useful approach to identifying multiple TD effects is by forward selection:

1. Determine the prognostic model with time-fixed effects (already described in chapter 6). Call this the current model.
2. Select a significance level, α, for testing TD effects.
3. For each (remaining) variable that has a time-fixed effect in the current model, find the p-value for including it as a TD effect in the current model according to a likelihood-ratio test. Find the variable whose p-value, $P_{\min}$ say, is the lowest.
4. If $P_{\min} < \alpha$, then add a TD effect of the corresponding variable to the current model and return to step 3. Otherwise, stop.

Two issues deserve consideration: the significance level (α) and the complexity (number of d.f.) of the putative TD effects. Because there is multiple testing of TD effects, to guard against overfitting we suggest that α should be small—no larger than 0.01, say. TD effects may be simple or complex in form. For maximum flexibility, we suggest applying the above selection algorithm using the same d.f. for the TD effects as for the baseline spline function. Once TD effects have been identified, the AIC or BIC criterion may be applied to all combinations of TD d.f. for all such variables to choose a single final model.

7.10.1 Example

We continue the development of the prognostic model, based on multivariable FPs, for relapse-free survival time in the Rotterdam breast cancer data. The multivariable FP model is described in section 6.4.2. It comprises variables `age`(1), `enodes`(2), `pr`(0), `size` (2 dummies), `grade`, `chemo`, and `hormon`. Values in parentheses denote powers in FP transformations of continuous variables; thus `enodes`(2) denotes the square of `enodes`, and `pr`(0) denotes the log of `pr` (in fact, of `pr` + 1, to avoid zeros). A PO RP model with 2 baseline d.f. was selected for the time-fixed effects of the covariates (prognostic factors).

According to the above scheme, we include each covariate as TD with 2 d.f. and test it. As a result, `pr`(0) is found to be highly significantly TD ($P < 0.001$). At the second round, `chemo` is also found to be TD ($P = 0.006$). At the third round, no further variable is selected as significantly TD at the $P < 0.01$ level. The code and results for this analysis are as follows:

```
. use rott2, clear
(Rotterdam breast cancer data, truncated at 10 years)
. generate enodes = exp(-0.12 * nodes)
. fracgen enodes 2
-> gen double enodes_1 = enodes^2
. fracgen pr 0
-> gen double pr_1 = ln(X)
   (where: X = (pr+1)/1000)
```

```
. // Select time-varying effects significant at 1% level
. // by forward stepwise selection.
. xi: stpm2t age enodes_1 pr_1 (i.size) (i.grade) chemo hormon,
> tvselect(0.01) scale(odds) df(2) dftvc(2) detail
i.size            _Isize_1-3         (naturally coded; _Isize_1 omitted)
i.grade           _Igrade_2-3        (naturally coded; _Igrade_2 omitted)
Variable        Deviance      P-value   Final
name(s)        difference     vs null   deviance
---------------------------------------------------
[none]                                  6661.275
age                 7.381     0.0250        add?
enodes_1            3.895     0.1426        add?
pr_1               65.087     0.0000        add?
_Isize_2 ...        3.721     0.4450        add?
_Igrade_3           1.289     0.5249        add?
chemo              12.407     0.0020        add?
hormon              5.650     0.0593        add?
pr_1               65.087     0.0000    6596.188
age                 7.382     0.0249        add?
enodes_1            4.654     0.0976        add?
_Isize_2 ...        2.279     0.6847        add?
_Igrade_3           1.416     0.4925        add?
chemo              10.314     0.0058        add?
hormon              8.191     0.0167        add?
chemo              10.314     0.0058    6585.874
age                 3.185     0.2034        add?
enodes_1            2.763     0.2512        add?
_Isize_2 ...        3.088     0.5432        add?
_Igrade_3           1.333     0.5136        add?
hormon              8.703     0.0129        add?
---------------------------------------------------

-> stpm2  age enodes_1 pr_1 _Isize_2 _Isize_3 _Igrade_3 chemo hormon if
> e(sample), scale(odds) df(2) tvc( pr_1 chemo) dftvc(2)
Log likelihood = -3292.9369                    Number of obs   =       2982

------------------------------------------------------------------------------
             |      Coef.   Std. Err.      z    P>|z|     [95% Conf. Interval]
-------------+----------------------------------------------------------------
xb           |
         age |  -.0189295   .0031774    -5.96   0.000    -.0251571   -.0127019
    enodes_1 |  -2.479077   .1264016   -19.61   0.000    -2.726819   -2.231334
        pr_1 |  -.0836695   .0165862    -5.04   0.000    -.1161779   -.0511612
    _Isize_2 |   .3908022   .0786344     4.97   0.000     .2366816    .5449227
    _Isize_3 |   .6691492   .1289807     5.19   0.000     .4163516    .9219468
   _Igrade_3 |   .5122867   .0856633     5.98   0.000     .3443897    .6801837
       chemo |  -.7501744   .1048362    -7.16   0.000    -.9556495   -.5446992
      hormon |  -.7037152   .1197052    -5.88   0.000    -.9383329   -.4690974
       _rcs1 |   1.522782   .0640972    23.76   0.000     1.397154     1.64841
       _rcs2 |   .1333842   .0472964     2.82   0.005      .040685    .2260834
   _rcs_pr_11 |   .0717717   .0125451     5.72   0.000     .0471838    .0963596
   _rcs_pr_12 |  -.0248937   .0093679    -2.66   0.008    -.0432544    -.006533
_rcs_chemo1 |   .2372396   .0768244     3.09   0.002     .0866665    .3878127
_rcs_chemo2 |   .0826296   .0601394     1.37   0.169    -.0352415    .2005007
       _cons |   1.253865   .2413714     5.19   0.000     .7807861    1.726945
------------------------------------------------------------------------------

. // Get AIC and BIC with different d.f. for time-varying effects
```

```
. forvalues i = 1 / 2 {
  2.         forvalues j = 1 / 2 {
  3.                 quietly xi: stpm2 age enodes_1 pr_1 i.size i.grade chemo
>                 hormon, df(2) sc(o) tvc(pr_1 chemo)
>                 dftvc(pr_1:`i´ chemo:`j´)
  4.                 di "df for pr = " `i´ " df for chemo = " `j´
>                 " AIC = " %8.3f e(AIC) " BIC = " %8.3f e(BIC)
  5.         }
  6. }
df for pr = 1 df for chemo = 1 AIC = 6620.218 BIC = 6689.089
df for pr = 1 df for chemo = 2 AIC = 6620.853 BIC = 6695.022
df for pr = 2 df for chemo = 1 AIC = 6615.797 BIC = 6689.966
df for pr = 2 df for chemo = 2 AIC = 6615.874 BIC = 6695.340
```

We use the ado-file `stpm2t` to do forward selection of significant TD effects. The lines in the output marked `add?` show `stpm2t` considering (and in most cases, rejecting) the next TD effect for inclusion in the final model. In the first round, the most significant TD effect is `pr_1` and the second most significant is for `chemo`. The latter is duly selected in the second round. In the third round, no variable is significant at the 1% level (although `hormon` comes close, with $P = 0.013$). Nothing further can be added and the process terminates at the third round. The final model is then fit and displayed.

We now consider the four possible models with TD d.f. of 1 and 2 for `pr`(0) and `chemo`, respectively. As we can see from the output above, the model with the lowest AIC and BIC has 2 d.f. for log(`pr` + 1) and 1 d.f. for `chemo`. Figure 7.27 shows the estimated HRs for these two variables as functions of time.

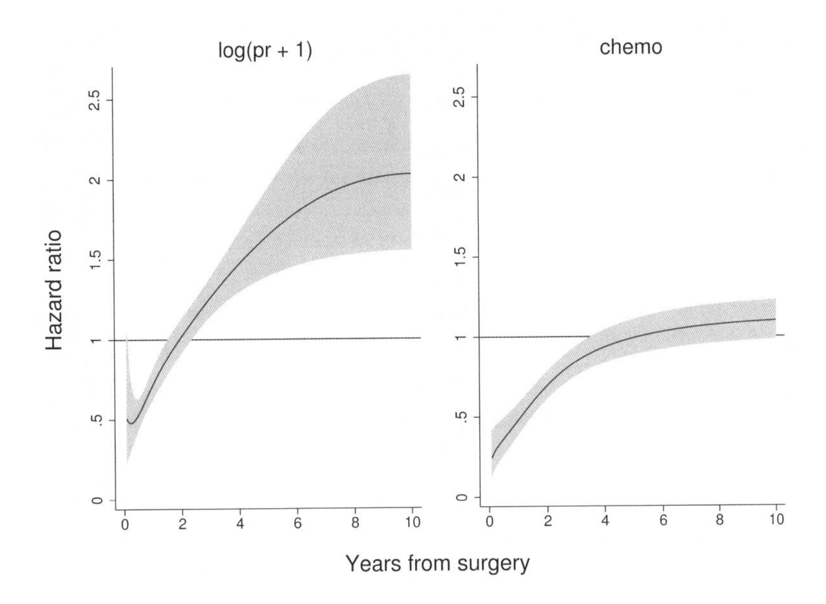

Figure 7.27. Rotterdam breast cancer data. TD HRs for log(`pr` + 1) and `chemo`. The HR for the former is for the median compared with the minimum value.

The code for figure 7.27 is as follows:

```
. use rott2
(Rotterdam breast cancer data, truncated at 10 years)
. generate enodes = exp(-0.12 * nodes)
. fracgen enodes 2
-> gen double enodes_1 = enodes^2
. fracgen pr 0
-> gen double pr_1 = ln(X)
   (where: X = (pr+1)/1000)
. // Fit final model (dftvc = 2 for pr_1, 1 for chemo)
. quietly xi: stpm2 age enodes_1 pr_1 i.size i.grade chemo hormon, df(2) sc(o)
> tvc(pr_1 chemo) dftvc(pr_1:2 chemo:1)
. // Predict HR and ci for each TV variable.
. // For pr, compare HR between median and minimum values.
. quietly sum pr_1, detail
. local min = r(min)
. local median = r(p50)
. predict hrpr, hrnum(pr_1 `median') hrden(pr_1 `min') ci
. predict hrchemo, hrnum(chemo 1) ci
. // Plot HRs against time
. quietly bysort _t: keep if _n == 1
```

```
. twoway (rarea hrpr_lci hrpr_uci _t, sort pstyle(ci))
> (line hrpr _t, sort lstyle(refline)), yline(1)
> title("log(pr + 1)") xtitle("") ytitle("") name(g1, replace) legend(off)
. twoway (rarea hrchemo_lci hrchemo_uci _t, sort pstyle(ci))
> (line hrchemo _t, sort lstyle(refline)), yline(1)
> title("chemo") xtitle("") ytitle("") name(g2, replace) legend(off)
. graph combine g1 g2, l1title("Hazard ratio")
> b2title("Years from surgery") ycommon
```

The function for pr(0) is interesting in that high pr appears to have a protective effect for $t < 2$ years and a reversal of that effect thereafter. The effect of chemo is quite large near $t = 0$ but dwindles to nothing (HR $\simeq 1$) after about 4 years or so. This seems a plausible outcome for the effect of a treatment given over a relatively short period soon after $t = 0$.

We recall that a PO model already has the property that HRs tend to 1 as $t \to \infty$. That chemo exhibits a significant TD effect superimposed on this tendency suggests that the effect of treatment is more short-lived than the effect of the other prognostic variables.

7.11 Discussion

In this chapter, we have covered a range of approaches to modeling TD effects. Within the Cox modeling framework, it is possible to estimate piecewise HRs or to assume a linear or some other function of (log) time. However, the reasons why we advocated the use of parametric approaches for PH models apply equally well to models with TD effects.

In section 7.4, we showed that proportionality on one scale leads to nonproportionality on another scale. For example, the PO model implies that hazard rates converge as follow-up time increases. The analyst needs to make a choice here; is it best to choose a model with a potentially hard-to-interpret scale but which seems to fit the data (for example, an RP model with the general Aranda-Ordaz link function and its parameter θ), or a model with a TD effect that is reported on the HR scale? In general, our preference would be for the latter because researchers are more used to interpreting HRs, and this would probably lead to less confusion. However, the choice depends on the research question. If interest lies in development of a prognostic model and we are not particularly interested in the interpretation of individual coefficients, then (from the viewpoint of interpretation) the choice of scale is less important. This is similar to the PO prognostic model developed in chapter 6, in which little emphasis was placed on the odds ratio of each of the individual model parameters.

In this chapter, we have also considered some ideas for alternative presentation of data. In particular, we believe that quantifying effects as hazard differences as well as HRs is particularly important when assessing the impact of some factor on the population. To calculate CIs for these measures, we apply the delta method, which is implemented in the postestimation `predict` command of `stpm2`. It uses Stata's `predictnl` command to obtain SEs and hence CIs. CIs derived by the delta method and by the bootstrap are similar. See section 1.9 for a comparison.

When extending a model on the log cumulative-hazard scale to include TD effects, the TD is modeled on the log cumulative-hazard scale. This introduces two issues. First, it is possible to transform to (log) HRs, but when deriving CIs the SE needs to be obtained using the delta method. The comparison with the bootstrap in section 1.9 shows this not to be a problem, but it should perhaps be investigated in smaller samples. However, with very small samples there would be little power to detect TD. The second issue is that if there is more than one TD variable, even if there is no interaction, the TD HR for one variable depends on the value of the other variable(s). This principle was illustrated in figure 7.19 where the difference between the two TD HRs was very small. This small difference is what we have found in most examples, but it is always something that should be checked.

In this chapter, we have not gone into much detail regarding selection of the number and location of the knots, but the approach is similar to that discussed in chapters 4 and 5—that is, use of the AIC and BIC. With large sample sizes, including one or two extra knots makes little difference to inferences.

8 Relative survival

Summary

1. Relative survival is a measure of patient survival corrected for the effect of other causes of death by utilizing patients' expected survival.
2. Relative survival is traditionally estimated in life tables, but there is growing use of models for relative survival. These models give an estimate of the excess mortality rate—that is, how much higher the mortality rate is in a group of patients with a particular disease or condition compared with the mortality rate expected in the general population.
3. Both Poisson models and Royston–Parmar (RP) models can be extended to relative survival by incorporating information on expected survival or mortality.
4. Nonproportional excess hazards is extremely common in population-based cancer studies, and thus the modeling of time-dependent effects is crucial.
5. Continuous variables such as age are often categorized with a potential loss of information. Modeling relative survival at the individual level allows more realistic investigation of associations with continuous variables.

8.1 Introduction

In this chapter, we consider relative survival, an extension of the Poisson and RP models described in the previous chapters. We initially concentrate on the description of what relative survival is, when it is used, and how to interpret it, because once these concepts are understood, the models and their interpretations are very similar to those of "standard" survival models.

8.2 What is relative survival?

Relative survival is the most common method for the analysis of survival data in population-based cancer studies. In such studies, interest lies in mortality associated with a diagnosis of a particular type of cancer (for example, breast or lung cancer). In general, cancer is a disease of old age. Although a person may be diagnosed with a particular cancer, they may die of another, unrelated cause—for example, heart disease, or even an unrelated type of cancer. If we analyze only overall survival, we are not distinguishing between those patients who die of their cancer and those who die from other causes. This distinction is important, because not only are we interested in the effect of age on the prognosis of a particular type of cancer, but also age is usually one of the commonest and strongest confounding variables. We often want to adjust for age in an analysis, but the effect of age on all-cause mortality and mortality associated with a particular type of cancer may actually be different.

One solution is to use cause-specific survival, where deaths not due to the cancer are treated as censored observations at the event time. Use of cause-specific survival assumes that the underlying cause of death is accurately recorded, but unfortunately this is often not the case. Cause of death is usually obtained from a death certificate, and doctors are notoriously bad at completing these correctly. The accuracy of death certification varies over time and among countries, making temporal comparisons and international comparisons of survival problematic (Begg and Schrag 2002). Further problems of cause-specific analysis include the fact that a death is regarded as either definitely due to or definitely not due to the particular cancer. In reality, it is hard to be so specific; for example, in some instances the cancer may only be a contributing factor to the death. A further issue is that a cause-specific analysis may not be possible, because many cancer registries do not have access to information on the cause of death.

Relative survival overcomes the problems of the inaccurate recording of cause of death by comparing observed overall survival with expected survival. Expected survival is usually available from routine sources, such as national life tables. Although most of the application and development of relative survival methods has been in cancer, it has recently been applied in other areas, including heart disease (Nelson et al. 2008) and human immunodeficiency virus (Bhaskaran et al. 2008).

8.3 Excess mortality and relative survival

In previous chapters, we have seen how we can summarize time-to-event data with either hazard functions or survival functions. In relative survival, the equivalent to the hazard rate is called the excess hazard rate or the excess mortality rate. The excess mortality rate tells us how much higher the mortality rate is in the patients with the disease in question compared with the expected mortality rate in the general population.

8.3.1 Excess mortality

For patients diagnosed with a particular disease, usually cancer, the total mortality (hazard) rate, $h(t)$, can be considered as the sum of two components. These components are the mortality rate associated with the disease of interest, $\lambda(t)$; and the expected mortality rate due to other causes, $h^*(t)$:

$$h(t) = h^*(t) + \lambda(t) \tag{8.1}$$

The expected mortality rate is usually obtained from national or regional life tables stratified by age, sex, calendar year, and potentially other variables—for example, deprivation group or social class (Coleman et al. 1999). In relative survival, t is nearly always time from diagnosis of the disease of interest. An example of expected mortality rates is shown in figure 8.1, which shows how the all-cause mortality rate for females with age and varies by deprivation group (Coleman et al. 1999). Note the initial higher mortality rate in the first year of life, and the hump at about 20 years of age. This hump is mainly due to an increase in accidents and suicides.

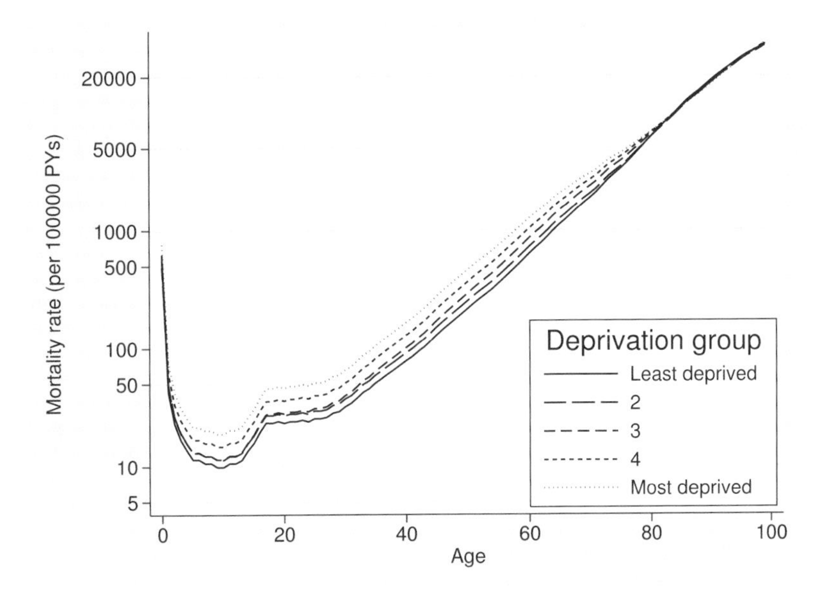

Figure 8.1. Population mortality rates for females in North and Yorkshire region of England in 1995 by deprivation group. PYs stands for person-years.

Relative survival is related to the concept of competing risks (Gamel and Vogel 2001). We assume that an individual is at risk of either dying of their cancer or dying of another cause. The main difference between relative survival and standard competing-risks analysis is that we do not actually observe the cause of death in the individual, but rely on the assumption that we can estimate the expected mortality rate due to other causes accurately from routine data sources.

8.3.2 Relative survival is a ratio

If we transform the hazard function to the survival scale, we find that overall survival is the product of the expected survival, $S^*(t)$, and the relative survival, $R(t)$:

$$S(t) = S^*(t)R(t) \tag{8.2}$$

Rearranging, we find that relative survival is the ratio of overall survival to expected survival.

$$R(t) = \frac{S(t)}{S^*(t)}$$

If the mortality rate of those patients diagnosed with the disease of interest was no different from that expected in the general population, then $\lambda(t) = 0$, $h(t) = h^*(t)$, and $S(t) = S^*(t)$. We would observe a relative survival estimate of $R(t) = 1$. It is, of course, unlikely that our relative survival curve would be constant at 1, because we generally study diseases where we expect mortality to be higher than in the general population. It is worthwhile to note here that it is possible in theory to have an estimate of relative survival greater than 1. This would occur in the unlikely situation where the group of diseased individuals had a lower mortality rate than that expected—that is, there was negative excess mortality. An example where relative survival was estimated to be greater than 1 was in an analysis investigating relative survival in patients having elective surgery for abdominal aortic aneurysm who were aged 80 and over (Norman et al. 1998). The reason for the increased survival is that only patients who were well enough to undergo surgery would have been selected. Such a group is likely to be healthier than a similarly aged group in the general population.

Relative survival, like cause-specific survival, is an estimate of *net survival*, which is survival in a hypothetical world where it is impossible to die of anything other than the disease under study; that is, it is survival in the absence of death due to other causes. Although this hypothetical world may at first seem a strange concept, when making comparisons between regions or countries or over time it is important to adjust for the fact that mortality due to other causes may also be different. The interpretation of relative survival as the probability of surviving in the absence of other causes depends on an assumption of independence between mortality due to the disease (for example, cancer) under study and mortality due to other causes (Gamel and Vogel 2001). If the presence of cancer alters the rate of death due to other causes, this assumption is violated. An alternative way to think about violation of this assumption is if the type of person who gets a particular type of cancer has an increased or decreased rate of mortality due to other causes. The use of relative survival for lung cancer has been criticized because smoking is the primary cause of lung cancer, but people who smoke are at increased risk for a number of other diseases, and so the independence assumption is violated.

8.4 Motivating example

We return to the England and Wales breast cancer data used in chapter 7. Rather than restrict the analysis to those under 50 years of age, we now include all ages, giving 115,331 observations. Because there are now older women included in the analysis, mortality from other causes plays a greater role. If we are interested in mortality associated with breast cancer, we need relative survival. A cause-specific analysis is not possible here, because there is no information in the dataset on cause of death. However, even if cause of death was recorded, we would be reluctant to use it because of the problems of death certification discussed above.

We initially define five age groups, < 50, 50–59, 60–69, 70–79, and 80 +. In section 8.9, we show how age can be modeled as a continuous variable. Kaplan–Meier estimates of overall survival by age group are shown in figure 8.2. There is clear separation among the survival estimates of the five groups, with the oldest age group having lowest survival. However, because we have not separated mortality from breast cancer from mortality due to other causes, we do not know how much of the observed difference is due to breast cancer mortality and how much is because older women are far more likely to die of other causes.

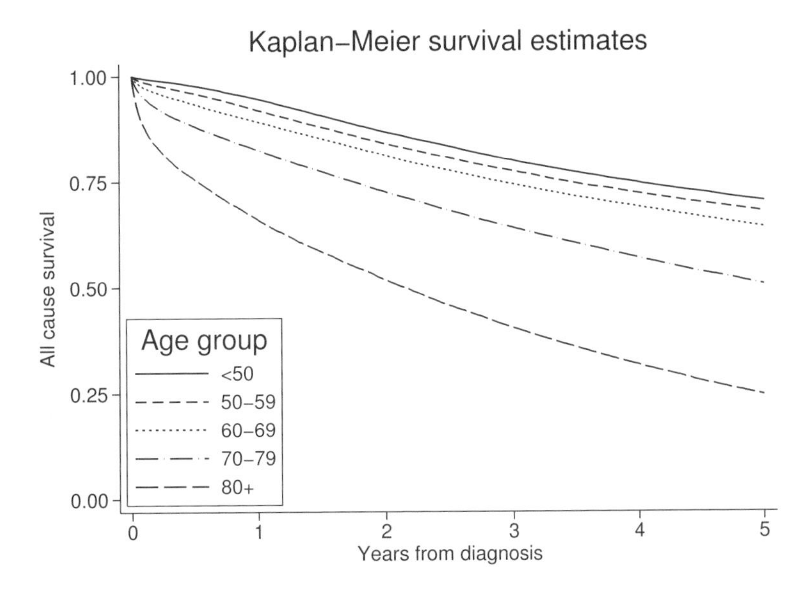

Figure 8.2. England and Wales breast cancer data. Kaplan–Meier estimate of overall survival by age group.

A proportional hazards (PH) RP model with 7 degrees of freedom (d.f.) for the baseline can be fit with age group < 50 years as the reference, as follows:

```
. use ew_breast_ch8
(England and Wales Breast Cancer: All ages)
. stset survtime, failure(dead==1) exit(time 5) id(ident)
                id:  ident
     failure event:  dead == 1
obs. time interval:  (survtime[_n-1], survtime]
 exit on or before:  time 5

------------------------------------------------------------------------------
   115331  total obs.
        0  exclusions
------------------------------------------------------------------------------
   115331  obs. remaining, representing
   115331  subjects
    47692  failures in single failure-per-subject data
 432458.2  total analysis time at risk, at risk from t =         0
                             earliest observed entry t =         0
                                  last observed exit t =         5
. stpm2 agegrp2-agegrp5, df(7) scale(hazard) eform nolog
Log likelihood = -139289.55                       Number of obs   =     115331

------------------------------------------------------------------------------
             |     exp(b)   Std. Err.      z    P>|z|     [95% Conf. Interval]
-------------+----------------------------------------------------------------
xb           |
     agegrp2 |   1.116183   .0183251     6.69   0.000     1.080838    1.152684
     agegrp3 |   1.284478    .019533    16.46   0.000     1.246759    1.323338
     agegrp4 |   1.979577    .029436    45.92   0.000     1.922716    2.038119
     agegrp5 |   4.155222   .0631774    93.68   0.000     4.033224    4.280911
       _rcs1 |   2.454866   .0106054   207.88   0.000     2.434168    2.475741
       _rcs2 |   .9625049   .0029487   -12.47   0.000     .9567428    .9683017
       _rcs3 |   .9534433   .0016509   -27.53   0.000     .9502129    .9566846
       _rcs4 |   1.017265   .0011238    15.49   0.000     1.015065     1.01947
       _rcs5 |   1.002373    .000697     3.41   0.001     1.001008     1.00374
       _rcs6 |   1.001476   .0004642     3.18   0.001     1.000567    1.002386
       _rcs7 |   1.000059   .0003113     0.19   0.850      .999449    1.000669
       _cons |   .2124442   .0025008  -131.60   0.000     .2075989    .2174026
------------------------------------------------------------------------------
```

We used 7 d.f. for the baseline for comparison with the relative survival models fit later in this chapter. It is an all-cause mortality model, because we use `stset` with the option `failure(dead==1)` and we do not know cause of death for the women. Not surprisingly, given what we have seen in the Kaplan–Meier graph, the hazard ratios (HRs) increase with age group, with those women aged over 80 years having more than a fourfold higher mortality rate compared with those aged under 50. We could also have fit a Cox model here, but we hope by now you would have gotten the message that the HRs would be virtually the same. Because this is an analysis of all-cause mortality, we have not yet accounted for the fact that older people are more likely to die of other causes. We aim, therefore, to fit models for relative survival, but before doing this, we explain the traditional life-table method of calculating relative survival in separate subgroups.

8.5 Life-table estimation of relative survival

The most common method of estimating relative survival is to determine it separately in groups of interest using life tables. Relative survival is not a standard survival analysis methodology, and none of the major statistical packages have official commands that enable relative survival to be estimated or modeled. However, several user-written programs are available. Stata is probably the best-equipped of the major packages for the estimation and modeling of relative survival. The user-written command for the estimation of relative survival in life tables is `strs`. It was developed by Paul Dickman and is available from his website (http://www.pauldickman.com/rsmodel/stata_colon/). To estimate relative survival, we need access to a data file containing expected mortality and survival by age group, sex, and calendar year, so that the expected survival for each individual in the study can be calculated. This file is known as a population mortality file. An example of such data for England and Wales is shown below:

```
. use popmort_uk
(England and Wales Population Mortality)
. list if region == 1 & sex == 2 & dep == 1 & inrange(age,70,79) & year == 1990,
> noobs
```

sex	age	rate	dep	region	survprob	year
2	70	0.018627	1	N & York	.9815449	1990
2	71	0.020727	1	N & York	.9794856	1990
2	72	0.023674	1	N & York	.976603	1990
2	73	0.026983	1	N & York	.9733762	1990
2	74	0.029958	1	N & York	.9704841	1990
2	75	0.033198	1	N & York	.967344	1990
2	76	0.037211	1	N & York	.9634687	1990
2	77	0.042244	1	N & York	.9586298	1990
2	78	0.047933	1	N & York	.9531889	1990
2	79	0.054568	1	N & York	.9468813	1990

The output shows the probability of surviving 1 year (`survprob`) for females (`sex == 2`) aged between 70 and 79 and living in the most affluent areas (`dep == 1`) in the North and Yorkshire regions of England (`region == 1`) in 1990. Also shown is the mortality rate (`rate`), which is just a transformation of the survival probability—that is, `rate = -ln(survprob)` because it is assumed that the mortality rate is constant for each age within each calendar year. The rates are needed for the extension of RP models to relative survival. The probability a 70-year old woman will survive one year is 0.9815, whereas for a 79-year old woman the figure has reduced to 0.9469.

We do not go into details here, but the general approach to estimating relative survival using life tables is as follows:

1. Split survival time into a number of intervals. Traditionally, these are yearly intervals—that is, zero to one year, one to two years, etc., from diagnosis.

2. Calculate the attained age of each subject and attained year of follow-up within each interval and merge in the expected survival from the population mortality file.

3. Collapse the data over the time intervals and any categorical covariates of interest, calculating for each interval the number of subjects at risk (n), the number of deaths (d), the number of censored observations (w), and the interval-specific expected survival (p_star). With this information, it is possible to obtain the conditional probability of surviving an interval (p), the cumulative probability of surviving to the end of each interval (cp), the cumulative expected survival (cp_e2), the interval-specific relative survival (r), and cumulative relative survival (cr_e2). The variable names in parentheses are those calculated by the strs command. The e2 subscript refers to the fact that Ederer II method (the default) was used to estimate expected survival (Ederer and Heise 1959). Other options for calculating expected survival are available; the Ederer I (Ederer et al. 1961) and Hakulinen approaches (Hakulinen 1982).

8.5.1 Using strs

In the following output, the strs command is applied to the England and Wales breast cancer data.

```
. use ew_breast_ch8
(England and Wales Breast Cancer: All ages)
. stset survtime, failure(dead==1) exit(time 5) id(ident)
  (output omitted)
. strs using popmort_uk if inlist(agegroup,1,5), breaks(0(1)5) noshow
> diagage(agediag) diagyear(yeardiag) attage(age) attyear(year)
> mergeby(sex region dep year age) survprob(survprob) by(agegroup)
> list(end n d p p_star r cp cp_e2 cr_e2)
No late entry detected - p is estimated using the actuarial method
```

-> agegroup = <50

end	n	d	p	p_star	r	cp	cp_e2	cr_e2
1	24889	1356	0.9455	0.9986	0.9469	0.9455	0.9986	0.9469
2	23529	1957	0.9168	0.9984	0.9182	0.8668	0.9970	0.8694
3	21554	1680	0.9220	0.9983	0.9236	0.7993	0.9953	0.8030
4	19857	1322	0.9334	0.9981	0.9352	0.7460	0.9934	0.7510
5	18519	1051	0.9432	0.9979	0.9452	0.7037	0.9913	0.7098

```
-> agegroup = 80+
```

end	n	d	p	p_star	r	cp	cp_e2	cr_e2
1	14110	4790	0.6605	0.9006	0.7335	0.6605	0.9006	0.7335
2	9319	2022	0.7830	0.8969	0.8730	0.5172	0.8077	0.6403
3	7296	1597	0.7811	0.8905	0.8771	0.4040	0.7193	0.5616
4	5696	1234	0.7834	0.8824	0.8878	0.3164	0.6347	0.4986
5	4462	1001	0.7756	0.8739	0.8875	0.2454	0.5547	0.4425

Only the life tables for the oldest and youngest age groups have been calculated. The interval-specific probability of survival is denoted by `p`. For the youngest age group, this is 0.9455 in the first year after diagnosis, whereas for the oldest age group it is 0.6605. The expected survival is denoted by `p_star` and is higher at 0.9986 in the youngest age group than at 0.9006 in the oldest age group. This should not be surprising because a woman aged over 80 has a greatly reduced chance of survival when compared with a woman under 50. Also the interval-specific expected survival reduces over follow-up time, which is to be expected because the study population is aging as follow-up time increases. The interval-specific relative survival, `r`, is calculated as `p/p_star`. Under the assumption of independence of mortality due to cancer and other causes, `r` can be interpreted as the conditional probability of not dying of breast cancer in the hypothetical world where it is impossible to die from another cause. The (cumulative) relative survival is calculated as `cp/cp_e2`. There is a greater difference between the relative survival (`cr_e2`) and overall survival (`cp`) estimates for the oldest age groups, which is to be expected because those under 50 are unlikely to die from other causes. From the relative survival estimates, we can state that at five years from diagnosis the probability of surviving breast cancer (under the assumption that it is not possible to die of other causes) is 0.71 in the youngest age group and 0.44 in the oldest age group.

Life tables are a useful aid for summarizing cancer survival. There are, however, many advantages to modeling relative survival. Advantages include simultaneously investigating a number of different factors, quantification of differences between groups, significance testing, and prediction. We therefore now switch to different approaches to modeling relative survival.

8.6 Poisson models for relative survival

8.6.1 Piecewise models

Traditionally, models for relative survival have been based on life tables as calculated in the previous section. We concentrate on the Poisson-based models described by Dickman et al. (2004b). Alternative, but similar, models include those of Hakulinen and Tenkanen (Hakulinen and Tenkanen 1987) and Estève (Estève et al. 1990). Dickman showed that the estimates from the different modeling approaches are very similar, and in some cases, identical (Dickman et al. 2004b). Traditionally, a relative survival model is fit on the (log) excess-hazard scale. As a starting point, proportional excess hazards are assumed, and thus a model can be written as

$$h(t) = h^*(t) + \lambda_0(t) \exp(\mathbf{x}\boldsymbol{\beta})$$

where $\lambda_0(t)$ is the baseline excess-hazard function. We use the term excess mortality rate rather than excess hazard rate because the former gives a better description of what the function is estimating. The model looks similar to a standard PH model, with the exception that an extra term, the expected mortality rate, $h^*(t)$, is included. In Poisson-based relative survival models, the baseline excess-mortality rate is estimated in a piecewise fashion. Traditionally, one year intervals have been used. Dickman et al. (2004b) showed that this model can be fit in a generalized linear modeling framework with a Poisson likelihood. The theory is similar to that explained in chapter 4. However, because we need to incorporate expected mortality, we use a modified link function.

Let d_{ik} be a censoring indicator for the ith subject in the kth interval, where 1 indicates that the subject died in the interval and 0 indicates that the subject survived at least part of the interval. We can then write

$$d_{ik} \sim \text{Poisson}(\mu_{ik}) \text{ where } \mu_{ik} = h_{ik} y_{ik}$$

Here h_{ik} is the total mortality rate and y_{ik} is the person-time at risk for the ith subject in the kth interval. Because $h_{ik} = h^*_{ik} + \exp(\mathbf{x}\boldsymbol{\beta})$ and $h^*_{ik} = d^*_{ik}/y_{ik}$, where d^*_{ik} is the expected number of deaths, we can write

$$\frac{\mu_{ik}}{y_{ik}} = \frac{d^*_{ik}}{y_{ik}} + \exp(\mathbf{x}\boldsymbol{\beta})$$

Rearranging and taking logs gives

$$\ln(\mu_{ik} - d^*_{ik}) = \ln(y_{ik}) + \mathbf{x}\boldsymbol{\beta}$$

The usual link function for a Poisson model is $\ln(\mu_{ik})$. To fit a relative survival model, we need to change the link function to $\ln(\mu_{ik} - d^*_{ik})$. This is not a standard link function, but the `glm` command enables user-defined link functions by writing an appropriate ado-file. When installing `strs`, a file called `rs.ado` is also installed, which enables this special link function to be used. The subscript ik for d^*_{ik} indicates that the link function may be different for each observation in the model.

It chapter 4, we discussed that there were computational advantages in collapsing the data. The same applies to relative survival models. When collapsing, we essentially obtain the estimates from the life table, and thus we can use `strs` to generate the collapsed data needed for modeling. Unlike standard survival models, relative survival models do not give identical estimates when fitting models to the individual and collapsed level data. This difference is because the expected survival is likely to vary within each covariate pattern. However, in practice the estimates from models based on the individual and collapsed data are very similar (Dickman et al. 2004b). This is particularly so if age is modeled, because the greatest variation in expected survival is due to age. The `strs` command enables both the individual and collapsed level data to be saved using the `savind()` and `savgroup()` options, respectively. A dataset collapsed by age group can be generated as follows:

```
. use ew_breast_ch8
(England and Wales Breast Cancer: All ages)
. stset survtime, failure(dead==1) exit(time 5) id(ident)
  (output omitted)
. strs using popmort_uk, breaks(0(1)5) noshow diagage(agediag)
> diagyear(yeardiag) attage(age) attyear(year) mergeby(sex region dep year age)
> survprob(survprob) by(agegroup) notables savgroup(breast_grouped, replace)
No late entry detected - p is estimated using the actuarial method
```

Note the inclusion of the `notables` option, which suppresses output of the tables. The grouped data have been saved in `breast_grouped.dta`. Because the data have been collapsed over time interval and age group, we have 25 rows of data, as shown below:

```
. use breast_grouped
(Collapsed (or grouped) survival data)
. list agegroup end n_prime d d_star y, noobs
```

agegroup	end	n_prime	d	d_star	y
<50	1	24887.0	1356	34.3	24267.3
<50	2	23520.0	1957	35.2	22545.0
<50	3	21545.5	1680	35.8	20693.8
<50	4	19849.0	1322	36.7	19158.7
<50	5	18516.0	1051	38.0	17974.1
50-59	1	23243.0	1882	104.9	22268.1
50-59	2	21357.5	1850	106.6	20424.5
50-59	3	19502.0	1519	108.4	18715.8
50-59	4	17977.0	1231	111.2	17330.2
50-59	5	16737.0	993	115.5	16233.6
60-69	1	29269.0	3172	361.0	27376.8
60-69	2	26091.0	2361	359.8	24917.6
60-69	3	23723.5	1977	359.1	22696.7
60-69	4	21741.0	1596	363.5	20906.8
60-69	5	20139.5	1367	372.2	19446.8
70-79	1	23814.5	4176	733.4	21133.2
70-79	2	19633.5	2364	703.5	18425.5
70-79	3	17262.5	2012	683.4	16224.0
70-79	4	15247.0	1709	667.3	14373.4
70-79	5	13534.0	1473	652.4	12771.9
80+	1	14109.5	4790	1105.2	10848.6
80+	2	9318.5	2022	893.0	8266.5
80+	3	7294.5	1597	748.0	6467.0
80+	4	5696.0	1234	630.9	5055.0
80+	5	4461.5	1001	529.6	3937.2

The observed number of deaths within each interval can be compared with the expected number of deaths. For example, for those aged less than 50, the effective number at risk (`n_prime`) at diagnosis was 24,887, with 1,356 of these woman dying within the first year, compared with only 34.3 who were expected to die. A relative survival model can be fit using `glm` with the `rs` user-defined link function to incorporate the expected number of deaths.

```
. glm d ibn.end i.agegroup, family(poisson) link(rs d_star) lnoffset(y) eform
> nocons nolog baselevels

Generalized linear models                         No. of obs      =         25
Optimization     : ML                             Residual df     =         16
                                                  Scale parameter =          1
Deviance         =  1272.329853                   (1/df) Deviance =   79.52062
Pearson          =  1227.530867                   (1/df) Pearson  =   76.72068

Variance function: V(u) = u                       [Poisson]
Link function    : g(u) = log(u-d*)               [Relative survival]

                                                  AIC             =   60.92002
Log likelihood   = -752.500207                    BIC             =   1220.828

------------------------------------------------------------------------------
             |                 OIM
           d |     exp(b)   Std. Err.      z    P>|z|     [95% Conf. Interval]
-------------+----------------------------------------------------------------
         end |
           1 |   .0913214   .0013257  -164.87   0.000     .0887597    .0939571
           2 |   .0716402   .0011346  -166.44   0.000     .0694506    .0738989
           3 |   .0658234   .0011071  -161.77   0.000     .0636889    .0680294
           4 |    .056892   .0010464  -155.86   0.000     .0548777    .0589803
           5 |   .0495787   .0010035  -148.43   0.000     .0476505     .051585
             |
    agegroup |
           1 |          1  (base)
           2 |   1.060791   .0183518     3.41   0.001     1.025425    1.097377
           3 |   1.093422   .0183589     5.32   0.000     1.058025    1.130003
           4 |   1.455602   .0255592    21.38   0.000     1.406359    1.506569
           5 |   2.766525   .0529771    53.14   0.000     2.664616    2.872331
       ln(y) |          1  (exposure)
------------------------------------------------------------------------------
```

The effects of `end` (interval) and `agegroup` (age group) are modeled using factor variables. The `glm` command fits the relative survival model. It is a relative survival model because of use of the `link(rs d_star)` option, which states that `glm` should use the `rs.ado` program for the link function and that the expected number of deaths are stored in `d_star`. If the `link()` option was not included or it was the default (`link(log)`), an overall survival model would be fit. The factor variables for `end` estimate the excess mortality rate in the reference group, which is the youngest age group (< 50); that is, this is the baseline excess-mortality rate. In the first year after diagnosis, there were 91.3 excess deaths per 1,000 person-years when compared with the expected mortality rate. In the fifth year after diagnosis, the rate had reduced to 49.6 excess deaths per 1,000 person-years. This is a proportional excess-hazards model because there is no interaction between the covariates and the time scale. The reference group is `agegroup=1`, and excess mortality-rate ratios are estimated for the other age groups. We prefer the term excess mortality-rate ratio to excess HR. An alternative name sometimes used is *relative excess risk*, which we regard as confusing. There is a clear gradient with increasing age, with the oldest age group having an excess mortality rate 2.77 times that of the youngest age group. Because we are accounting for the fact that older people are more likely to die of other causes through the inclusion of the expected number of deaths, `d_star`, we can state that older people diagnosed with breast cancer are at greater risk of dying from their cancer. In an all-cause analysis, we would not be able to disentangle this information.

Nonproportional excess hazards are extremely common in population-based cancer studies, and thus the proportional excess-hazards model above is likely to be too simple. Because the model is a GLM and there are many observations within each cell, we can use the deviance as a measure of model fit. The deviance is 1272.3 with 16 d.f. A well-fitting model would have a deviance similar to the d.f. As was shown in chapter 7, nonproportional models can be fit by including an interaction between the covariates of interest and the time scale. A nonproportional excess-hazards model is fit below:

```
. glm d ibn.end ibn.end#ib1.agegroup, family(poisson) link(rs d_star)
> lnoffset(y) eform nocons nolog noheader allbaselevels
```

d	exp(b)	OIM Std. Err.	z	P>|z|	[95% Conf.	Interval]
end						
1	.0544624	.0015174	-104.45	0.000	.051568	.0575192
2	.0852414	.0019622	-106.96	0.000	.081481	.0891753
3	.0794541	.0019807	-101.59	0.000	.0756653	.0834325
4	.0670884	.0018978	-95.51	0.000	.06347	.070913
5	.0563593	.0018037	-89.87	0.000	.0529328	.0600076
end#agegroup						
1 1	1	(base)				
1 2	1.465279	.0542796	10.31	0.000	1.362663	1.575622
1 3	1.885286	.0646993	18.48	0.000	1.762649	2.016456
1 4	2.991051	.1004855	32.61	0.000	2.800447	3.194628
1 5	6.236595	.2095595	54.47	0.000	5.839099	6.661151
2 1	1	(base)				
2 2	1.001361	.0337887	0.04	0.968	.9372784	1.069824
2 3	.9421687	.0315232	-1.78	0.075	.8823666	1.006024
2 4	1.057258	.0393781	1.49	0.135	.9828285	1.137325
2 5	1.602167	.0737055	10.25	0.000	1.464028	1.75334
3 1	1	(base)				
3 2	.9486068	.0353006	-1.42	0.156	.8818819	1.02038
3 3	.8971789	.0332887	-2.92	0.003	.8342501	.9648545
3 4	1.030688	.0432548	0.72	0.471	.9493027	1.11905
3 5	1.652229	.0880071	9.43	0.000	1.488437	1.834046
4 1	1	(base)				
4 2	.9631636	.0406571	-0.89	0.374	.8866846	1.046239
4 3	.8787022	.0378037	-3.01	0.003	.8076462	.9560097
4 4	1.080232	.0526467	1.58	0.113	.981821	1.188506
4 5	1.778356	.1151521	8.89	0.000	1.566397	2.018997
5 1	1	(base)				
5 2	.959085	.0461343	-0.87	0.385	.872795	1.053906
5 3	.907651	.0445168	-1.98	0.048	.8244622	.9992336
5 4	1.140011	.0646059	2.31	0.021	1.020164	1.273936
5 5	2.124373	.157962	10.13	0.000	1.836276	2.45767
ln(y)	1	(exposure)				

Interactions between `end` and `agegroup` have been fit. The model has been parameterized in such a way that the excess mortality-rate ratios for `agegroup` are given for each of the five time intervals with the youngest `agegroup` as the reference group. Because there are five age groups and five time intervals, the model has a total of 25 parameters. In the first year following diagnosis, the excess mortality-rate ratios for the other age groups are 1.47, 1.89, 2.99, and 6.24, with the youngest age group as the reference. For all the age groups, the largest excess mortality-rate ratios are seen in the first year after diagnosis. For example, the oldest group has an excess mortality-rate ratio of 6.24 in the first year after diagnosis, which reduces to 1.60, 1.65, 1.78, and 2.12 in the four subsequent years.

The piecewise models suffer from the same problems as those described in chapter 4. The choice of cutpoints is subjective, and using intervals that are too wide may miss important features of the data. Modeling time-dependent effects is possible, but may lead to overfitting if we include interactions between the time-dependent covariates and the time-intervals. We thus now move on to estimating smooth functions of the baseline excess-mortality rate and any time-dependent effects.

8.6.2 Restricted cubic splines

In chapter 5, we described how Poisson models could be extended by finely splitting the time scale and using either splines or fractional polynomials (FPs) to model the baseline hazard and any time-dependent effects as smooth functions. Exactly the same procedure is possible for relative survival models. First, the data must be split into a large number of small intervals. Because we also need the expected number of deaths, we use the `strs` command to split the time scale, merge in the expected survival, and collapse over the covariate patterns.

```
. use ew_breast_ch8
(England and Wales Breast Cancer: All ages)
. stset survtime, failure(dead==1) exit(time 5) id(ident)
  (output omitted)
. strs using popmort_uk, breaks(0(`=1/12')5) noshow diagage(agediag)
> diagyear(yeardiag) attage(age) attyear(year) mergeby(sex region dep year age)
> survprob(survprob) by(agegroup) notables
> savgroup(breast_grouped_narrow, replace)
No late entry detected - p is estimated using the actuarial method
```

The time scale is split into monthly intervals by use of the `breaks(0(‘=1/12’)5)` option, and the data are saved to a new dataset called `breast_grouped_narrow.dta`. We load this dataset and generate the restricted cubic-spline variables using `rcsgen`.

```
. use breast_grouped_narrow, clear
(Collapsed (or grouped) survival data)
. generate midtime = (start + end)/2
. generate lnmidtime = ln(midtime)
. rcsgen lnmidtime, gen(rcs) df(5) fw(d) orthog
Variables rcs1 to rcs5 were created
```

The splines are calculated on the log time scale, and 6 knots (5 d.f.) are used because this gives the lowest Akaike information criterion (AIC). Because we are using collapsed data, we make use of the `fw()` option as described in section 4.8.3. A proportional excess-hazards model can be fit by including the restricted cubic-spline variables in the model together with the dummy covariates for age group.

```
. glm d rcs* i.agegroup, family(poisson) link(rs d_star) lnoffset(y) eform
> nolog noheader
```

d	exp(b)	OIM Std. Err.	z	P>|z|	[95% Conf.	Interval]
rcs1	.8071378	.0042601	-40.59	0.000	.7988312	.8155308
rcs2	.9412534	.0044385	-12.84	0.000	.9325942	.949993
rcs3	1.127323	.0061382	22.01	0.000	1.115356	1.139418
rcs4	1.019196	.0061491	3.15	0.002	1.007215	1.031319
rcs5	.9991478	.0065186	-0.13	0.896	.986453	1.012006
agegroup						
2	1.055627	.0183351	3.12	0.002	1.020296	1.092182
3	1.081396	.0182671	4.63	0.000	1.04618	1.117799
4	1.430751	.0252913	20.26	0.000	1.38203	1.481189
5	2.728909	.0520415	52.64	0.000	2.628792	2.832838
_cons	.0638819	.000778	-225.86	0.000	.0623751	.0654251
ln(y)	1	(exposure)				

The excess mortality-rate ratios for the age groups are similar to those obtained for the piecewise model. The small differences are mainly due to the crude splitting of the time scale for the piecewise model. The predicted values of the excess mortality rates can be obtained by use of the `predict` command:

```
. predict log_eh_ph, xb nooffset
. generate eh_ph = exp(log_eh_ph)*1000
```

The predicted values have been multiplied by 1,000 so that they are expressed as a rate per 1,000 person-years. The predicted values are plotted by age group in figure 8.3. There appears to be a noticeable difference for the oldest two age groups when compared with the youngest age group. However, although the excess mortality-rate ratios are smaller for the 50–59-year-olds and the 60–69-year-olds (at 1.06 and 1.08, respectively), they are still significant at the 1% level because of the large sample size.

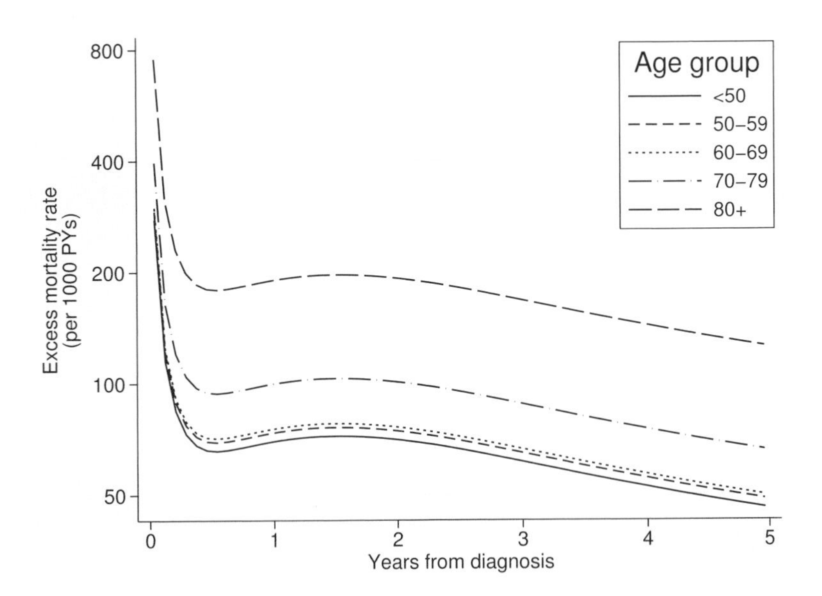

Figure 8.3. England and Wales breast cancer data. Excess mortality rates (log scale) from a proportional excess-hazards relative-survival Poisson model incorporating restricted cubic splines. PYs stands for person-years.

There was clear evidence of nonproportional excess hazards in the piecewise model, so we should extend the model to allow for time-dependent effects. Here we take the view that the number of knots for time-dependent effects is generally fewer than those needed for the baseline, so we initially choose 2 interior knots (3 d.f.). Again we calculate the restricted cubic-spline variables on the log time scale.

```
. rcsgen lnmidtime, gen(rcstvc) df(3) fw(d) orthog
Variables rcstvc1 to rcstvc3 were created
. tabulate agegroup, generate(agegrp) nofreq
. forvalues i = 2/5 {
  2.         forvalues j = 1/3 {
  3.                 gen age`i'rcs`j' = agegrp`i'*rcstvc`j'
  4.         }
  5. }
```

The model incorporating these time-dependent effects is shown below:

```
. glm d rcs1-rcs5 agegrp2-agegrp5 age?rcs?, family(poisson) link(rs d_star)
> lnoffset(y) nolog noheader
```

d	Coef.	OIM Std. Err.	z	P>|z|	[95% Conf.	Interval]
rcs1	.0551923	.0130978	4.21	0.000	.0295211	.0808636
rcs2	.0856464	.0123887	6.91	0.000	.0613651	.1099278
rcs3	.1653102	.0113062	14.62	0.000	.1431504	.18747
rcs4	.0373546	.007464	5.00	0.000	.0227254	.0519839
rcs5	-.0026072	.0066376	-0.39	0.694	-.0156166	.0104023
agegrp2	.0437359	.0180165	2.43	0.015	.0084241	.0790476
agegrp3	.0197955	.0180916	1.09	0.274	-.0156635	.0552545
agegrp4	.2169832	.0204492	10.61	0.000	.1769036	.2570629
agegrp5	.7244779	.0263588	27.49	0.000	.6728156	.7761401
age2rcs1	-.1783091	.0176363	-10.11	0.000	-.2128756	-.1437425
age2rcs2	-.056696	.0167396	-3.39	0.001	-.0895049	-.023887
age2rcs3	-.0211089	.0176936	-1.19	0.233	-.0557877	.0135699
age3rcs1	-.3008078	.0170512	-17.64	0.000	-.3342276	-.267388
age3rcs2	-.114347	.0162135	-7.05	0.000	-.1461249	-.082569
age3rcs3	-.0372897	.0174339	-2.14	0.032	-.0714596	-.0031199
age4rcs1	-.3822193	.0181502	-21.06	0.000	-.417793	-.3466456
age4rcs2	-.1776453	.0173777	-10.22	0.000	-.211705	-.1435857
age4rcs3	-.1018443	.0189519	-5.37	0.000	-.1389892	-.0646993
age5rcs1	-.4100838	.0215608	-19.02	0.000	-.4523421	-.3678254
age5rcs2	-.2584767	.0208533	-12.39	0.000	-.2993485	-.2176049
age5rcs3	-.1545944	.0227939	-6.78	0.000	-.1992696	-.1099191
_cons	-2.700436	.0123028	-219.50	0.000	-2.724549	-2.676323
ln(y)	1	(exposure)				

Rather than use Stata's factor variables, we have created our own interactions between age group and the new spline variables. The individual parameter estimates have very little meaning. It is best to examine the predicted values graphically, as shown in figure 8.4.

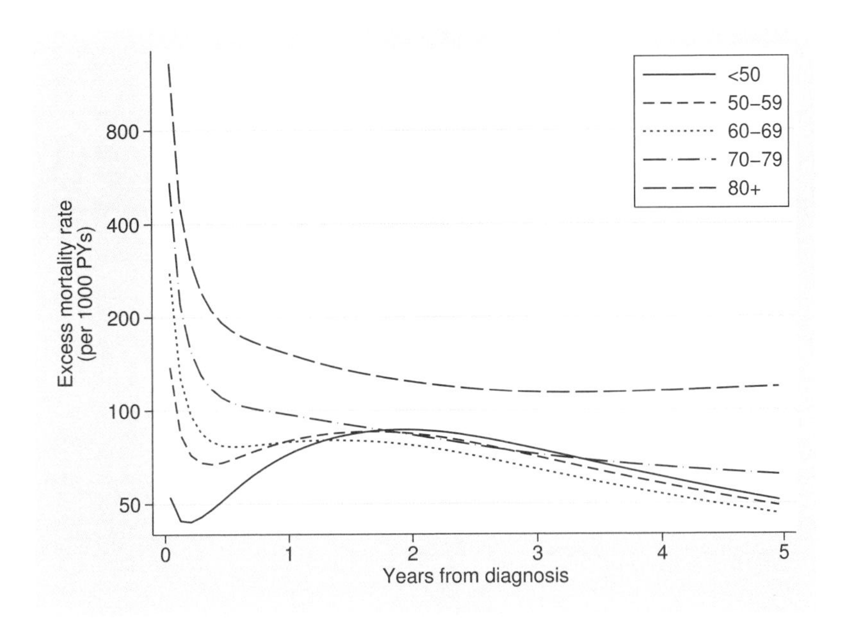

Figure 8.4. England and Wales breast cancer data. Excess mortality rates (log scale) from nonproportional excess-hazards Poisson model incorporating restricted cubic splines. PYs stands for person-years.

The excess mortality rate is shown on the log scale. If proportional excess hazards was a reasonable assumption, there would be an approximately constant difference between the lines. This is clearly not the case. The finding is backed up by the fact that the change in deviance gives $\chi^2_{12} = 2093.86$ ($P < 0.001$) when compared with the proportional excess-hazards model. To compare the age groups, we can calculate the time-dependent excess mortality-rate ratios using the `predictnl` command. The following loop calculates four time-dependent excess mortality-rate ratios, with age < 50 as the reference group.

```
forvalues i = 2/5 {
     predictnl lhr`i´ = _b[agegrp`i´] + _b[age`i´rcs1] * age`i´rcs1 +   ///
          _b[age`i´rcs2] * age`i´rcs2 + _b[age`i´rcs3] * age`i´rcs3,  ///
          ci(lhr`i´_lci lhr`i´_uci)
     gen hr`i´ = exp(lhr`i´)
     gen hr`i´_lci = exp(lhr`i´_lci)
     gen hr`i´_uci = exp(lhr`i´_uci)
}
```

The estimated functions are shown in figure 8.5. The four graphs show a similar pattern with a high initial excess mortality-rate ratio that reduces over time. This is to be expected from the graph of the excess hazard rates shown in figure 8.4, which showed that the youngest age group had an initial rate much lower than the other age groups. The excess mortality-rate ratio for the oldest age group increases near two and one-half years from diagnosis. This is due to a reduction in the excess mortality rate for the denominator, those patients aged less than 50, rather than an increase in the numerator, as is clear from figure 8.4.

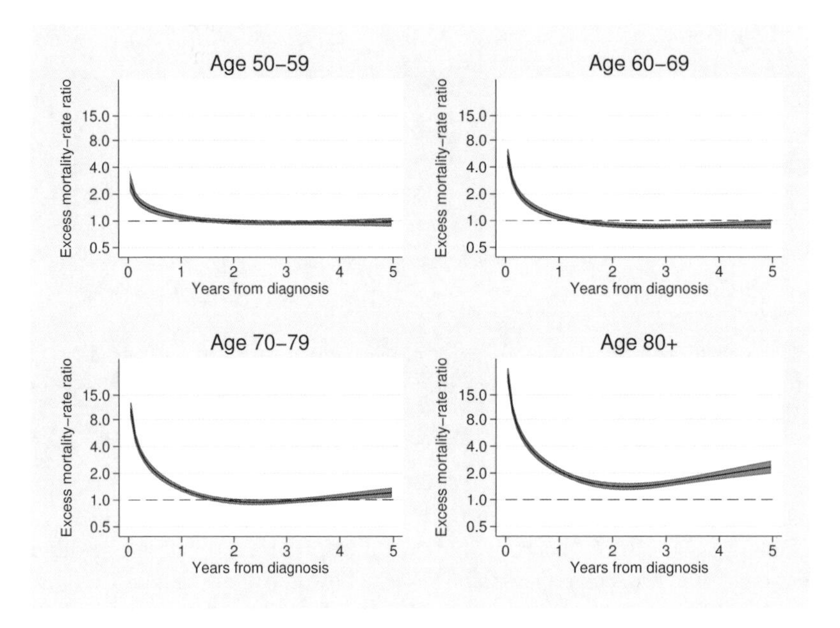

Figure 8.5. England and Wales breast cancer data. Estimated excess mortality-rate ratios with a 95% confidence interval (CI) with age less than 50 as the reference.

There is still, of course, the issue of how many knots to use for both the baseline excess-mortality rate and any time-dependent effects. In section 8.8, we discuss a sensitivity analysis for an RP model extended to relative survival. However, the model selection issues are similar to those for the Poisson model.

8.7 RP models for relative survival

The RP models discussed in chapters 5 and 7 can be extended to relative survival, as was first described by Nelson et al. (2007). One of the key advantages of extending RP models to relative survival is that all-cause, cause-specific, and relative survival can all be analyzed within the same framework.

8.7.1 Likelihood for relative survival models

We can substitute the definitions of the overall hazard and survival functions in (8.1) and (8.2) into the general log-likelihood function for survival data in (1.1). This substitution gives the contribution to the log likelihood for the ith subject as

$$\ln L_i = \ln\{h^*(t_i) + \lambda(t_i)\} + \ln S^*(t_i) + \ln R(t_i) \tag{8.3}$$

The term $\ln S^*(t_i)$ does not depend on any of the model parameters, and so can be excluded when maximizing the likelihood. This is important because it is computationally intensive to calculate the expected survival at the time of death or censoring, $S^*(t_i)$, because it is a cumulative measure. Obtaining the expected mortality rate at the time of death, $h^*(t_i)$, is much simpler, because we just need to merge in the population mortality file on attained age, sex, calendar year, etc. When calculating relative survival in life tables, the expected survival, $S^*(t_i)$, was calculated for each person by splitting the time scale. If we can write down analytical expressions for the excess mortality rate, $\lambda(t)$, and the relative survival function, $R(t)$, we can fit a relative survival model without the need to split the time scale. Given that relative survival models are often fit to very large datasets, we gain a big advantage in computational time.

8.7.2 Proportional cumulative excess hazards

Covariate effects in most relative survival models are fit on the log excess hazard scale

$$h(t) = h^*(t) + \lambda_0 \exp(\boldsymbol{x\beta})$$

For example, the Poisson approach in the previous section was modeled on this scale. RP models are usually fit on the log cumulative-hazard scale. We fit RP models extended to relative survival on the log *cumulative* excess-hazard scale. The overall cumulative hazard, $H(t)$, can be written as

$$H(t) = H^*(t) + \Lambda(t)$$

where $H^*(t)$ is the cumulative expected hazard and $\Lambda(t)$ is the cumulative excess hazard. The cumulative excess hazard is modeled on the log scale as

$$\ln\Lambda(t) = \ln\Lambda_0(t) + \boldsymbol{x\beta}$$

where $\Lambda_0(t)$ is the baseline cumulative excess hazard. Just as proportional cumulative hazards implies PH, so too proportional cumulative excess hazards implies proportional excess hazards. Restricted cubic splines can be used to model the log baseline excess-hazard rate, as before. Thus if $s(\ln t; \boldsymbol{\gamma})$ denotes the restricted cubic spline function of $\ln t$, the relative survival function can be written as

$$R(t) = \exp[-\exp\{s(\ln t; \gamma) + \boldsymbol{x\beta}\}] \tag{8.4}$$

and the excess hazard function can be written as

$$\lambda(t) = \frac{ds(\ln t; \boldsymbol{\gamma})}{dt} \exp\{s(\ln t; \gamma) + \boldsymbol{x\beta}\} \tag{8.5}$$

These are exactly the same expressions we used in standard RP models, but now we use the terms relative survival function rather than survival function and excess hazard function rather than hazard function. If we substitute (8.4) and (8.5) into the definition of the likelihood for relative survival models in (8.3), we get the general likelihood for the extension of RP models to relative survival models on the log cumulative-hazard scale.

8.7.3 RP models on other scales

In chapter 5, we showed that by using different link functions, we could fit models on scales alternative to the more usual cumulative hazard scale. Relative survival models can also be fit on the log cumulative odds and probit scales. In addition, we can extend the Aranda-Ordaz (AO) family of link functions to relative survival. We can fit all of these models with the `stpm2` command. We demonstrate the proportional odds (PO) model and use the AO link function in section 8.7.5. We omit the mathematical details here because the survival and hazard functions for all these alternative scales given in chapter 5 can also be written as relative survival and excess hazard functions and substituted into (8.3).

8.7.4 Application to England and Wales breast cancer data

Before we can fit an RP model extended to relative survival, we need to merge in the expected mortality at death. This can be done as follows:

```
. use ew_breast_ch8, clear
(England and Wales Breast Cancer: All ages)
. stset survtime, failure(dead==1) exit(time 5) id(ident)
  (output omitted)
. generate age = int(min(agediag + _t,99))
. generate year = int(year(datediag) + _t)
. merge m:1 sex region dep year age using popmort_uk, keepusing(rate)
> keep(match)
    Result                           # of obs.
    -----------------------------------------
    not matched                             0
    matched                           115,331  (_merge==3)
    -----------------------------------------
```

First, the data are `stset` with the event defined as death from any cause. We then need to calculate the attained age and calendar year at death so that we can merge in the expected mortality rates. The attained age and calendar year at death are simply the sum of age at diagnosis and `_t` and year of diagnosis and `_t`, respectively, provided that our time variable is stored in years. The expected rates are then merged in from the population mortality file.

We can now fit a relative survival model. The only difference from fitting an overall survival model is the inclusion of the **bhazard()** option. A proportional excess-hazards model for age group is shown below:

```
. stpm2 agegrp2-agegrp5, scale(hazard) df(7) eform bhazard(rate) nolog
Log likelihood = -133767.97                     Number of obs   =     115331

------------------------------------------------------------------------------
             |     exp(b)   Std. Err.      z    P>|z|     [95% Conf. Interval]
-------------+----------------------------------------------------------------
xb           |
     agegrp2 |   1.051629   .0182862     2.90   0.004     1.016393    1.088087
     agegrp3 |   1.072436    .018162     4.13   0.000     1.037424    1.108631
     agegrp4 |   1.410387   .0250455    19.36   0.000     1.362143     1.46034
     agegrp5 |   2.649869   .0510512    50.58   0.000     2.551676    2.751841
       _rcs1 |   2.343311   .0111576   178.85   0.000     2.321544    2.365282
       _rcs2 |   .9680121   .0032421    -9.71   0.000     .9616784    .9743875
       _rcs3 |   .9520213   .0018722   -25.00   0.000     .9483589    .9556979
       _rcs4 |   1.024994   .0013508    18.73   0.000      1.02235    1.027645
       _rcs5 |   1.004471   .0008377     5.35   0.000     1.002831    1.006115
       _rcs6 |   1.002511   .0005577     4.51   0.000     1.001419    1.003605
       _rcs7 |   1.000378   .0003745     1.01   0.312     .9996448    1.001113
       _cons |   .2110661   .0025578  -128.36   0.000      .206112    .2161393
------------------------------------------------------------------------------

. estimates store rs_hazard
```

We have used 7 d.f. for the baseline excess-mortality rate because it gives the lowest Bayes information criterion (BIC) when comparing models with 1 to 10 d.f. The excess mortality-rate ratios are very similar to those excess mortality-rates estimated using the Poisson approach in section 8.6.2. The Poisson approach is only an approximation because we had to define monthly time intervals. With the extension of RP models to relative survival, no splitting of the time scale is required.

The predicted excess mortality rates for each age group can be obtained as follows:

```
. range temptime 0.003 5 200
(115131 missing values generated)

. predict eh_ph1, hazard per(1000) zeros timevar(temptime)

. forvalues i = 2/5 {
  2.        predict eh_ph`i´, hazard per(1000) at(agegrp`i´ 1)
>                   timevar(temptime) zeros
  3. }
```

The resulting estimates are shown in figure 8.6. The general shapes of the excess hazard rate functions are broadly similar to those obtained from the Poisson model using restricted cubic splines (see figure 8.3), but possibly with more of a dip at around half a year. The excess hazard mortality rate is higher initially in all age groups than with the Poisson model because the extension to the RP model is based on individual data as opposed to monthly intervals. The initial prediction for the Poisson model is an average of the excess mortality rate in the first month, a time when the excess mortality rate predicted by the extended RP model is rapidly changing.

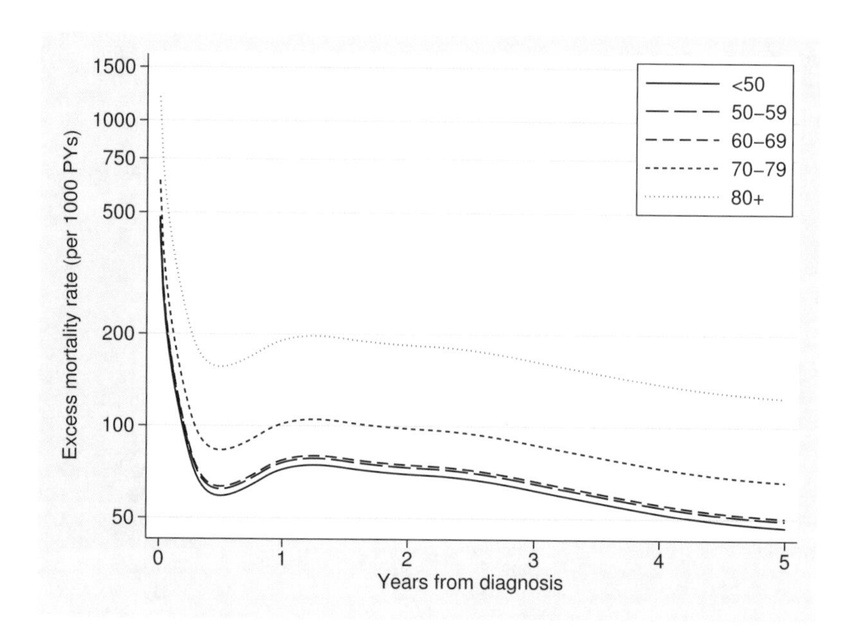

Figure 8.6. England and Wales breast cancer data. Predicted excess mortality rates by age groups from a proportional excess-hazards model. PYs stands for person-years.

8.7.5 Relative survival models on other scales

In chapter 5, we showed that alternative link functions could be used, so that covariate effects were assumed constant on alternative scales. Given that we know that the excess mortality rates are nonproportional, we can try to apply these alternative scales so that the excess mortality-rate ratios become a function of time. We first fit a PO model:

```
. stpm2 agegrp2-agegrp5, scale(odds) df(7) eform bhazard(rate) nolog
Log likelihood = -133560.82                    Number of obs   =     115331
```

	exp(b)	Std. Err.	z	P>|z|	[95% Conf.	Interval]
xb						
agegrp2	1.075605	.0216612	3.62	0.000	1.033977	1.118909
agegrp3	1.118832	.0219419	5.73	0.000	1.076643	1.162675
agegrp4	1.58167	.0331317	21.89	0.000	1.518048	1.647958
agegrp5	3.601549	.087144	52.96	0.000	3.434737	3.776463
_rcs1	2.518479	.0123705	188.04	0.000	2.494349	2.542842
_rcs2	.940196	.0032375	-17.91	0.000	.933872	.9465627
_rcs3	.9394548	.0019535	-30.04	0.000	.9356338	.9432913
_rcs4	1.022296	.0014561	15.48	0.000	1.019446	1.025154
_rcs5	1.003905	.0009332	4.19	0.000	1.002078	1.005736
_rcs6	1.002429	.0006381	3.81	0.000	1.001179	1.00368
_rcs7	1.000291	.0004394	0.66	0.507	.9994306	1.001153
_cons	.2332407	.0032439	-104.66	0.000	.2269685	.2396861

```
. estimates store rs_odds
. predict ehr5_po, hrnum(agegrp5 1) timevar(temptime) ci
```

The odds ratios are in the expected direction, getting larger with increasing age. We can compare the proportional excess-hazard model with the PO model using the AIC and BIC, as follows:

```
. estimates stats rs_hazard rs_odds, n(47692)

-----------------------------------------------------------------------------
       Model |    Obs    ll(null)   ll(model)     df          AIC         BIC
-------------+---------------------------------------------------------------
   rs_hazard |  47692           .     -133768     12     267559.9    267665.2
     rs_odds |  47692           .   -133560.8     12     267145.6    267250.9
-----------------------------------------------------------------------------
               Note:  N=47692 used in calculating BIC
```

Note that n()'s the number of events, not the number of subjects. The PO model has a much lower AIC and BIC, indicating that it is a much better fit. We can also fit the more general AO link function.

```
. stpm2 agegrp2-agegrp5, scale(theta) df(7) bhazard(rate) nolog
Log likelihood = -132941.85                     Number of obs   =     115331

------------------------------------------------------------------------------
             |      Coef.   Std. Err.      z    P>|z|     [95% Conf. Interval]
-------------+----------------------------------------------------------------
xb           |
     agegrp2 |   .4687334   .0523386     8.96   0.000     .3661516    .5713151
     agegrp3 |   .9482299   .0633837    14.96   0.000     .8240002     1.07246
     agegrp4 |   1.950532   .0784701    24.86   0.000     1.796734    2.104331
     agegrp5 |   3.364705   .0891609    37.74   0.000     3.189953    3.539457
       _rcs1 |   2.056262   .0646924    31.79   0.000     1.929467    2.183057
       _rcs2 |  -.5480185   .0301029   -18.20   0.000    -.6070191   -.4890179
       _rcs3 |  -.3047498   .0160757   -18.96   0.000    -.3362577   -.2732419
       _rcs4 |   -.044905    .005773    -7.78   0.000    -.0562199   -.0335901
       _rcs5 |  -.0144737   .0028868    -5.01   0.000    -.0201317   -.0088157
       _rcs6 |  -.0030217   .0020755    -1.46   0.145    -.0070896    .0010462
       _rcs7 |  -.0020584   .0015738    -1.31   0.191     -.005143    .0010262
       _cons |   .4325026   .1276457     3.39   0.001     .1823215    .6826836
-------------+----------------------------------------------------------------
ln_theta     |
       _cons |   2.614265   .0472525    55.33   0.000     2.521652    2.706878
------------------------------------------------------------------------------

. estimates store rs_theta
. predict ehr5_theta, hrnum(agegrp5 1) timevar(temptime) ci
```

Again we can compare the AIC and BIC:

```
. estimates stats rs_hazard rs_odds rs_theta, n(47692)
```

Model	Obs	ll(null)	ll(model)	df	AIC	BIC
rs_hazard	47692	.	-133768	12	267559.9	267665.2
rs_odds	47692	.	-133560.8	12	267145.6	267250.9
rs_theta	47692	.	-132941.8	13	265909.7	266023.7

Note: N=47692 used in calculating BIC

The AIC and BIC for the AO link function are even lower than for the PO model. The parameter $\theta = \exp(2.614) = 13.6$, a long way from either a proportional excess-hazards model ($\theta = 0$) or PO model ($\theta = 1$). However, the big disadvantage of using this link function is that it is difficult to interpret the model parameters. We can, however, plot the predicted excess mortality-rate ratios from each model. These ratios are shown in figure 8.7, which compares the oldest age group (80 +) with the youngest (< 50). The horizontal reference line shows the estimated excess mortality-rate ratio from the proportional excess-hazards model. Both the PO model and the model with the AO link function show a declining excess mortality-rate ratio as a function of time. The model using the AO link function shows a much more rapidly decreasing function. The CIs are very narrow because of the large number of subjects in the analysis.

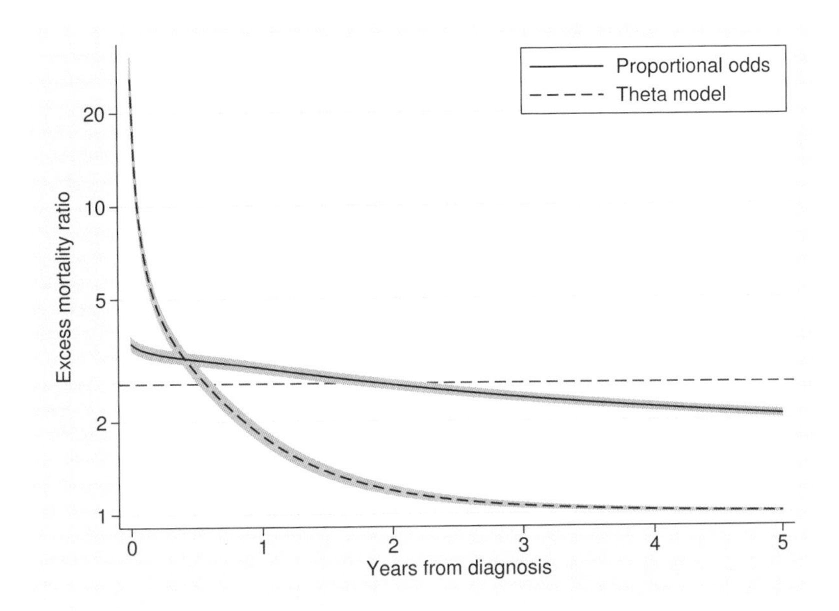

Figure 8.7. England and Wales breast cancer data. Excess mortality-rate ratios for age group 80 + compared with those aged < 50 from a PO model and a model using the AO link function. The corresponding estimate from a proportional excess-hazards model is denoted by the horizontal reference line.

Although it is possible to model time-dependence of the excess mortality-rate ratios by modeling on the PO or using the AO link function, we feel it is generally better in these large datasets to model on the log cumulative excess-hazard scale; this is because we generally want to report differences as excess mortality-rate ratios. Researchers are more used to seeing and being able to interpret HRs. When we are modeling several covariates, we can probably assume proportional excess hazards for at least some of them. With models on the log cumulative excess-hazard scale, we can conveniently make that assumption.

8.7.6 Time-dependent effects

The extension to time-dependent effects follows the same principles as for standard RP models. The following code uses 7 d.f. for the baseline excess-mortality rate and 3 d.f. for each of the four time-dependent effects for age group. We discuss some model selection issues in section 8.8.

```
. stpm2 agegrp2-agegrp5, scale(hazard) df(7) bhazard(rate)
> tvc(agegrp2-agegrp5) dftvc(3) nolog
Log likelihood = -132695.39                       Number of obs   =     115331
```

	Coef.	Std. Err.	z	P>|z|	[95% Conf.	Interval]
xb						
agegrp2	.1570058	.0198093	7.93	0.000	.1181803	.1958313
agegrp3	.2443474	.0189302	12.91	0.000	.2072448	.2814499
agegrp4	.5389824	.0195635	27.55	0.000	.5006387	.5773261
agegrp5	1.116983	.0216114	51.68	0.000	1.074625	1.15934
_rcs1	1.276374	.0246041	51.88	0.000	1.228151	1.324597
_rcs2	-.0551114	.0172072	-3.20	0.001	-.088837	-.0213858
_rcs3	.012761	.0041103	3.10	0.002	.0047049	.0208171
_rcs4	.0533987	.0027366	19.51	0.000	.048035	.0587624
_rcs5	.012423	.0010691	11.62	0.000	.0103275	.0145184
_rcs6	.0033881	.0005763	5.88	0.000	.0022586	.0045176
_rcs7	.0002432	.0003847	0.63	0.527	-.0005108	.0009972
_rcs_ageg~21	-.2459719	.0291705	-8.43	0.000	-.303145	-.1887988
_rcs_ageg~22	.002394	.0199957	0.12	0.905	-.0367968	.0415848
_rcs_ageg~23	-.0277671	.0065719	-4.23	0.000	-.0406477	-.0148865
_rcs_ageg~31	-.4132617	.0267016	-15.48	0.000	-.4655959	-.3609274
_rcs_ageg~32	.0288664	.0184079	1.57	0.117	-.0072124	.0649452
_rcs_ageg~33	-.0563371	.0061226	-9.20	0.000	-.0683372	-.044337
_rcs_ageg~41	-.5315413	.0260559	-20.40	0.000	-.5826099	-.4804727
_rcs_ageg~42	.0590587	.0180795	3.27	0.001	.0236236	.0944938
_rcs_ageg~43	-.0837796	.0061977	-13.52	0.000	-.0959268	-.0716324
_rcs_ageg~51	-.6173929	.0260023	-23.74	0.000	-.6683565	-.5664292
_rcs_ageg~52	.0686192	.0181099	3.79	0.000	.0331243	.104114
_rcs_ageg~53	-.1054197	.006716	-15.70	0.000	-.1185828	-.0922565
_cons	-1.730399	.0143465	-120.62	0.000	-1.758517	-1.70228

The predicted excess mortality rates can be obtained as follows:

```
predict eh_tvc1, hazard per(1000) timevar(temptime) zeros
predict rs_tvc1, survival timevar(temptime) zeros
forvalues i = 2/5 {
     predict eh_tvc`i´, hazard per(1000) at(agegrp`i´ 1) ///
          timevar(temptime) zeros
     predict rs_tvc`i´, survival at(agegrp`i´ 1) timevar(temptime) zeros
}
```

The resulting estimates are shown in figure 8.8. The general pattern is similar to the corresponding excess mortality rates obtained from the Poisson model. As with the proportional excess-hazards models, there is an initially higher excess mortality rate compared with the Poisson models, because the extended RP model uses individual-level data.

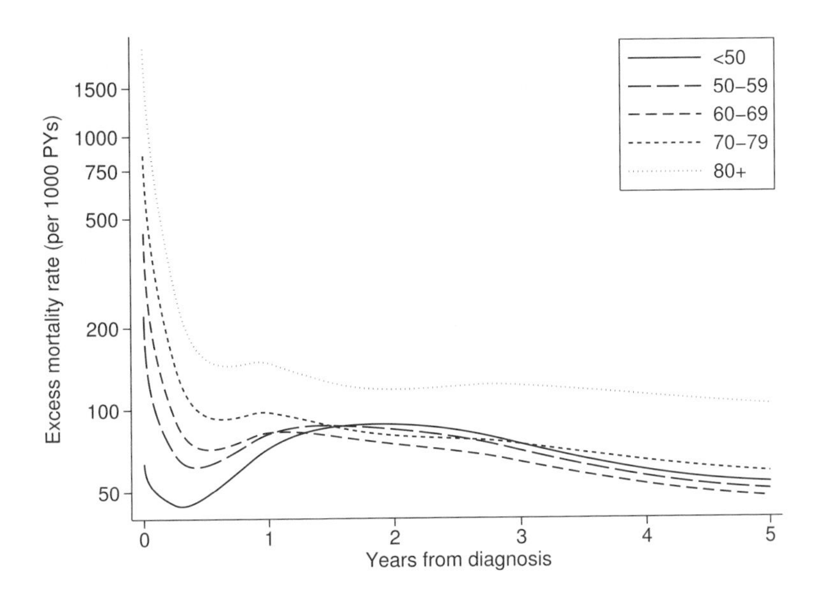

Figure 8.8. England and Wales breast cancer data. Predicted excess mortality rates by age group from a nonproportional excess-hazards model. PYs stands for person-years.

We now want to quantify differences between the groups. The usual way to do so is through the excess mortality-rate ratio. However, as we showed in chapter 7, there are also advantages to quantifying absolute differences. In a relative survival model, this can be achieved by estimating differences in the excess mortality rate and differences in the relative survival function of the groups of interest. We can use the **hrnumerator()**, **hdiff1()**, and **sdiff1()** options to predict the excess mortality-rate ratios, the difference in excess mortality rates, and the difference in relative survival, respectively, for each age group, with the youngest age group (< 50) as the reference group. We do not need to use the **hrdenominator()**, **hdiff2()**, and **sdiff2()** options because by default these set all covariate values to zero, which is what we want, to make the youngest age group the reference.

The predictions of the excess mortality-rate ratios, the difference in excess mortality rates, and the difference in relative survival can be calculated in a loop.

```
forvalues i = 2/5 {
     predict ehr`i´_tvc, hrnum(agegrp`i´ 1) timevar(temptime) ci
     predict ehdiff`i´_tvc, hdiff1(agegrp`i´ 1) timevar(temptime) per(1000) ci
     predict rsdiff`i´_tvc, sdiff1(agegrp`i´ 1) timevar(temptime) ci
}
```

Figure 8.9 shows the estimated excess mortality-rate ratios by age group. These are similar to the time-dependent excess mortality-rate ratios obtained from the Poisson model using restricted cubic splines (see figure 8.5). This should not be too surprising because both models are attempting to estimate the same thing; we should be concerned if we came to different conclusions. The main difference is that the excess mortality-rate ratios start from a higher level than in the Poisson model for the same reason as stated above; that is, we have individual data, and thus the initial prediction is at one day for the extended RP model and 0.5 months for the Poisson model.

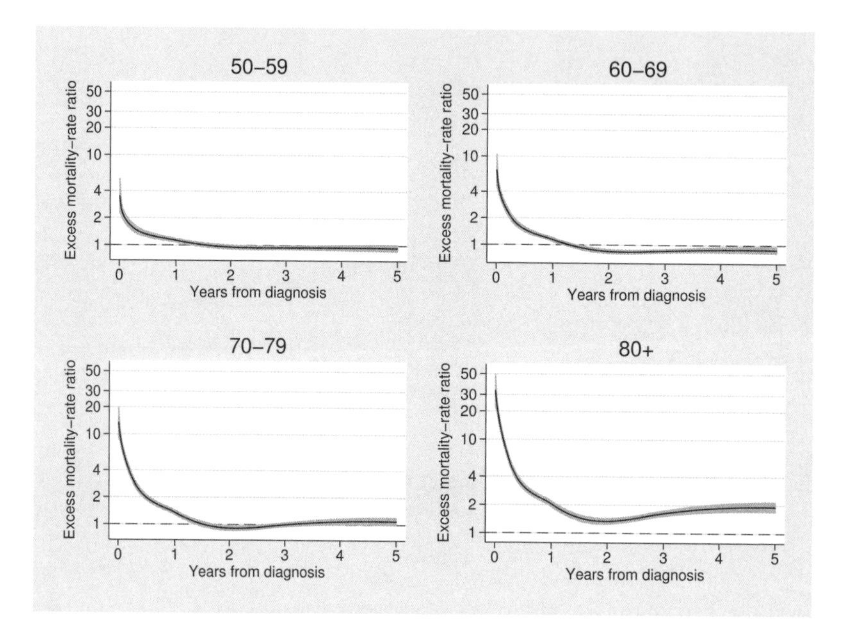

Figure 8.9. England and Wales breast cancer data. Excess mortality-rate ratios by age group from a nonproportional excess-hazards model.

Figure 8.10 shows the difference in the excess mortality rates by age group. There is a problem in plotting these graphs because there is a very high initial excess mortality rate for the oldest age groups, which makes visualizing the difference difficult if we want to show the graphs on the same scale (which we should!). For this reason, we have chosen not to plot the difference in excess mortality rates for the first month for the oldest age group. It is important to make clear to the reader that such a decision to exclude some observations has been made.

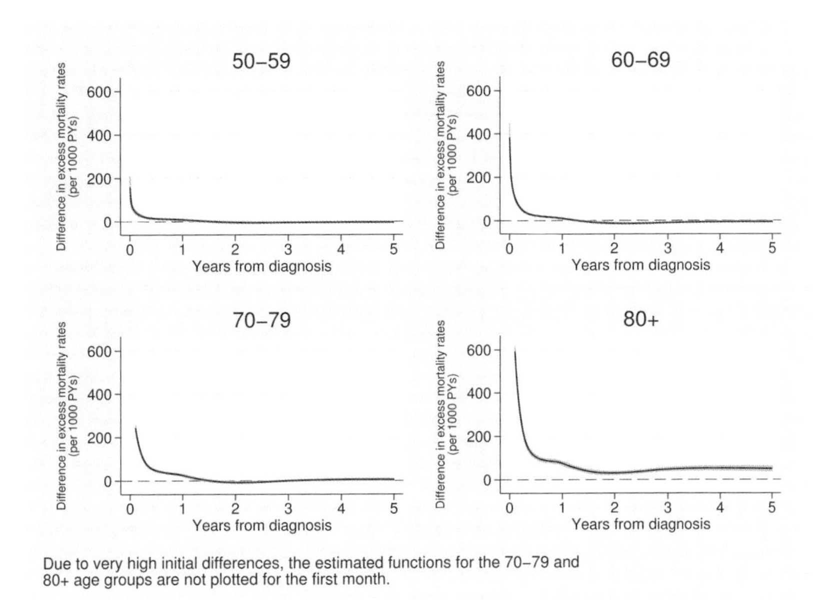

Figure 8.10. England and Wales breast cancer data. Difference in excess mortality rates by age group from a nonproportional excess-hazards model. PYs stands for person-years.

Figure 8.11 shows the predicted relative-survival function for each age group. The oldest age group has a much steeper initial decline in the relative survival function than the other groups. This is to be expected from the high excess HR in the first half-year after diagnosis, as shown in figure 8.9. Also shown on the graph are the estimated values of relative survival obtained from the life-table based approach described in section 8.5. The estimates from the two approaches are in good agreement.

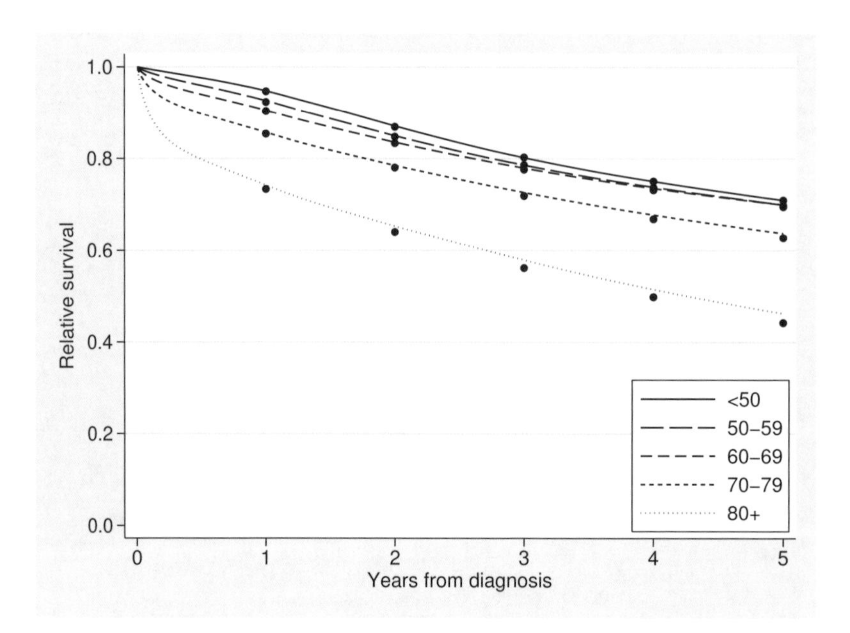

Figure 8.11. England and Wales breast cancer data. Predicted relative survival by age group from a nonproportional excess-hazards model. The dots show life-table estimates.

We can quantify differences in relative survival by obtaining the difference between any two relative survival curves. These are shown in figure 8.12 with the youngest age group as the baseline. The steep initial reduction for the older age groups is clear.

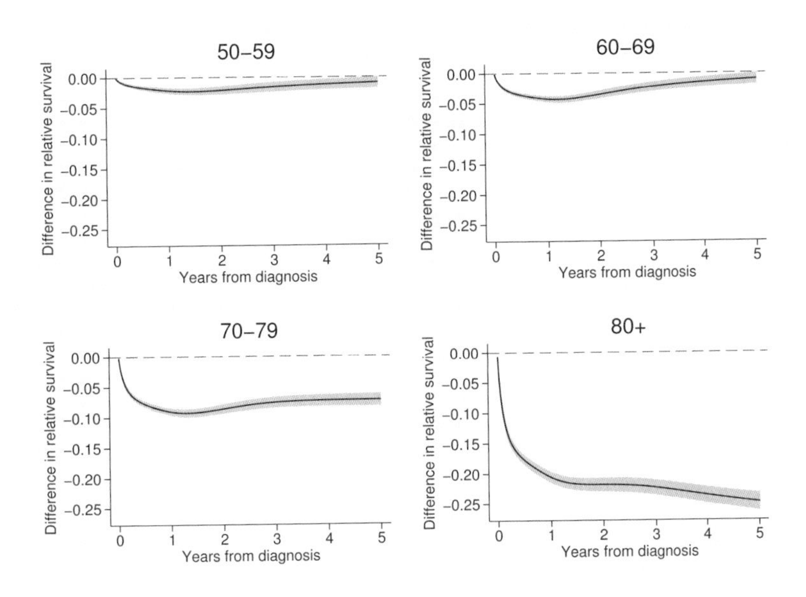

Figure 8.12. England and Wales breast cancer data. Difference in relative survival by age group from a nonproportional excess-hazards model. The comparison group is women aged < 50.

8.8 Some comments on model selection

Because most analyses of relative survival include all cases of a particular cancer within a country or large region, they tend to involve large datasets. Analysis of such large datasets raises some interesting model selection issues. For example, nearly everything will be significant at the 5% level. The extremely narrow CIs from the England and Wales breast cancer data illustrate this well. The issue here is that having something statistically significant at the 5% level does not mean a difference is important from a subject-matter point of view. For example, we would probably not be too concerned with a relative survival difference of 0.5% at five years between males and females, even if it were statistically significant. Analysis of population-based cancer studies are often used for descriptive purposes. The analyst generally needs to incorporate background medical knowledge into which covariates are included and how those covariates should be modeled.

When using splines (as we have done for modeling baseline distributions and time-dependent effects), a key question is clearly how many knots to use. It is important that we regard the spline functions not as some kind of truth in themselves but as a useful tool to provide an approximation to some truth, given that various modeling assumptions are correct. A sensitivity analysis can be an effective means of persuading both ourselves and others that our conclusions are not sensitive to our choice of knots. An example of a small sensitivity analysis is shown below.

We fit 10 different models to the England and Wales breast cancer data using a variety of knots for the baseline and time-dependent effects. The number of d.f. for the baseline and time-dependent effects are shown in table 8.1.

Table 8.1. Degrees of freedom used for the baseline excess hazard and the time-dependent effect of age group for a sensitivity analysis.

Model	degrees of freedom	
	Baseline	Time-dependent
1	3	3
2	5	3
3	5	5
4	7	3
5	7	5
6	7	7
7	9	3
8	9	5
9	9	7
10	9	9

We could have made things more complicated by having different d.f. for the TD effect each age group, but our main aim is to see if using different d.f. leads to different conclusions. The models were fit in a loop using the following code:

```
local model1 df(3) dftvc(3) tvc(agegrp2-agegrp5)
local model2 df(5) dftvc(3) tvc(agegrp2-agegrp5)
local model3 df(5) dftvc(5) tvc(agegrp2-agegrp5)
local model4 df(7) dftvc(3) tvc(agegrp2-agegrp5)
local model5 df(7) dftvc(5) tvc(agegrp2-agegrp5)
local model6 df(7) dftvc(7) tvc(agegrp2-agegrp5)
local model7 df(9) dftvc(3) tvc(agegrp2-agegrp5)
local model8 df(9) dftvc(5) tvc(agegrp2-agegrp5)
local model9 df(9) dftvc(7) tvc(agegrp2-agegrp5)
local model10 df(9) dftvc(9) tvc(agegrp2-agegrp5)
forvalues i = 1/10 {
      stpm2 agegrp2-agegrp5, scale(hazard) `model`i'' bhazard(rate) nolog
      estimates store model`i'
      predict eh0_m`i', hazard zeros per(1000)
      predict rs0_m`i', survival zeros
      predict ehr5_m`i', hrnum(agegrp5 1) ci
      predict ehdiff5_m`i', hdiff1(agegrp5 1) per(1000) ci
      predict rsdiff5_m`i', sdiff1(agegrp5 1) ci
}
```

The baseline excess-mortality rate and relative survival functions are estimated together with the excess mortality-rate ratio, excess mortality-rate difference, and relative survival difference, comparing the most deprived group with the least deprived group.

As an initial model selection guide, we can inspect the AIC and BIC. These are shown in the output below:

```
. qui count if _d == 1
. estimates stats model*, n(`r(N)')
```

Model	Obs	ll(null)	ll(model)	df	AIC	BIC
model1	47692	.	-132948.5	20	265937	266112.5
model2	47692	.	-132815.9	22	265675.7	265868.7
model3	47692	.	-132785.1	30	265630.2	265893.4
model4	47692	.	-132695.4	24	265438.8	265649.3
model5	47692	.	-132694.5	32	265453	265733.7
model6	47692	.	-132683.5	40	265447.1	265798
model7	47692	.	-132659	26	265370	265598.1
model8	47692	.	-132651.5	34	265371	265669.3
model9	47692	.	-132643.4	42	265370.8	265739.2
model10	47692	.	-132639.2	50	265378.3	265817

Note: N=47692 used in calculating BIC

The lowest AIC and BIC is for model 7, which has 9 d.f. for the baseline excess-mortality rate and 3 d.f. for the time-dependent effects. The AIC and BIC do not always agree in these large datasets. Because BIC has a much larger penalty term for each additional d.f., AIC usually selects a more complicated model. This is illustrated by inspection of models 8 and 9, which also have 9 d.f. for the baseline excess-mortality rate, but have 5 and 7 d.f., respectively, for the time-dependent effects. The AIC values for models 8 and 9 are only slightly higher than for model 7, whereas the BIC is substantially higher.

To rely solely on the AIC or BIC is inadvisable. We want to see how the shapes of our excess mortality rates, relative survival functions, and any of the other measures used to quantify differences between groups change with differing d.f.

Figure 8.13 shows the baseline excess-mortality rates for the 10 different models. Model 1 has the darkest line, and model 10 the lightest. We have distinguished model 1 with a thick line because it provides a poor fit when it comes to comparing groups. The general shape of the baseline excess-mortality rate is similar among the models. There is some variation in the location of the two turning points. For example, the models with 9 d.f. for the baseline have the first turning point at about three months, whilst the models with 3 d.f. for the baseline have the first turning point before one month.

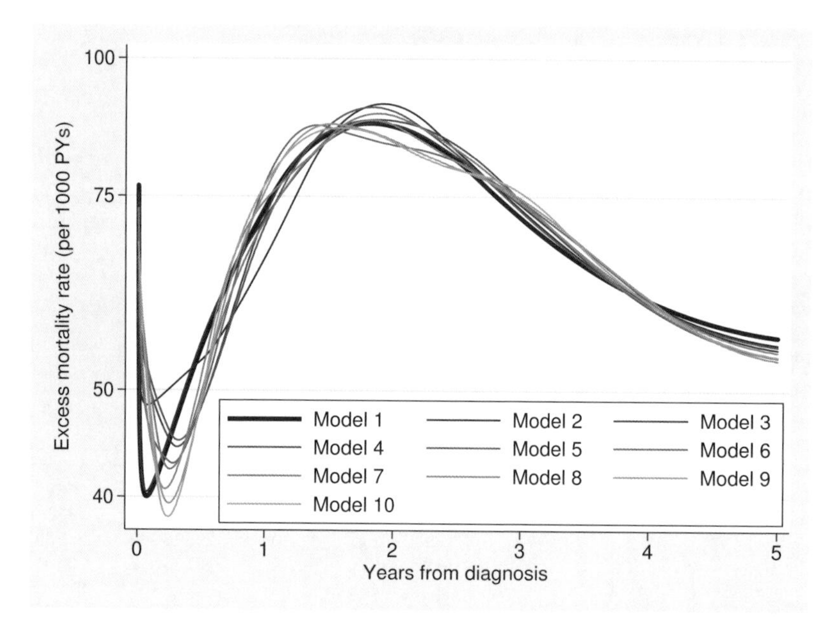

Figure 8.13. England and Wales breast cancer data. Baseline excess-mortality rate for the 10 models in the sensitivity analysis. PYs stands for person-years.

Figure 8.14 shows the estimated baseline relative-survival function for the 10 different models. The agreement is so good among the different models that it appears that there is only one line drawn (there are actually 10). Because relative survival is a cumulative measure, we would expect that the agreement would be better than for the excess mortality rate. The implication of this is that if interest lies solely in estimation of relative survival, then the choice of number and location of the knots is less important than if interest lies in estimation of the excess mortality rate.

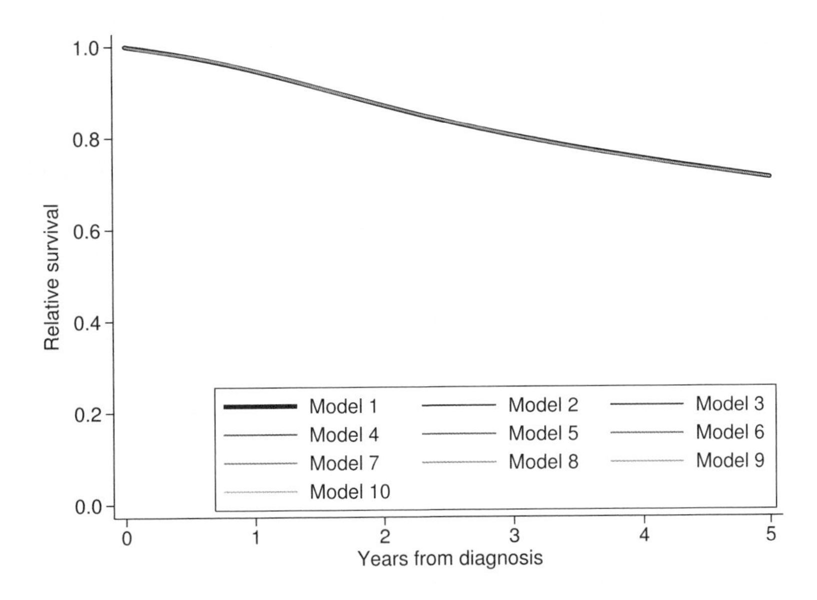

Figure 8.14. England and Wales breast cancer data. Baseline relative survival for the 10 models in the sensitivity analysis.

Figure 8.15 shows the time-dependent excess mortality-rate ratio for age group 5 (compared with age group 1). The shapes are similar among the different models. As the number of d.f. increases for the time-dependent effect, there are more humps and bumps in the estimated function. It is also of interest to compare the 95% CIs. Figure 8.16 shows the models with 9 d.f. for the baseline excess-mortality rate and 3, 5, 7, and 9 d.f. for the time-dependent effect. The extra humps and bumps can be seen for model 10 (9 d.f. for the time-dependent effect), but although this model is likely to be overfitted, our conclusions would be very similar. The width of the 95% CIs increases as we use more parameters to model the time-dependent effect.

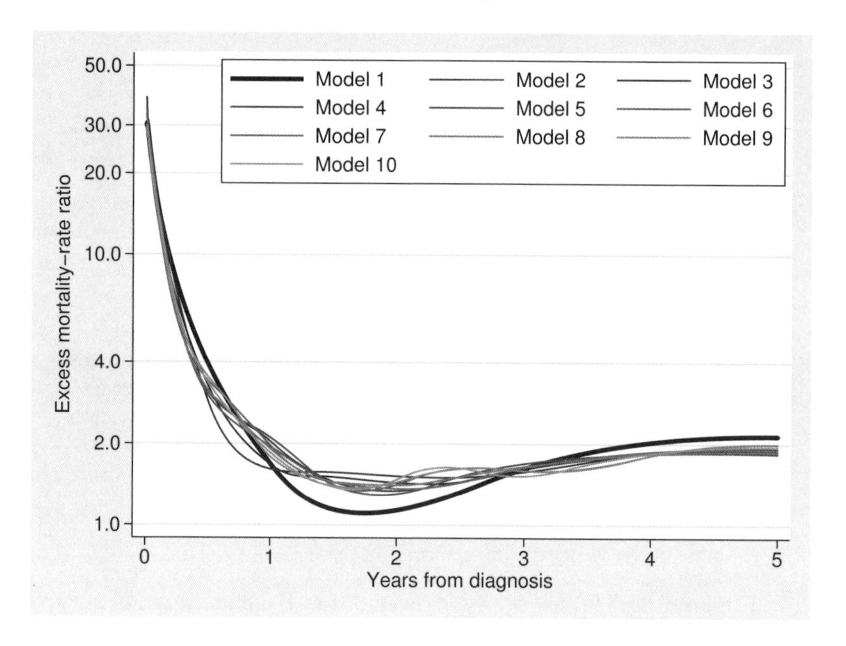

Figure 8.15. England and Wales breast cancer data. Excess mortality-rate ratios from 10 models using different numbers of knots.

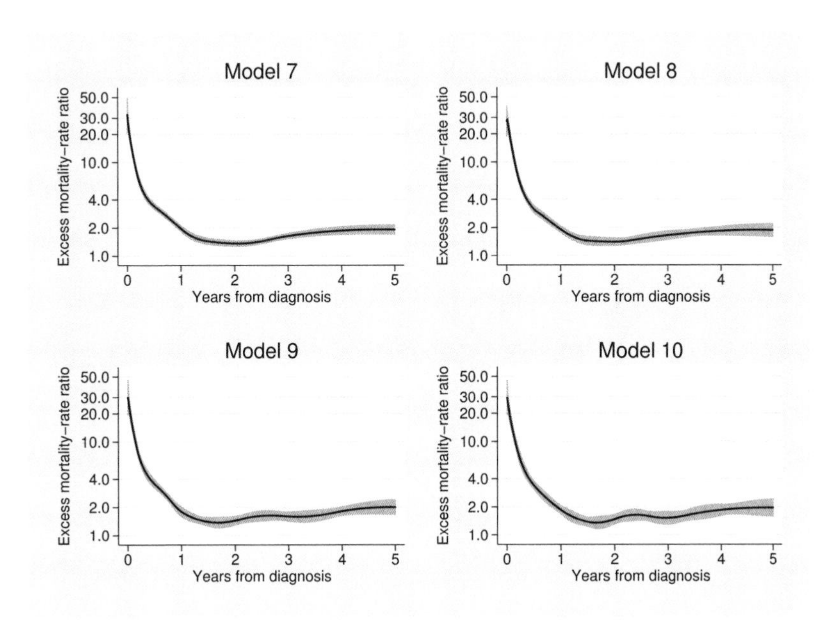

Figure 8.16. England and Wales breast cancer data. Excess mortality-rate ratios for models with 9 d.f. for the baseline excess-mortality rate and 3, 5, 7, or 9 d.f. for the time-dependent effects.

Figure 8.17 shows the estimated difference in the excess mortality rate comparing the oldest age group with the youngest age group. With the exception of model 1 (3 d.f. for baseline and 3 d.f. for time-dependent effects), the general pattern is similar across the models. Overfitting is apparent from the humps and bumps seen in the models with higher d.f.

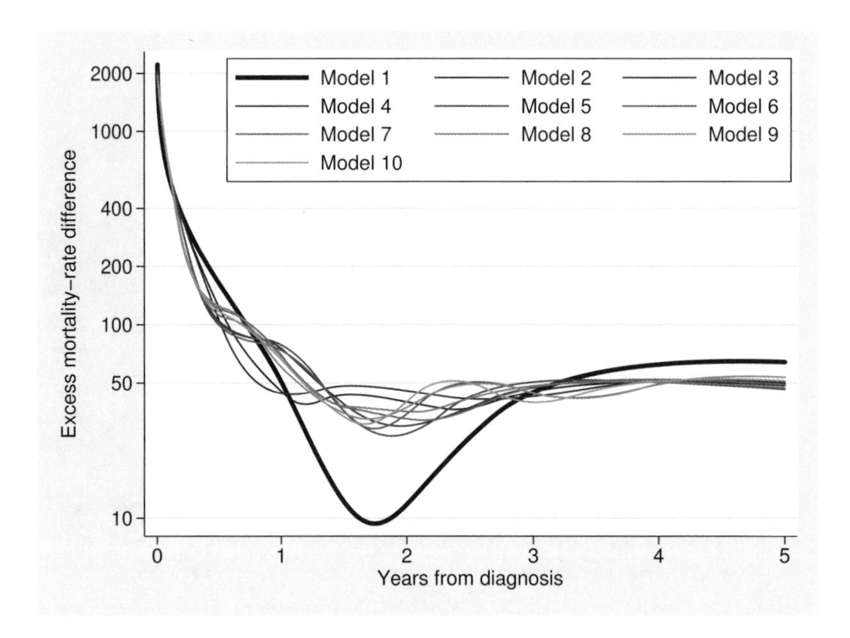

Figure 8.17. England and Wales breast cancer data. Excess mortality-rate differences for the 10 different models in the sensitivity analysis.

Figure 8.18 shows the difference in the estimated relative-survival curves. Again, with the exception of model 1, there is fairly good agreement among the various models.

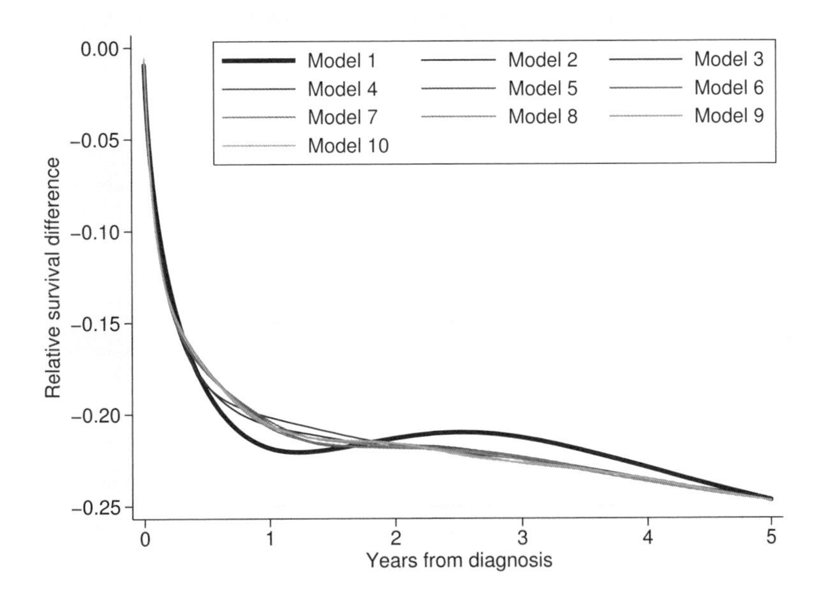

Figure 8.18. England and Wales breast cancer data. Differences in relative survival for the 10 different models in the sensitivity analysis.

In summary, the sensitivity analysis has shown us that we do not get exactly the same functions when we vary the number of knots. We should not be surprised by this. What is important is the similarity in our conclusions. If splines provide us with an approximation to some true effect, then having a few extra wiggles, and humps, and bumps should not be too much of problem. We should of course be careful not to overinterpret some of these minor features, and perhaps more importantly, we should guide our collaborators not to overinterpret them, either.

8.9 Age as a continuous variable

So far in this chapter, we have treated age as a categorical variable by categorizing it into five groups. By doing this, we implicitly assume that the excess mortality rate and predicted relative survival are constant within each of the five groups. Relative survival generally depends on age. Often both younger and older patients are at increased risk. Cancer is often more aggressive in younger patients, and older patients tend to be more frail and suffer from greater comorbidity. By analyzing the effect of age in groups, we may potentially miss some important features of our data. It is also statistically more efficient to treat age as a continuous variable. In section 7.7, we used splines to model the time-dependent effect of age in an all-cause analysis. In this section, we use FPs to investigate the nonlinear effect of age on the excess mortality rate and relative survival.

We start by fitting a proportional excess-hazards model, but we extend it to include a time-dependent effect later in this section. We use the `fracpoly` "prefix" command, which fits 44 different models with all combinations of first-order FPs and second-order fractional polynomial (FP2) models using the default set of powers.

```
. fracpoly, center(60): stpm2 agediag, df(7) scale(hazard) bhazard(rate)
........
-> gen double Iaged__1 = X^2-36 if e(sample)
-> gen double Iaged__2 = X^3-216 if e(sample)
   (where: X = agediag/10)
Iteration 0:   log likelihood = -134281.11
Iteration 1:   log likelihood = -133525.11
Iteration 2:   log likelihood = -133521.09
Iteration 3:   log likelihood = -133521.09
Log likelihood = -133521.09                     Number of obs   =     115331

------------------------------------------------------------------------------
             |      Coef.   Std. Err.      z    P>|z|     [95% Conf. Interval]
-------------+----------------------------------------------------------------
xb           |
    Iaged__1 |  -.0672357   .0024638   -27.29   0.000    -.0720645   -.0624068
    Iaged__2 |   .0085039   .0002474    34.37   0.000      .008019    .0089889
       _rcs1 |   .8554534   .0047402   180.47   0.000     .8461627     .864744
       _rcs2 |  -.0328773   .0033371    -9.85   0.000    -.0394179   -.0263366
       _rcs3 |  -.0493122   .0019622   -25.13   0.000    -.0531579   -.0454664
       _rcs4 |   .0244528   .0013153    18.59   0.000     .0218749    .0270308
       _rcs5 |   .0044998   .0008343     5.39   0.000     .0028646    .0061351
       _rcs6 |   .0024569   .0005574     4.41   0.000     .0013645    .0035494
       _rcs7 |   .0003821   .0003757     1.02   0.309    -.0003542    .0011185
       _cons |  -1.556453   .0076264  -204.09   0.000    -1.571401   -1.541506
------------------------------------------------------------------------------
Deviance:267042.18. Best powers of agediag among 44 models fit: 2 3.
```

The `center(60)` option centers the age at diagnosis at 60 years, thereby setting 60 as the reference age. The best-fitting model is an FP2 model with powers of 2 and 3. The parameters are difficult to interpret individually, so we need to make some predictions.

```
. generate ageround = round(agediag)
. bysort ageround: gen ageflag = _n==1
. predict hr_age if ageflag, hrnum(Iaged__1 . Iaged__2 .) ci
```

Because this is a large dataset, we do not want a separate prediction for every single observation, and so we have rounded age at diagnosis. We created a flag so that we obtain only one prediction for each unique rounded age at diagnosis. Note the use of the `hrnum(Iaged__1 . Iaged__2 .)` option. `Iaged__1` and `Iaged__2` are the FP variables created by `fracpoly`—that is, transformations of age with powers 2 and 3. The use of `.` tells Stata to use the observed values of `Iaged__1` and `Iaged__2`. The predicted excess mortality-rate ratio is shown in figure 8.19. The graph shows that both younger patients and older patients are at increased risk compared with those aged 60. The CIs are narrow because of the large size of the dataset.

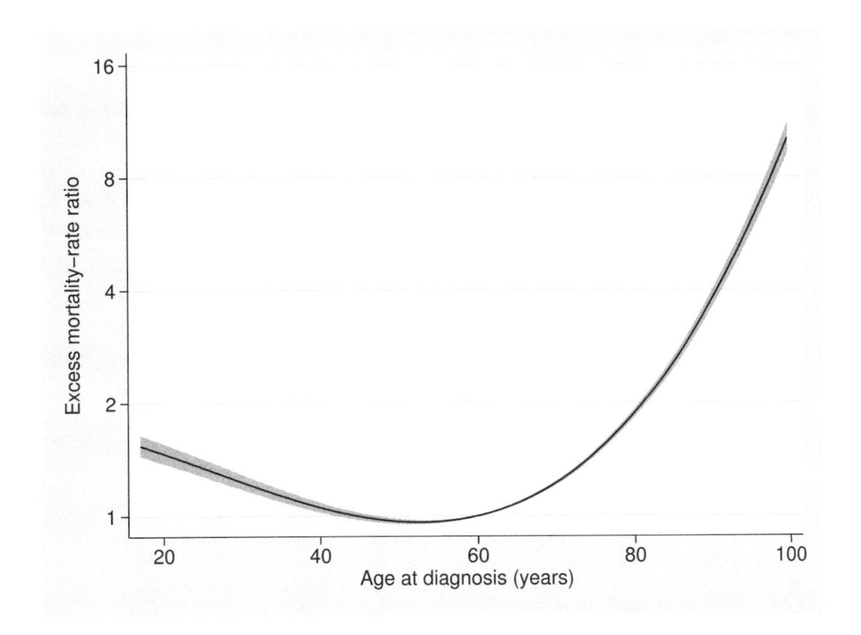

Figure 8.19. England and Wales breast cancer. Excess mortality-rate ratio for age at diagnosis from a proportional excess-hazards model. The effect of age is modeled using FPs.

We now wish to extend the model to include time-dependent effects. We keep the FP2 model with powers $(2,3)$. We form interactions between the two FP variables and some restricted cubic-spline variables by specifying the FP variables in the `tvc()` option.

```
. gen age_fp1 = Iaged__1

. gen age_fp2 = Iaged__2

. stpm2 age_fp1 age_fp2, df(7) scale(hazard) bhazard(rate) nolog
> tvc(age_fp1 age_fp2) dftvc(3)

Log likelihood = -132486.13                     Number of obs   =     115331

------------------------------------------------------------------------------
             |      Coef.   Std. Err.      z    P>|z|     [95% Conf. Interval]
-------------+----------------------------------------------------------------
xb           |
     age_fp1 |  -.0407644   .0026383   -15.45   0.000    -.0459354   -.0355935
     age_fp2 |   .0060757   .0002647    22.96   0.000      .005557    .0065945
       _rcs1 |   .9501846   .0073354   129.53   0.000     .9358075    .9645617
       _rcs2 |  -.0308951   .0051743    -5.97   0.000    -.0410365   -.0207536
       _rcs3 |  -.0214897   .0024564    -8.75   0.000    -.0263041   -.0166753
       _rcs4 |   .0298028   .0014904    20.00   0.000     .0268817     .032724
       _rcs5 |   .0055425   .0008638     6.42   0.000     .0038495    .0072354
       _rcs6 |   .0023264   .0005756     4.04   0.000     .0011982    .0034545
       _rcs7 |   .0002911   .0003862     0.75   0.451    -.0004659     .001048
_rcs_age_~11 |  -.0378008   .0025692   -14.71   0.000    -.0428363   -.0327653
_rcs_age_~12 |   .0039975   .0018113     2.21   0.027     .0004474    .0075476
_rcs_age_~13 |  -.0055942   .0008159    -6.86   0.000    -.0071934    -.003995
_rcs_age_~21 |   .0027428   .0002344    11.70   0.000     .0022833    .0032023
_rcs_age_~22 |  -.0002396   .0001665    -1.44   0.150     -.000566    .0000868
_rcs_age_~23 |   .0003639   .0000799     4.55   0.000     .0002073    .0005206
       _cons |  -1.582153   .0077879  -203.15   0.000    -1.597417   -1.566889
------------------------------------------------------------------------------
```

We have used 3 d.f. for the time-dependent effects for each of the FP variables. Interpretation of individual parameters is difficult (perhaps impossible), so we need to obtain some useful predictions.

```
local ref1 = (60/10)^2 - 36
local ref2 = (60/10)^3 - 216
foreach age in 30 40 50 70 80 90 {
     local c1 = (`age´/10)^2 - 36
     local c2 = (`age´/10)^3 - 216
     predict hr_age_`age´, hrnum(age_fp1 `c1´ age_fp2 `c2´) ///
          hrdenom(age_fp1 `ref1´ age_fp2 `ref2´) ci
}
```

We have defined the values of the two FP variables at the reference age of 60. **fracpoly** has automatically rescaled age at diagnosis by dividing it by 10. We can estimate the time-dependent excess mortality-rate ratios, with 60 as the reference age, through use of the **hrnum()** and **hrdenom()** options. Because there is a separate excess mortality ratio for each unique age at diagnosis, we select some ages of interest, these are 30, 40, 50, 70, 80, and 90.

The predicted time-dependent excess mortality-rate ratios for the selected ages are shown in figure 8.20. As before, all comparisons are with a woman aged 60. The pattern is similar for women aged 30, 40, and 50. Up to one year, their excess mortality-rate ratio is less than 1. After that, women aged 30 and 40 have a higher excess mortality rate, whereas women aged 50 have an excess mortality rate similar to that of a 60-year-old. Women of 70 and older have an initially higher excess mortality rate than 60-year-old women. Their excess mortality rate ratio remains above 1 and gets larger with increasing age.

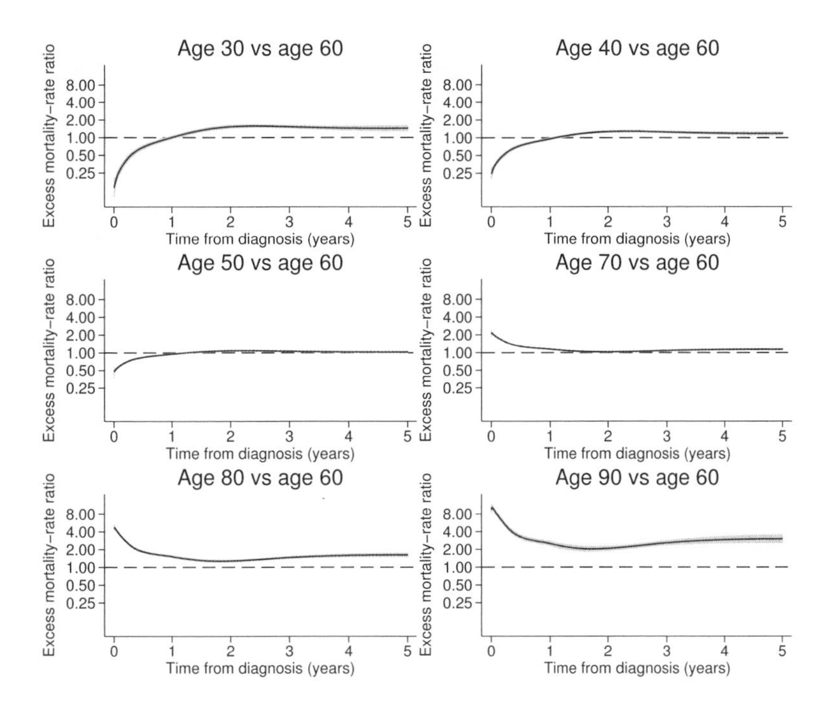

Figure 8.20. England and Wales breast cancer data. Excess mortality-rate ratios for a selection of ages, with age 60 as the reference. The effect of age is modeled using FPs with time-dependent effects.

8.10 Concluding remarks

Relative survival is often considered separately from more standard survival analysis. In population-based studies, for example, it has been common for descriptive analyses to be based on life-table based estimates of relative survival, with the modeling using an all-cause Cox model. We have aimed to show in this chapter that the modeling issues in relative survival are extremely similar to those encountered in the previous chapters in the book. A key advantage of using RP models is that it is easy to fit models for overall, cause-specific, and relative survival in the same analytical framework.

9 Further topics

9.1 Introduction

In this chapter, we describe the application of flexible parametric modeling in seven disparate topic areas:

- estimating the number needed to treat from clinical trials data
- modeling entire distributions using Royston–Parmar (RP) models
- modeling data with multiple events per patient
- fitting Bayesian RP models
- modeling data with competing risks
- performing period analysis
- estimating the crude probability of death in a relative survival context

Each topic is of interest in its own right. Our main aim is to show how parametric approaches may be helpful in these areas and how we can use the `stpm2` software to fit the required models. We conclude the chapter and the book with some remarks about further extensions and applications of flexible parametric models.

9.2 Number needed to treat

The number of patients who need to be treated to prevent one additional event is known as the number needed to treat (NNT) (Cook and Sackett 1995). It is widely used in clinical trials to quantify treatment benefit when there is a binary outcome. The NNT for a binary outcome is simply the reciprocal of the risk difference. Let p_0 denote the probability of the event in the control arm, and p_1 the probability of the event in the experimental arm. The risk difference is $p_0 - p_1$, and thus

$$\text{NNT} = \frac{1}{p_0 - p_1}$$

The NNT varies according to the length of follow-up. For example, we would expect to see a different NNT if follow-up were one or five years. In the analysis of time-to-event data, the risk difference is the difference in survival curves, and it will clearly vary over follow-up time (Altman 1998). If $S_0(t)$ is the survival function for the control arm, and $S_1(t)$ is the survival function for the experimental arm, then the difference in the survival curves is $S_1(t) - S_0(t)$. The NNT is a function of time; that is,

$$\text{NNT}(t) = \frac{1}{S_1(t) - S_0(t)}$$

Calculation of the difference in survival curves is simple using RP models (see sections 6.5.6 and 7.6.2), and thus it is simple to also calculate NNT(t).

9.2.1 Example

An example using the kidney cancer data (Medical Research Council RE01 trial) is shown below. We adopt the graphical approach of Altman (1998). Figure 9.1 shows the risk difference and NNT on the same graph.

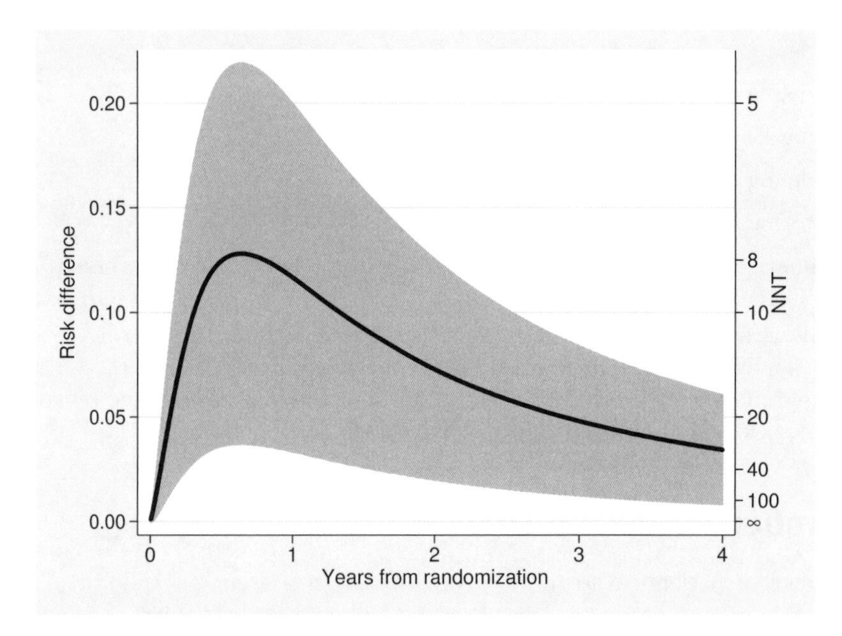

Figure 9.1. Kidney cancer data. Survival (risk) difference and NNT plotted against follow-up time. Shaded area shows the 95% pointwise confidence interval (CI) for the risk difference and NNT.

The code used to generate the graph is shown below:

```
. use kidney_ca
(kidney cancer data)
. // Truncate follow-up at 4 years
. stset survtime, failure(cens) scale(365.24) exit(time 4 * 365.24)

     failure event:  cens != 0 & cens < .
obs. time interval:  (0, survtime]
 exit on or before:  time 4 * 365.24
    t for analysis:  time/365.24

------------------------------------------------------------------------------
      347  total obs.
        0  exclusions
------------------------------------------------------------------------------
      347  obs. remaining, representing
      320  failures in single record/single failure data
 362.7685  total analysis time at risk, at risk from t =         0
                             earliest observed entry t =         0
                                  last observed exit t =         4
. quietly stpm2 trt, df(2) scale(odds)
. predict sd, sdiff(trt 1) ci
. foreach num in 100 40 20 10 8 5 {
  2.          local tmp = 1 / `num´
  3.          local ylab `ylab´ `tmp´
  4.          local ylab `ylab´ "`num´"
  5. }
. twoway (rarea sd_lci sd_uci _t, sort pstyle(ci) yaxis(1 2))
> (line sd _t, sort lpattern(solid) clwidth(thick) yaxis(1 2)),
> ylab(,angle(horizontal) format(%3.2f))
> ylab(`ylab´ 0 "{&infinity}", axis(2) angle(horizontal))
> ytitle("Risk difference", axis(1))
> ytitle("NNT", axis(2)) xtitle("Years from randomization") legend(off)
```

We plot on the risk difference scale, but also show a second y axis with the reciprocal of the risk difference (that is, the NNT). The maximum benefit of the experimental treatment is seen about two-thirds of one year after randomization (that is, start of treatment), with an NNT of about 8 (95% CI; [5, 27]). Over a longer time scale, the NNT increases considerably.

9.3 Average and adjusted survival curves

When comparing survival between two or more groups, the Kaplan–Meier graph of the survival function is usually shown. For example, the results of nearly every clinical trial with a time-to-event outcome show a Kaplan–Meier graph. A problem arises if there is a need to adjust for potential confounding variables. For example, if interest lies in comparing two groups but there is the need to adjust for one or more confounding variables, then a regression model is usually fit, such as a Cox proportional hazards (PH) model or an RP model. In this situation, an adjusted hazard ratio (HR) is usually reported, but it is less common to show adjusted survival curves.

In fact, it is not always clear what adjusted actually means in the context of survival curves. One approach is the mean covariate method, which obtains predictions of the survival function for each group of interest at the mean values of other covariates (Cupples et al. 1995). The prediction is for a hypothetical individual who happens to have the mean values for the covariates. This is what is done when using the `stcurve` command. The method has been criticized, particularly if there are categorical variables in the analysis (Nieto and Coresh 1996). For example, the predicted survival curve could be for a hypothetical individual of mean age who is half male and half female.

An alternative to the mean covariate method is to obtain a directly adjusted survival curve. In this approach, a survival curve is estimated for all subjects, and the curves are averaged (Makuch 1982; Nieto and Coresh 1996). With categorical variables, rather than estimate a separate survival curve for each individual, a survival curve is estimated for each combination of covariates. These are then combined with weights defined by the frequency of each covariate pattern.

The difference between the two approaches can be explained algebraically. If interest lies in a dichotomous covariate, z_i, with two confounding covariates, x_{1i} and x_{2i}, then the following RP model could be fit:

$$\ln\{H_i(t)\} = s\{\ln(t)\,|\gamma\} + \beta_1 z_i + \beta_2 x_{1i} + \beta_2 x_{2i}$$

The adjusted survival curve using the mean covariate method when $z_i = 0$ is

$$\exp\left(-\exp\left[s\{\ln(t)\,|\gamma\} + \beta_2\overline{x}_1 + \beta_2\overline{x}_2\right]\right)$$

and for $z_i = 1$,

$$\exp\left(-\exp\left[s\{\ln(t)\,|\gamma\} + \beta_1 + \beta_2\overline{x}_1 + \beta_2\overline{x}_2\right]\right)$$

Thus in the mean covariate method, we are obtaining the predicted survival function in each group for a hypothetical individual who has the mean values of all the confounding variables. As stated above, there is a problem in interpretation when the confounding variables are categorical. In contrast, the directly adjusted survival curve when $z_i = 0$ is

$$N^{-1}\sum_{i=1}^{N}\exp\left(-\exp\left[s\{\ln(t)\,|\gamma\} + \beta_2 x_{1i} + \beta_2 x_{2i}\right]\right)$$

and for $z_i = 1$,

$$N^{-1}\sum_{i=1}^{N}\exp\left(-\exp\left[s\{\ln(t)\,|\gamma\} + \beta_1 + \beta_2 x_{1i} + \beta_2 x_{2i}\right]\right)$$

Here we are asking the question "if each group has the distribution of covariates in the study population as a whole, what is the average survival curve?". Thus there are N predicted survival curves for each group, with the adjusted curve being the average of these N curves.

9.3.1 Renal data

To illustrate how adjusted survival curves can be calculated, we use a small study of 252 patients who entered a renal dialysis program in Leicestershire, England, between 1982 and 1991. Follow-up continued to December 1994. For some types of renal disease, there are known ethnic differences in incidence. At the time of the study, Leicester had approximately 25% of its population of South Asian origin, and thus there was interest in potential differences in survival by ethnicity. A Kaplan–Meier plot of the survival function of South Asian and non–South Asian patients can be seen in figure 9.2.

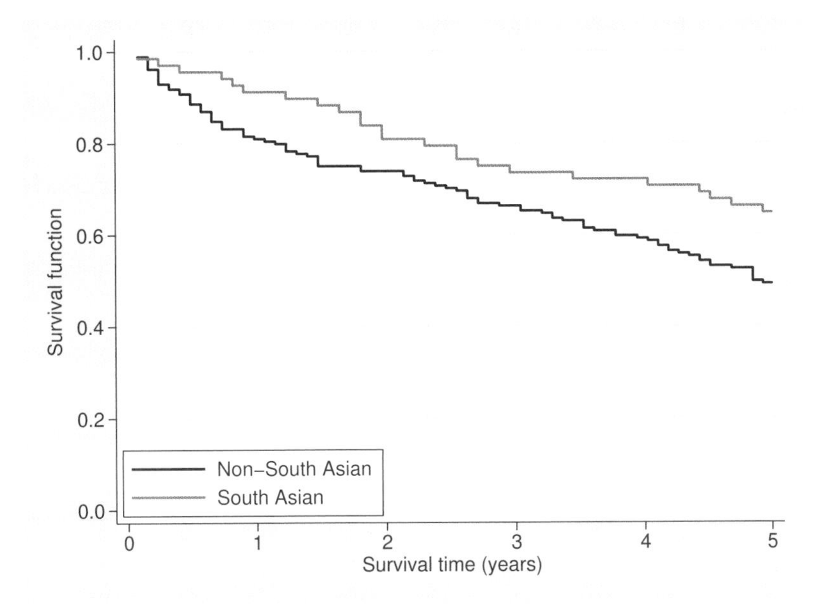

Figure 9.2. Renal disease study. Kaplan–Meier survival curves of all-cause mortality by ethnic status.

The plot indicates that the South Asian patients have better survival than the non–South Asian patients. Fitting an RP survival curve, including only the binary covariate `s_asian` gives

```
. stpm2 s_asian, df(3) scale(hazard) eform nolog
Log likelihood = -313.15269                     Number of obs   =        252
```

	exp(b)	Std. Err.	z	P>|z|	[95% Conf.	Interval]
xb						
s_asian	.6116469	.1400791	-2.15	0.032	.3904442	.9581702
_rcs1	2.484988	.2077101	10.89	0.000	2.109482	2.927337
_rcs2	1.096045	.0588939	1.71	0.088	.9864856	1.217772
_rcs3	.9400925	.0234175	-2.48	0.013	.8952975	.9871289
_cons	.410308	.044542	-8.21	0.000	.3316696	.5075915

The mortality rate for the South Asian group is 39% lower than for the non–South Asian group. However, this is an observational study and the comparison may not be a fair one if there is imbalance for important confounders between the two groups. In any study of mortality, the most obvious potentially confounding variable is age. The output below shows the mean age in the two groups:

```
. table s_asian, c(n age mean age sd age) format(%9.2f)
```

s_asian	N(age)	mean(age)	sd(age)
Non-Asian	184	62.93	16.48
Asian	68	55.46	13.62

There is a notable difference in age, with patients in the South Asian group being almost seven and one-half years younger on average than those in the non–South Asian group. Given that mortality is likely to increase with age, we should adjust for age. The model below includes `age` as a continuous covariate, assuming a linear effect.

```
. stpm2 s_asian age, df(3) scale(hazard) eform nolog
Log likelihood = -276.74248                     Number of obs   =        252
```

	exp(b)	Std. Err.	z	P>|z|	[95% Conf.	Interval]
xb						
s_asian	1.098929	.270559	0.38	0.702	.678269	1.780482
age	1.064484	.0090539	7.35	0.000	1.046885	1.082378
_rcs1	2.644969	.2268688	11.34	0.000	2.235682	3.129186
_rcs2	1.074259	.0598434	1.29	0.198	.9631445	1.198193
_rcs3	.9273007	.0249322	-2.81	0.005	.8796998	.9774773
_cons	.0060964	.0038145	-8.15	0.000	.0017885	.0207811

The effect for `age` indicates that there is a 6.4% increase in the mortality rate for each yearly increase in age. Including `age` in the model has an important effect on the HR for `s_asian` because the HR is now greater than one, indicating that the patients in the South Asian group are at increased risk. However, this adjusted HR is not statistically significant ($P = 0.7$).

For these data, it is clearly sensible to adjust for the effect of age because of the imbalance in the age distribution between the two groups. The problem is that our graphical display of the Kaplan–Meier curves is unadjusted.

To obtain the mean covariate-adjusted survival curves, we need to obtain predictions at the mean age. This can be done by use of the `at()` option.

```
. summ age, meanonly
. local mean_age = `r(mean)´
. predict s0_meancov, survival at(s_asian 0 age `mean_age´)
. predict s1_meancov, survival at(s_asian 1 age `mean_age´)
```

The resulting curves can be seen in figure 9.3, together with the original Kaplan–Meier estimates. The adjusted survival curves are more similar than the unadjusted curves. The adjusted survival curve is slightly higher for the non–South Asian group, which is to be expected because the adjusted HR is now greater than one.

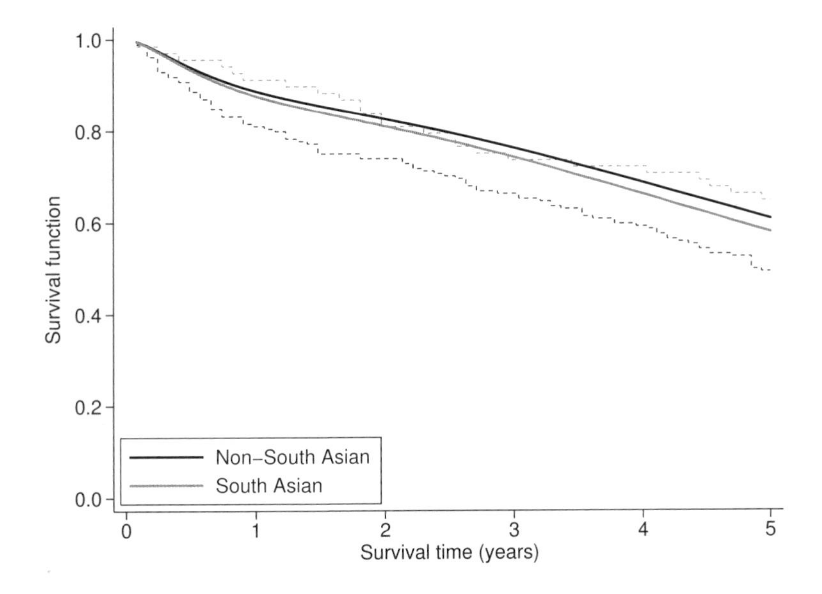

Figure 9.3. Renal disease study. Kaplan–Meier survival curves of all-cause mortality by ethnic status with mean covariate adjusted curves from an RP model.

We now move on to directly adjusted survival curves. These can be obtained by use of the `meansurv` option of the `predict` command after using `stpm2`.

```
. predict s0_diradj_all, meansurv at(s_asian 0)
. predict s1_diradj_all, meansurv at(s_asian 1)
```

What the **meansurv** option does is to obtain a predicted survival curve for each subject using their covariate pattern with the possibility of fixing certain covariates with the use of the `at()` option. In the code above, we are using the age distribution for the study population as a whole and applying this distribution to the two ethic groups separately. The predicted curves are plotted in figure 9.4. Again the adjusted curves are more similar than the unadjusted curves. The direct adjusted survival curves are lower than the adjusted survival curves using the mean covariate method. It can be shown that this will always be the case.

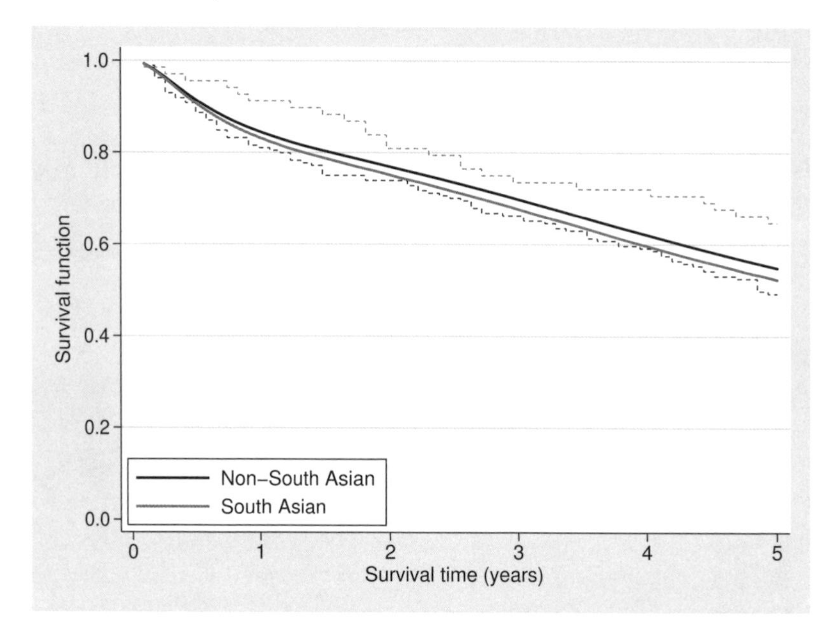

Figure 9.4. Renal disease study. Kaplan–Meier survival curves of all-cause mortality by ethnic status with direct adjusted survival curves from an RP model. The curves are adjusted for the age distribution for the study population as a whole.

These predictions are for the age distribution as a whole. It is possible to use any age distribution. For example, when comparing cancer survival between countries it is usual to standardize to an international standard age distribution so that the comparisons are fair (Coleman et al. 2008). The result would be an out-of-sample prediction.

The code below obtains directly adjusted survival curves first by applying the age distribution of the non–South Asians and then, the South Asians.

```
. /* Age distribution for non-South Asians */
. predict s0_diradj_nonasian if s_asian == 0, meansurv at(s_asian 0)
. predict s1_diradj_nonasian if s_asian == 0, meansurv at(s_asian 1)
. /* Age distribution for South Asians */
. predict s0_diradj_asian if s_asian == 1, meansurv at(s_asian 0)
. predict s1_diradj_asian if s_asian == 1, meansurv at(s_asian 1)
```

The resulting directly adjusted survival curves are shown in figure 9.5. In the left-hand graph, we are asking what if the South Asian population had the same age distribution as the non–South Asians, and in the right-hand graph we are asking what if the non–South Asians had the same age distribution as the South Asians. An important point here is that when presenting adjusted survival curves, one needs to be very clear regarding the covariate distribution being applied.

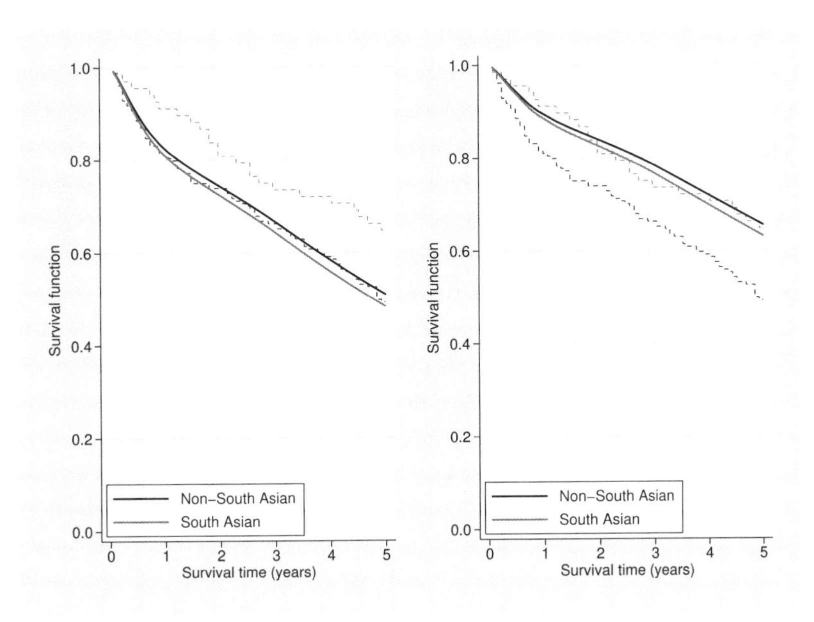

Figure 9.5. Renal disease study. Kaplan–Meier survival curves of all-cause mortality by ethnic status with directly adjusted survival curves from an RP model. The curves are adjusted for the age distribution for non–South Asians (left panel) and South Asians (right panel).

With large datasets, use of the `meansurv` option can be computationally intensive because the default is to obtain predictions for each individual at all values of the `_t` variable. Use of the `timevar()` option so that predictions are obtained for 100–200 time points over a suitable range can considerably improve computational time.

One of the advantages of using RP models to obtain directly adjusted survival curves is that it is simple to include time-dependent effects and continuous covariates. It is also possible to obtain out-of-sample predictions, which may be important when comparing survival between different studies.

It is not currently possible to use the `ci` option to obtain CIs of the directly adjusted survival curve. It is possible to use bootstrapping, but if interest just lies in a few points on the time scale, then the `margins` commands can be used (see [R] **margins**). For example, to obtain the directly adjusted estimates of survival at five years, we can use the following code:

```
. forvalues i = 1/3 {
  2.         summ _rcs`i´ if _t == 5, meanonly
  3.         local c`i´ `r(mean)´
  4. }
. margins, at(_rcs1 = `c1´ _rcs2 =`c2´ _rcs3 =`c3´ s_asian=(0 1))
> expression(predict(survival)) post
Predictive margins                               Number of obs   =        252
Model VCE      : OIM

Expression     : predict(survival)
1._at          : s_asian         =           0
                 _rcs1           =    .6132655
                 _rcs2           =   -.3933858
                 _rcs3           =   -.3666817
2._at          : s_asian         =           1
                 _rcs1           =    .6132655
                 _rcs2           =   -.3933858
                 _rcs3           =   -.3666817
```

	Margin	Delta-method Std. Err.	z	P>|z|	[95% Conf.	Interval]
_at						
1	.5485655	.0311873	17.59	0.000	.4874395	.6096916
2	.5233779	.0561099	9.33	0.000	.4134045	.6333514

First, we have obtained the values of the restricted cubic-spline variables at five years and stored these in local macros. We then make use of the `at()` option to obtain predictions for when `asian=0` and `asian=1` at the required values of the spline variables. The `expression` option shows that we want to obtain predictions of the survival function that average over the values of the remaining covariates (only `age` in this case). The estimates are identical to those obtained from `meansurv` and those shown in figure 9.4, but now we have CIs, as well. We have used the `post` option so we can obtain linear (or nonlinear) contrasts. For example, to obtain the difference in the directly adjusted survival curves at five years, we can use the following code:

```
. lincom _b[1._at] - _b[2._at]
 ( 1)  1bn._at - 2._at = 0
```

	Coef.	Std. Err.	z	P>|z|	[95% Conf.	Interval]
(1)	.0251876	.0653983	0.39	0.700	-.1029908	.153366

9.4 Modeling distributions with RP models

So far in our book, we have concentrated on modeling data from a survival analysis perspective. Working with censored time-to-event data, we have been interested mainly in the characteristics of the hazard function, survival function, and HR in relation to the covariates in the dataset. In chapter 8, we consider the same things in the relative survival context. In chapter 6, we go a bit further and explore the distributions of survival time that are estimated by RP models; see section 6.5.7—in particular, figure 6.8.

Although we have described RP models in survival analysis terms, in fact they are flexible estimators of quite general distribution functions. Much of their power and generality arises from two characteristics: a) the use of spline functions to model (cumulative) distributional form (chapter 5), and b) the extensions to time-dependent effects (chapter 7). Here we explore some wider uses of the models.

We approach the terrain of the normal-errors linear model and some of its generalizations and extensions. For that reason, in this section we work exclusively with the RP probit class. Recall that the simplest such model is the lognormal, which has 1 degree of freedom (d.f.) and no spline terms (see section 5.5). Its basic formulation is given by (5.10).

One basic point to remember here is that RP models work with the log of time. For the model to make sense, the outcome variable must be *positively bound*—no zero or negative values of time are allowed. The restriction is not in fact significant, because a variable with support of all the real numbers can be made positively bound by exponential transformation before analysis with RP models. Estimates of time-related outputs may be back-transformed to the correct scale. To avoid excessive skewness when a variable of interest, z, is exponentially transformed, we might prefer to work with $t = \exp(cz)$ for some suitable scale factor c—for example, the reciprocal of the standard deviation of the observed values of z.

9.4.1 Example 1: Rotterdam breast cancer data

We revisit the Rotterdam breast cancer data that we have already extensively analyzed, but from a slightly different perspective. As already mentioned, we work within the RP probit class. Here the probit(2) model minimizes the Akaike information criterion (AIC) among probit models with d.f. between 1 and 5. The estimated density function for log time from the probit(2) model is shown in the left panel of figure 9.6.

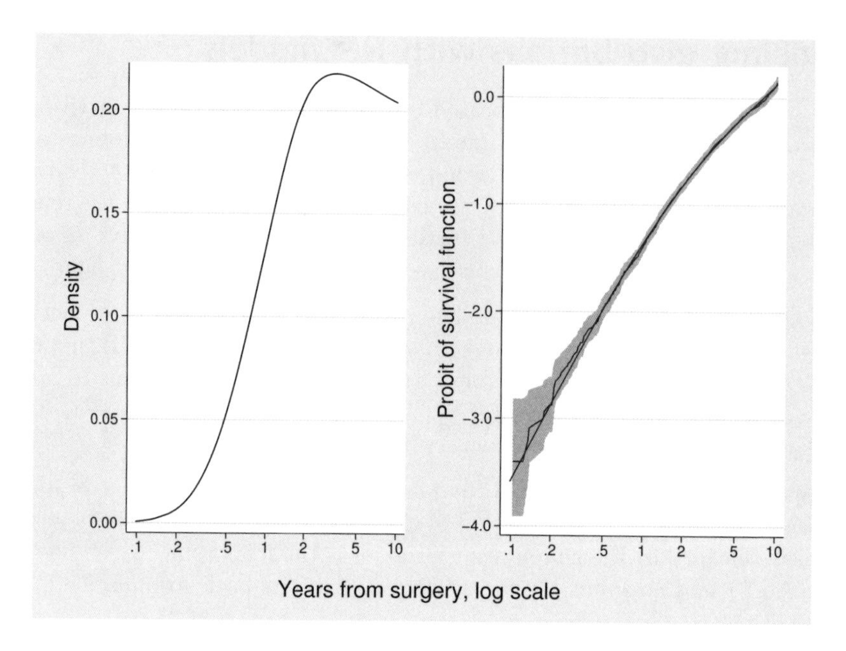

Figure 9.6. Rotterdam breast cancer data. Left panel: density function for log recurrence-free interval, estimated from a probit(2) model. Right panel: probit transformation of the survival function (jagged lines and pointwise 95% CI) and predicted probit function from `stpm2` (smooth curve).

We prefer to plot the density function of log time against time on a log scale, because under a lognormal model (1 d.f.), we obtain a normal (Gaussian) distribution.

To obtain the density of the log survival-time, we had to transform the output from the `predict, density` command following model fitting with `stpm2`, because the density of the survival time, not the log survival-time, is calculated. Denoting a density function by $f(.)$, we have, by definition,

$$
\begin{aligned}
f(t) &= -\frac{dS(t)}{dt} \\
f(\ln t) &= -\frac{dS(t)}{d\ln t} = -\frac{dS(t)}{dt}\frac{dt}{d\ln t} = -\frac{dS(t)}{dt}t \\
&= tf(t)
\end{aligned}
$$

We simply multiply the supplied density by `_t`.

The plot of the density function serves to remind us of our ignorance of the right-hand tail of the survival-time distribution. About half of the distribution is missing. We can glean no useful idea of what the right tail looks like from the data and the model. We could indeed extrapolate the model to much larger values of t, but the uppermost line in figure 6.8 reminds us of the nonsense that can be generated. Model-based extrapolation into the future is a dangerous game.

The right panel of figure 9.6 compares the empirical probit function (jagged lines) with the function estimated using `predict, normal` (smooth line). If the times to event were lognormally distributed, the lines would be straight; as it is, the slope diminishes as (log) time increases. The close agreement between the empirical and model-based curves shows that the probit(2) model fits the data very well.

9.4.2 Example 2: CD4 lymphocyte data

The cluster of differentiation #4 (CD4) lymphocyte counts of a sample of children born to women infected with human immunodeficiency virus (HIV) type 1 were recorded (European Collaborative Study 1991). The dataset consists of 610 measurements on children who were later diagnosed as not being infected with HIV type 1. Analysts took one randomly selected CD4 count per child. The outcome variable is the CD4 count; and there is one covariate, the age of the child. The aim of the analysis is to model the distribution of CD4, given age. There are no censored observations, and so we are moving away from a standard survival analysis here.

A solution to the problem was proposed by Royston and Wright (1998). We compare their results informally with those from a completely different approach, described below.

The CD4 counts are plotted against age in the left panel of figure 9.7.

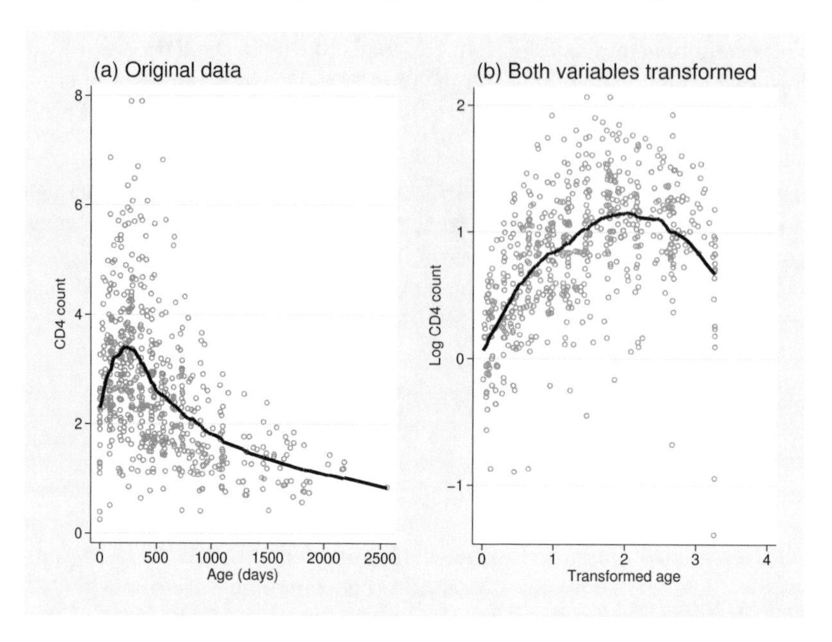

Figure 9.7. CD4 lymphocyte data. Relationship between CD4 count and age. (a) untransformed; (b) after log transformation of CD4 and scaled negative exponential transformation of age. Lines are running-line smooths.

Panel (b) shows the same data, but after transformation of both axes. The y axis is $y = \log$ CD4. The x axis is the negative exponential transformation

$$x = \exp\left(-\frac{\text{age} - \overline{\text{age}}}{s}\right)$$

where $\overline{\text{age}}$ is the sample mean age (539 days) and s is the standard deviation of age (456 days). The transformation draws the right-hand tail of the age distribution in toward the center, and is recommended by Royston and Sauerbrei (2008, 108–109) in situations in which a predictor has a skew distribution. It is also useful when the effect of the predictor appears to "tail off" at large values, as it does here. As can be seen in figure 9.7(b), the shape of the (y, x) relationship is much easier to model than that of (CD4, age), because the former resembles a quadratic—or more generally—a second-order fractional polynomial (FP2) curve, whereas the latter has a more complex shape with a point of inflection.

By inspecting figure 9.7(b) we see that the distribution of y given x is negatively skewed. There is also a hint that the skewness of y changes with x, suggesting that the distribution of y given x depends on x. To model such a situation, survival-time data need what we would call models with a time-dependent effect (see chapter 7). Here we are modeling CD4, not time, and we have no censoring. To generalize models with a time-dependent effect to a context wider than survival analysis, we talk about outcome-dependent models. Apart from the name, nothing else in the model structure changes.

Because the natural starting point for modeling complete (uncensored) distributions is the normal, we again work with RP probit models. To accommodate the possibly age-dependent skewness (that is, the changing distributional shape), we expect to need outcome-dependent models. The first step is to obtain the AIC for models with 0, 1, 2, and more knots for models without and with outcome-dependent effects. Having decided how many d.f. are needed overall, we can if necessary further refine the number of d.f. for the outcome-dependent part of the model.

Investigation shows that the mean of y given x is well approximated by an FP2 function of x with powers $(0.5, 3)$. Two variables, `x_1` and `x_2`, in the `cd4` dataset correspond to these two power terms. Before running `stpm2`, we `stset` the data omitting the event predictor, that is, `stset cd4`. Table 9.1 presents AIC values for various values of the d.f. in the spline component of probit models that include the predictor FP2(x)—that is, those that include `x_1` and `x_2` as covariates in the model. It also shows the AIC for outcome-dependent models with varying d.f. for the outcome-dependent component. The outcome-dependent component was fit by specifying the `tvc()` and `dftevc()` options of `stpm2`.

Table 9.1. CD4 data. Values of AIC for choosing appropriate d.f. for the main and outcome-dependent effects in a predictor that includes an FP2 function of x = transformed age. See text for details.

d.f.	Main effect	Outcome dependent (main effect d.f. = 2)
0	–	658.7
1	676.5	641.8
2	658.7	634.1
3	659.0	635.8
4	660.6	637.8
5	662.1	–

The clear choice for the main-effects model, according to AIC, is 2 d.f. The clear choice for the outcome-dependent component, given 2 d.f. for the main-effect component, is also 2 d.f. The code to generate the results in table 9.1 is as follows:

```
. use cd4
(CD4 lymphocyte data in HIV-infected children)
. stset cd4

     failure event:  (assumed to fail at time=cd4)
obs. time interval:  (0, cd4]
 exit on or before:  failure

------------------------------------------------------------------------------
      610  total obs.
        0  exclusions
------------------------------------------------------------------------------
      610  obs. remaining, representing
      610  failures in single record/single failure data
  1598.02  total analysis time at risk, at risk from t =         0
                             earliest observed entry t =         0
                                  last observed exit t =       7.9

. forvalues j = 1 / 5 {
  2.         quietly stpm2 x_1 x_2, scale(normal) df(`j´)
  3.         di `j´, e(AIC)
  4. }
1 676.50305
2 658.65567
3 658.99019
4 660.60007
5 662.06159
. // Best main effects model df(2). Check AIC for outcome-dependent models.
. forvalues j = 0 / 4 {
  2.         if `j´ == 0 local tvc
  3.         else local tvc dftvc(`j´) tvc(x_1 x_2)
  4.         quietly stpm2 x_1 x_2, scale(normal) df(2) `tvc´
  5.         di `j´, e(AIC)
  6. }
0 658.65567
1 641.76226
2 634.06243
3 635.76644
4 637.78019
```

Figure 9.8 shows the estimated density function for log CD4 count at the 10th, 50th, and 90th centiles of age.

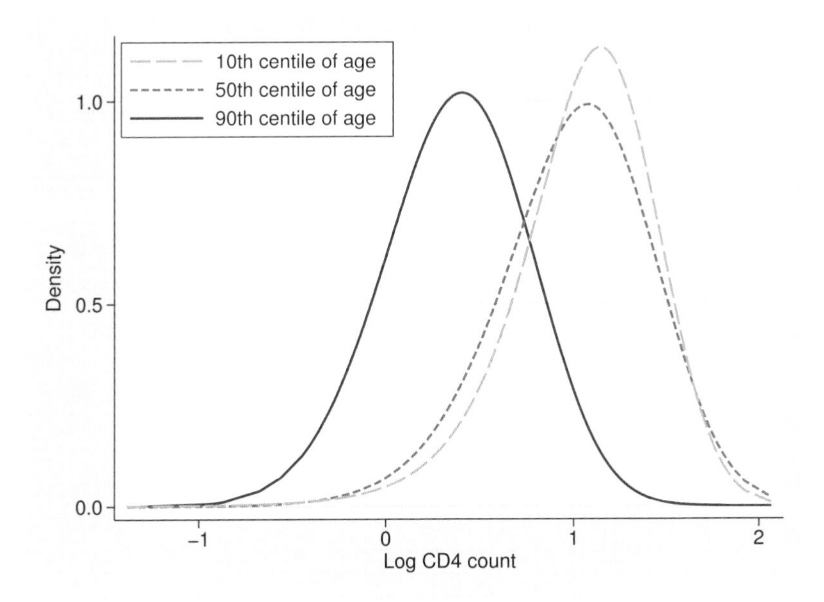

Figure 9.8. CD4 lymphocyte data. Density function of log CD4 count estimated at the 10th, 50th, and 90th centiles of the distribution of age.

The shape of the density function changes slightly with age, being negatively skewed (higher CD4 values) for the younger children (palest line in figure 9.8) and approximately symmetric for older ones (darkest line). The code to produce figure 9.8 is as follows:

```
. use cd4
(CD4 lymphocyte data in HIV-infected children)
. stset cd4
     failure event:  (assumed to fail at time=cd4)
obs. time interval:  (0, cd4]
 exit on or before:  failure
------------------------------------------------------------------------------
      610  total obs.
        0  exclusions
------------------------------------------------------------------------------
      610  obs. remaining, representing
      610  failures in single record/single failure data
  1598.02  total analysis time at risk, at risk from t =         0
                             earliest observed entry t =         0
                                  last observed exit t =       7.9
. quietly stpm2 x_1 x_2, scale(normal) df(2) dftvc(2) tvc(x_1 x_2)
. local ds
. local i 0
```

```
. forvalues j = 10(40)90 {
  2.           quietly centile x, centile(`j´)
  3.           local c = r(c_1)
  4.           // FP transformation of age centiles
  .          local x1 = `c´^0.5
  5.           local x2 = `c´^3
  6.           // Compute density for CD4 count
  .          local ++i
  7.           predict d`i´, density at(x_1 `x1´ x_2 `x2´)
  8.           // Compute density for log CD4 count
  .          quietly replace d`i´ = d`i´ * _t
  9.           local ds `ds´ d`i´
 10. }
. line `ds´ y, sort lcolor(gs4 gs8 gs12) clp(l - _)
> xtitle("log CD4 count") ytitle("Density") ylabel(,angle(horizontal))
> lwidth(medthick ..) legend(order(3 2 1) label(1 "90th centile of age")
> label(2 "50th centile of age")
> label(3 "10th centile of age") col(1) ring(0) pos(11))
```

We now turn to the estimation of age-specific reference intervals for CD4 count. The general idea is to compute age-specific extreme centiles (for example, 3rd and 97th) of a distribution of representative values of a variable y as a "norm" for judging a person's value of y. Typically, the sample is designed or believed to be of clinically normal people. Observing a new value of y lying outside of the reference interval—that is, either below the lower or above the upper centile—is a potential cause for concern and may trigger further testing or clinical intervention. Clearly, the sample we are analyzing now is not "normal" for the general population because it relates to children of HIV-infected mothers, but the same statistical principles apply as those that apply to the estimation of a reference interval for "normal" subjects.

As had others before them, Royston and Wright (1998) applied various types of transformation of the observed distribution toward normality to model such age-related distributions, and calculated reference intervals by back-transformation from theoretical normal values. We do not go into details here, but refer the interested reader to their article.

Estimating centiles, and hence reference intervals, within RP models is a simple matter of applying the `predict, centile()` command after fitting the relevant `stpm2` model. It is in fact easier to do than Royston and Wright's approach, because the latter involves determining fractional polynomials (FPs) in x for at least one and possibly as many as four moments of the distribution of y given x. The disadvantage of using `stpm2` is that RP models tend to produce relatively complex spline functions, which are less easy to write down and to transport for clinical use. However, in practical applications we need merely to graph and/or list the reference interval values for chosen values of x, which is straightforward enough. Splines have often been used to good effect for modeling reference intervals, particularly in studies of human growth where the shape of the mean of y given x (and sometimes of other conditional moments) is complex and therefore hard to model parsimoniously. Here we use splines for modeling the distributional shape, relying on FPs to represent the mean of y given x.

Figure 9.9 compares 3rd and 97th reference centile curves for log CD4 count, calculated by Royston and Wright's method (as reported for the same dataset in their article) using the `xriml` command and by the `stpm2` outcome-dependent probit(2) model, as described above.

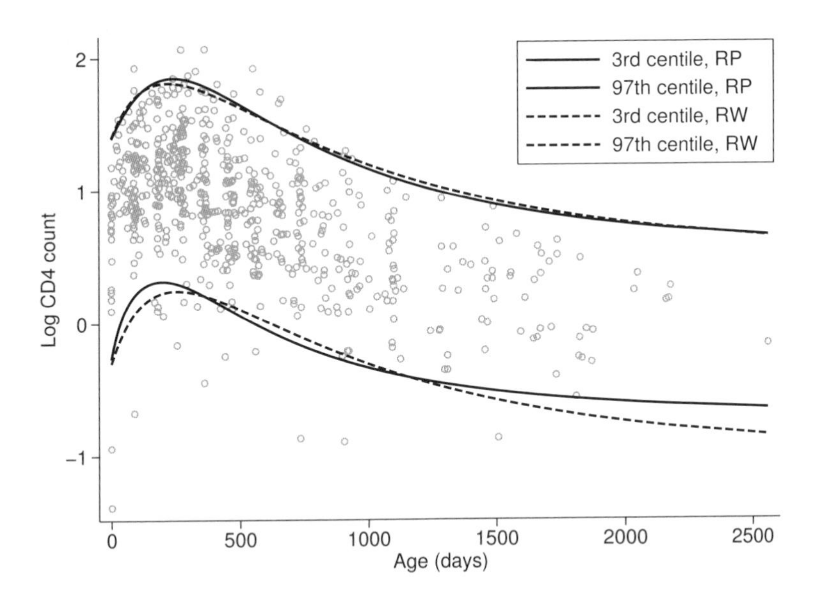

Figure 9.9. CD4 lymphocyte data. Ninety-four percent age-specific reference intervals according to an RP probit(2) model (solid lines) and the method of Royston and Wright (RW) (1998) (dashed lines).

The respective curves and the apparent fit to the data are similar, although the models that generated them are very different. The code for generating figure 9.9 is as follows:

```
. use cd4
(CD4 lymphocyte data in HIV-infected children)
. stset cd4
     failure event:  (assumed to fail at time=cd4)
obs. time interval:  (0, cd4]
 exit on or before:  failure
------------------------------------------------------------------------------
      610  total obs.
        0  exclusions
------------------------------------------------------------------------------
      610  obs. remaining, representing
      610  failures in single record/single failure data
  1598.02  total analysis time at risk, at risk from t =         0
                             earliest observed entry t =         0
                                  last observed exit t =       7.9
```

```
. stpm2 x_1 x_2, scale(normal) df(2) dftvc(2) tvc(x_1 x_2) nolog
Log likelihood = -308.03121                     Number of obs   =        610

------------------------------------------------------------------------------
             |      Coef.   Std. Err.      z    P>|z|     [95% Conf. Interval]
-------------+----------------------------------------------------------------
xb           |
         x_1 |  -2.958735   .2165747   -13.66   0.000    -3.383213   -2.534256
         x_2 |    .081194   .0087865     9.24   0.000     .0639728    .0984153
       _rcs1 |   1.647269   .1795104     9.18   0.000     1.295435    1.999103
       _rcs2 |  -.0484338   .1261677    -0.38   0.701     -.295718    .1988504
    _rcs_x_11 |  -.4647103   .1808821    -2.57   0.010    -.8192326   -.1101879
    _rcs_x_12 |  -.0612438   .1245441    -0.49   0.623    -.3053457    .1828581
    _rcs_x_21 |   .0143336   .0073418     1.95   0.051    -.0000561    .0287234
    _rcs_x_22 |  -.0053988   .0040699    -1.33   0.185    -.0133757    .0025782
       _cons |   2.827689   .2161215    13.08   0.000     2.404098    3.251279
------------------------------------------------------------------------------

. // Compute reference centiles
. predict c3, centile(3)
. replace c3 = ln(c3)
(610 real changes made)
. predict c97, centile(97)
. replace c97 = ln(c97)
(610 real changes made)
. // Royston & Wright (1998) method
. xriml y x, fp(m:0.5 3, g:1) dist(en) nograph
  (output omitted)
Exponential-Normal Regression                   Number of obs   =        610
                                                Wald chi2(2)    =     381.88
Log likelihood = -311.78444                     Prob > chi2     =     0.0000

------------------------------------------------------------------------------
           y |      Coef.   Std. Err.      z    P>|z|     [95% Conf. Interval]
-------------+----------------------------------------------------------------
M            |
        Xm_1 |   1.153304   .0640177    18.02   0.000     1.027832    1.278776
        Xm_2 |  -.0306443   .0030835    -9.94   0.000    -.0366878   -.0246007
       _cons |   1.068549   .0233816    45.70   0.000     1.022722    1.114376
-------------+----------------------------------------------------------------
S            |
       _cons |   .3980591   .0118113    33.70   0.000     .3749093    .4212089
-------------+----------------------------------------------------------------
G            |
        Xg_1 |   .0863987   .0308875     2.80   0.005     .0258602    .1469372
       _cons |   .1447552   .0297758     4.86   0.000     .0863957    .2031147
------------------------------------------------------------------------------

Final deviance =   623.569 (610 observations.)
. // Plot results
. twoway (scatter y age, ms(oh) mcolor(gs10))
> (line c3 c97 C3 C97 age, sort lpattern(l l - -) lwidth(medthick ..)),
> legend(label(2 "3rd centile, RP") label(3 "97th centile, RP")
> label(4 "3rd centile, RW") label(5 "97th centile, RW")
> ring(0) pos(1) col(1) order(2 3 4 5))
> xtitle("Age, days") ytitle("Log CD4 count") ylab(,angle(h))
> name(g1, replace)
```

The variables `x_1` and `x_2` that appear in the `stpm2` command are predefined in `cd4.dta` and are FP transformations of x used in modeling the conditional mean of log CD4 count. They are treated as time dependent in the `stpm2` fit, giving an outcome-dependent model. The command `xriml` fits a three-parameter transformed-normal model, as described by Royston and Wright (1998). The particular model used here again has an FP2 transformation of x with powers $(0.5, 3)$ for the location (conditional median) of y. The suboption `g:1` of the `fp()` option provides skewness that varies linearly with x (`1` denotes a linear function and `g` a particular parameter).

Assessment of the goodness of fit of reference interval models depends on deriving z scores, which (if the model is correct) have a standard normal distribution independent of x. We can easily calculate z scores for an RP model by using the command `predict` *varname*, `normal`. In the present example, both models generate z scores that appear to satisfy their assumptions adequately. Figure 9.10 shows running-line smooths of the first four central moments (powers) of the z scores from the probit(2) model, with the assumed expected values plotted as horizontal lines.

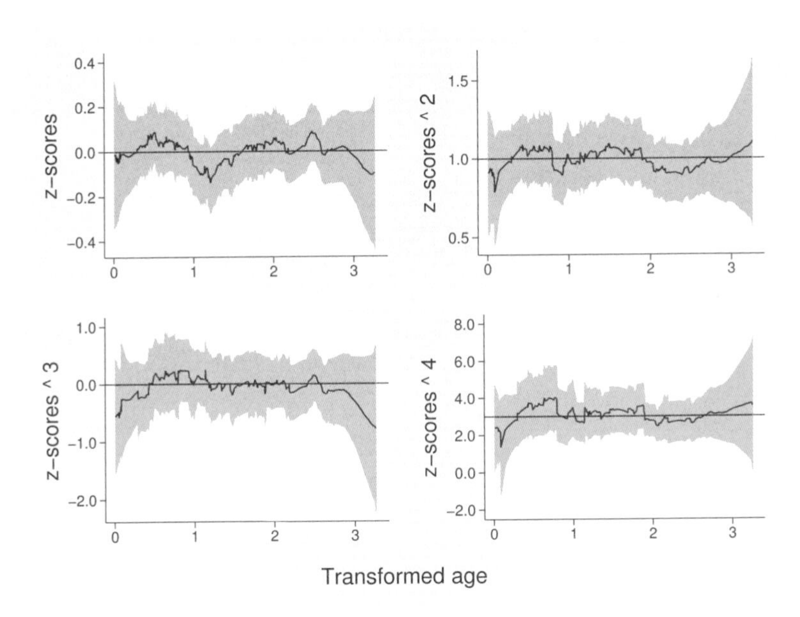

Figure 9.10. CD4 lymphocyte data. Smooths of the first four central moments of z scores from the probit(2) model plotted against x (transformed age). If the z scores are distributed as standard normal, the smooths should roughly follow the solid horizontal lines.

If the model fits well, we should see no obvious trends away from the horizontal lines that represent expected values. This appears to be the case.

9.4.3 Example 3: Prostate cancer data

Stamey et al. (1989) studied potential predictors of prostate specific antigen (PSA) in 97 patients with adenocarcinoma of the prostate. The aim was to see which factors or combinations of factors were associated with a raised PSA level. All observations were made around the time of radical prostatectomy, a surgical operation in which the entire prostate gland is removed. We use $y = \log$ PSA (`lpsa`) as the outcome variable. Further details are given by Royston and Sauerbrei (2008, 264–265).

Royston and Sauerbrei (2008) reported the following three-variable linear regression model for y, selected by the multivariable fractional polynomial modeling procedure:

$$y = 2.26 + 0.54 \times \ln(\texttt{cavol}) + 0.68 \times \texttt{svi} + 0.014 \times \texttt{weight} + 0.71 \times \mathrm{N}(0,1)$$

where `cavol` and `weight` are the volume and weight of the prostate gland, respectively, and `svi` is a binary variable indicating the presence or absence of seminal vessel invasion. To apply the present methods to analyze the data, we first `stset` PSA as the outcome variable with no censored observations, and we fit an RP probit model including ln(`cavol`), `svi`, and `weight` as covariates. We specify `scale(normal)` and initially fit outcome-dependent effects for ln(`cavol`), `svi`, and `weight`. The AIC values for models with $1, \ldots, 4$ d.f. are 203.3, 208.9, 215.1, and 220.4, respectively; so 1 d.f. is sufficient, and we use a probit(1) (that is, lognormal) model.

With the probit(1) model, the p-values for outcome-dependent effects of the three covariates are 0.09 for ln(`cavol`), 0.5 for `svi`, and 0.0001 for `weight`. We can therefore disregard outcome-dependent effects of ln(`cavol`) and `svi`, but we cannot do the same for `weight`.

The relationship between `lpsa` and `weight` is more intricate than just an additive effect of `weight` on the mean of `lpsa`, adjusted for ln(`cavol`) and `svi`. We explore it further by plotting the outcome-dependent regression coefficient for `weight` against `lpsa` (see figure 9.11). The output showing the calculations and creating figure 9.11 is shown below.

```
. use prostate_ca
(Prostate cancer data)
. rename lpsa y
. gen psa = exp(y)
. stset psa
     failure event:  (assumed to fail at time=psa)
obs. time interval:  (0, psa]
 exit on or before:  failure
------------------------------------------------------------------------------
         97  total obs.
          0  exclusions
------------------------------------------------------------------------------
         97  obs. remaining, representing
         97  failures in single record/single failure data
    2302.75  total analysis time at risk, at risk from t =         0
                             earliest observed entry t =         0
                                  last observed exit t =  265.8499
```

```
. gen lncavol = ln(cavol)
. stpm2 lncavol svi weight, dftvc(1) tvc(weight) df(1) scale(normal)
Iteration 0:   log likelihood = -103.62631
Iteration 1:   log likelihood = -96.973076
Iteration 2:   log likelihood = -96.917121
Iteration 3:   log likelihood = -96.917119
Log likelihood = -96.917119                    Number of obs   =        97
```

	Coef.	Std. Err.	z	P>|z|	[95% Conf.	Interval]
xb						
lncavol	-.767238	.1189826	-6.45	0.000	-1.00044	-.5340365
svi	-1.0642	.302829	-3.51	0.000	-1.657734	-.4706657
weight	-.0274903	.0061242	-4.49	0.000	-.0394935	-.015487
_rcs1	.9565805	.2372385	4.03	0.000	.4916015	1.42156
_rcs_weight1	.0199878	.0061408	3.25	0.001	.007952	.0320236
_cons	2.256768	.3012889	7.49	0.000	1.666252	2.847283

```
. predict tw, tvc(weight) ci
note: Confidence intervals calculated using Z critical values
. twoway (rarea tw_lci tw_uci y, pstyle(ci) sort)
> (line tw y, sort lstyle(refline) pstyle(p2)),
> ytitle("Outcome-dependent coefficient of weight")
> xtitle("Log PSA") ylab(, angle(h) format(%4.2f)) legend(off)
```

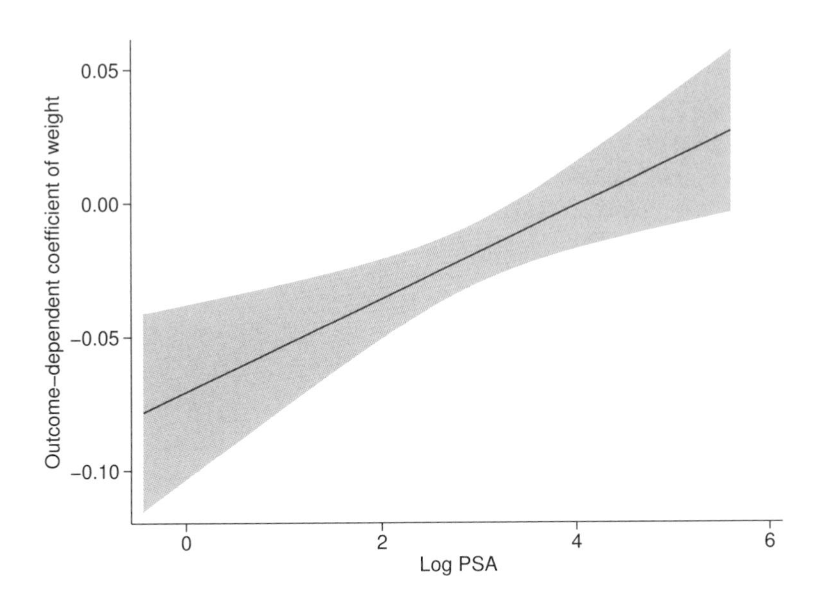

Figure 9.11. Prostate cancer data. Outcome-dependent coefficient of `weight` with pointwise 95% CI from a model for log PSA, adjusting for ln(`cavol`) and `svi`.

The coefficient for `weight` is negative for log PSA < 4 and positive but close to zero for higher values. This result suggests that `weight` influences log PSA differently at low and high values of log PSA. The probit(1) model that gauges the varying effect of `weight` on log PSA is a *varying-coefficient model*, as described by Hastie and Tibshirani (1993).

Finally, we can assess the variation explained by the varying-coefficient model by predicting the median PSA from the probit(1) model using `predict` *varname*, `centile(50)`. We then take logs to get an estimate of the mean log PSA, conditional on covariates and on the outcome-dependent effect of `weight`. The squared Pearson correlation between log PSA and its predicted mean is a measure of the explained variation, R^2. The probit(1) model shows a small increase in R^2 compared with the linear regression model without an outcome-dependent effect of `weight`: 65.3% versus 63.3%.

9.5 Multiple events

9.5.1 Introduction

So far in our book, we have considered situations where each individual can only have one event. If death is the outcome, then clearly it is not possible to have more than one event. However, if the event is recurrence of disease or admission to hospital, then it is possible for each individual to have repeated events. Here we are only concerned with events of the same type. With repeated events, we can expect correlation between the times to event of a given subject. For example, individuals with severe disease will tend to have more events and a shorter time between events than those with mild disease. The two main approaches for dealing with correlated data are to use random effects (frailty) models (Gutierrez 2002) or to use a marginal model where the correlation is dealt with using a robust sandwich-based estimator (Kelly and Lim 2000). In this section, we consider some different approaches to marginal models—namely, the Andersen–Gill (AG) (Andersen and Gill 1982); Wei, Lin, and Weissfeld (WLW) (Wei, Lin, and Weissfeld 1989); and Prentice, Williams, and Peterson (PWP) (Prentice, Williams, and Peterson 1981) models. These models have been developed as extensions of the Cox model. We show in section 9.5.5 that we can fit similar models within the RP framework. The descriptions of the different models are fairly brief because our aim here is to demonstrate that the models can be implemented in the flexible parametric approach. For more details of the approaches, see Therneau and Grambsch (2000) and Kelly and Lim (2000).

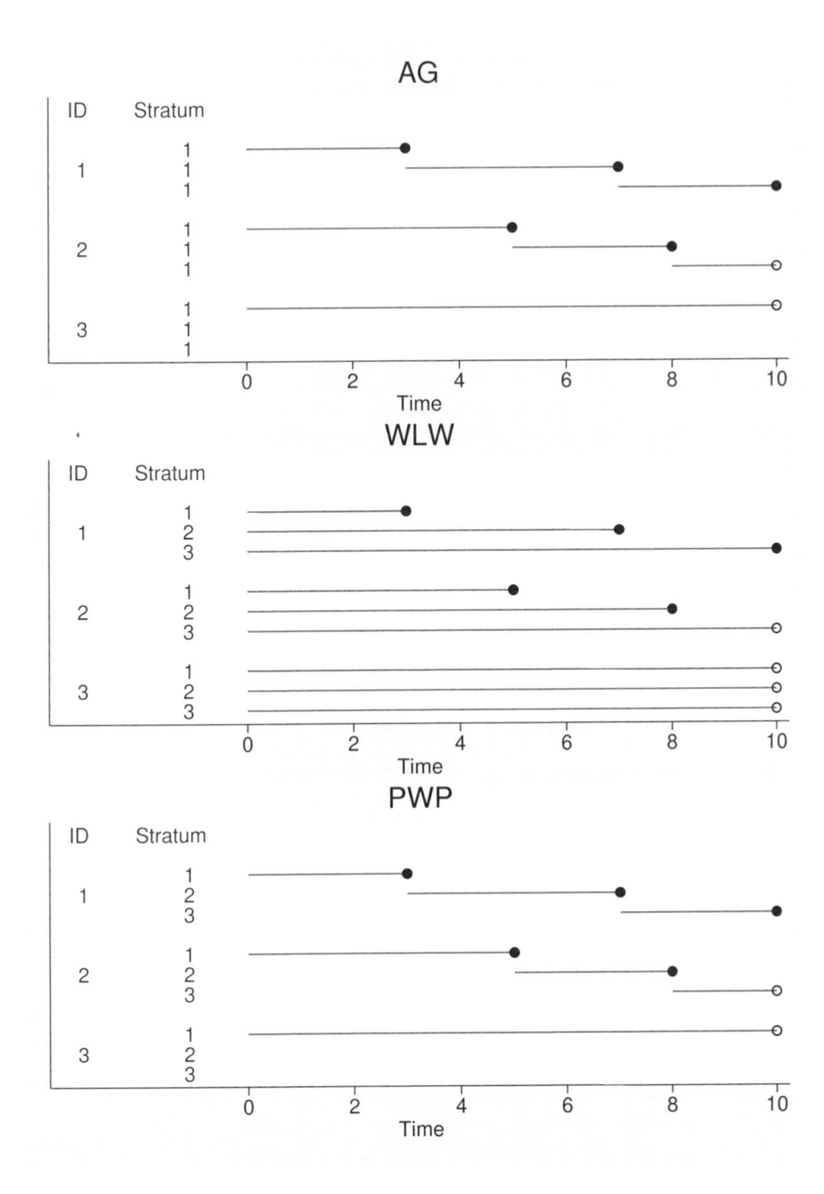

Figure 9.12. Schematic graph showing time at risk and stratum for three hypothetical patients for the AG, WLW, and PWP models.

9.5.2 The AG model

The AG model splits the time scale where the split points are defined by the events. The intervals are illustrated in the schematic diagram in figure 9.12. The time intervals are nonoverlapping; that is, the start time of a new event is the ending time of the preceding event. For example, subject 1 has 3 events at times 3, 7, and 10 and is not at risk of having the second and third event until after first and second events have occurred. In the AG model, the underlying shape of the baseline hazard is assumed to be the same for all events; that is, there is no stratification by event number. Although not used in the original article, cluster-based robust standard errors (SEs) are usually used.

9.5.3 The WLW model

In the WLW model, each subject is at risk for all possible events. For example, the schematic diagram in figure 9.12 shows that subject 3 is at risk of all three potential events, even though subject 3 did not even experience the first event. This means that time starts at zero for each event. A separate baseline hazard is estimated for each event through stratification. Usually, covariate effects are assumed to be constant across strata, but this assumption can be relaxed by including an interaction between the covariate and the event number. To account for the fact that there are multiple events per subject, robust SEs are used.

9.5.4 The PWP model

The PWP model is similar to the AG model in that it uses nonoverlapping time intervals for each subject. As for the AG model, it is not possible to be at risk of the second event before the first event has occurred. The PWP model differs from the AG model because the baseline hazard for each event is allowed to vary; that is, there is stratification by event number. This is shown in the schematic diagram in figure 9.12. To account for the clustering of events within subjects, robust SEs are used.

9.5.5 Multiple events in RP models

To fit marginal multiple-event models, we need to be able to have delayed entry (AG and PWP models) to calculate robust cluster SEs (AG, WLW, and PWP models) and to allow separate baseline hazards for the different events (WLW and PWP models). All three of these can be performed using `stpm2`. Recall from section 7.6.4 that stratification is the same as fitting time-dependent effects, and thus can be implemented using the `tvc()` and `dftvc()` options.

To illustrate the models, we use the bladder cancer data used by Wei, Lin, and Weissfeld (1989) and also by Therneau and Grambsch (2000). There are as many as four recurrence times for 86 subjects. We follow Therneau and Grambsch and drop the subject with 0 follow-up and 0 events because that subject does not contribute to the likelihood. Three covariates are included: `group`—a treatment code (1 = thiotepa, 0 = placebo); `size`—initial size of tumor; and `number`—the initial number of tumors. The Stata code used to fit multiple-event Cox models to the bladder cancer data is available as an FAQ on the Stata website at http://www.stata.com/support/faqs/stat/stmfail.html.

To fit the AG model, a dataset is constructed with each subject having a row of data for each event the subject is at risk for. The data for some selected individuals are shown below:

```
. list id start rec event strata if inrange(id,11,14), sepby(id) noobs
```

id	start	rec	event	strata
11	0	23	0	1
12	0	10	1	1
12	10	15	1	2
12	15	23	0	3
13	0	3	1	1
13	3	16	1	2
13	16	23	1	3
14	0	3	1	1
14	3	9	1	2
14	9	21	1	3
14	21	23	0	4

The variable `start` denotes when an individual starts to be at risk, and the variable `rec` denotes the time of the recurrence. The recurrence number is contained in the variable `strata`. The AG model does not stratify by event number, but this variable will be used in the PWP model below. Subject 11 has only one row of data because that subject did not have an event. Subject 12 has 3 rows of data because that subject had two events and was also at risk for the third event. Subject 13 has 3 rows of data because that subject had 3 events but was not followed up to be at risk of the fourth event. Subject 14 has four rows of data because that subject had 3 events and was also at risk for the fourth event.

The data can be `stset` as follows:

```
. stset rec, failure(event = 1) enter(start) id(id) exit(time .)
                id:  id
     failure event:  event == 1
obs. time interval:  (rec[_n-1], rec]
 enter on or after:  time start
 exit on or before:  time .
------------------------------------------------------------------------------
      178  total obs.
        0  exclusions
------------------------------------------------------------------------------
      178  obs. remaining, representing
       85  subjects
      112  failures in multiple failure-per-subject data
     2480  total analysis time at risk, at risk from t =         0
                                 earliest observed entry t =         0
                                      last observed exit t =        59
```

Note the use of the id() option, which is needed for computing cluster-based robust variances. Also note the exit(time .) option, which is needed because the default behavior of stset is to exit at the time of the first event. The enter(start) option gives the time when the record starts contributing to risk. The AG Cox model can be fit as follows:

```
. stcox group size number, nohr efron vce(cluster id) nolog noshow
Cox regression -- Efron method for ties
No. of subjects      =           85                Number of obs    =       178
No. of failures      =          112
Time at risk         =         2480
                                                   Wald chi2(3)     =     11.41
Log pseudolikelihood =   -449.98064                Prob > chi2      =    0.0097
                                   (Std. Err. adjusted for 85 clusters in id)
```

_t	Coef.	Robust Std. Err.	z	P>|z|	[95% Conf.	Interval]
group	-.464687	.2671369	-1.74	0.082	-.9882656	.0588917
size	-.0436603	.0780767	-0.56	0.576	-.1966879	.1093673
number	.1749604	.0634147	2.76	0.006	.0506699	.2992509

We have used the vce(cluster id) option so that robust SEs are calculated. Efron's correction for ties is used so that the results are directly comparable with Therneau and Grambsch (2000). The corresponding stpm2 model can be fit:

```
. stpm2 group size number, df(4) scale(hazard) vce(cluster id) nolog
note: delayed entry models are being fitted
Log pseudolikelihood = -170.21521                 Number of obs    =       178
                                   (Std. Err. adjusted for 85 clusters in id)
```

	Coef.	Robust Std. Err.	z	P>|z|	[95% Conf.	Interval]
xb						
group	-.4770162	.2631073	-1.81	0.070	-.9926969	.0386646
size	-.0414741	.0771663	-0.54	0.591	-.1927172	.109769
number	.1767393	.0627654	2.82	0.005	.0537213	.2997573
_rcs1	1.055811	.0908303	11.62	0.000	.8777867	1.233835
_rcs2	.1427236	.0542955	2.63	0.009	.0363063	.2491409
_rcs3	-.0675467	.0341353	-1.98	0.048	-.1344506	-.0006429
_rcs4	.0759846	.0262239	2.90	0.004	.0245868	.1273825
_cons	-.0336791	.4330642	-0.08	0.938	-.8824694	.8151111

The model uses 4 d.f. for the baseline hazard because it gives the lowest BIC. The vce(cluster id) option ensures that cluster-based robust SEs are calculated. The coefficients and their SEs are similar between the two models.

To fit the WLW model, we must restructure the data. An example of the required structure for selected individuals is shown below:

```
. list id  rec event strata if inrange(id,11,14), sepby(id) noobs

  ┌──────────────────────────┐
  │ id   rec   event   strata │
  ├──────────────────────────┤
  │ 11    23       0        1 │
  │ 11    23       0        2 │
  │ 11    23       0        3 │
  │ 11    23       0        4 │
  ├──────────────────────────┤
  │ 12    10       1        1 │
  │ 12    15       1        2 │
  │ 12    23       0        3 │
  │ 12    23       0        4 │
  ├──────────────────────────┤
  │ 13     3       1        1 │
  │ 13    16       1        2 │
  │ 13    23       1        3 │
  │ 13    23       0        4 │
  ├──────────────────────────┤
  │ 14     3       1        1 │
  │ 14     9       1        2 │
  │ 14    21       1        3 │
  │ 14    23       0        4 │
  └──────────────────────────┘
```

There are four rows of data for each subject because each subject is at risk for each of the events. For example, although subject 11 did not have any events, that subject was considered to be at risk for all four events from time 0. Similar patterns can be seen for the other subjects. The data are `stset` for the WLW model as follows:

```
. stset rec, failure(event = 1)

     failure event:  event == 1
obs. time interval:  (0, rec]
 exit on or before:  failure

------------------------------------------------------------------------------
      340  total obs.
        0  exclusions
------------------------------------------------------------------------------
      340  obs. remaining, representing
      112  failures in single record/single failure data
     8522  total analysis time at risk, at risk from t =         0
                             earliest observed entry t =         0
                                  last observed exit t =        59
```

The `id()` option is not used. There are $85 \times 4 = 340$ observations in total. The Cox WLW model is fit by clustering on `id` and stratifying on the failure occurrence variable `strata`.

```
. stcox group size number, nohr efron vce(cluster id) strata(strata) nolog
> noshow

Stratified Cox regr. -- Efron method for ties

No. of subjects      =          340                Number of obs   =        340
No. of failures      =          112
Time at risk         =         8522
                                                   Wald chi2(3)    =      15.35
Log pseudolikelihood =   -426.14683                Prob > chi2     =     0.0015

                                   (Std. Err. adjusted for 85 clusters in id)

------------------------------------------------------------------------------
             |               Robust
          _t |      Coef.   Std. Err.      z    P>|z|     [95% Conf. Interval]
-------------+----------------------------------------------------------------
       group |  -.5847935   .3097738    -1.89   0.059    -1.191939    .0223521
        size |   -.051617    .095148    -0.54   0.587    -.2381036    .1348697
      number |   .2102937   .0670372     3.14   0.002     .0789032    .3416842
------------------------------------------------------------------------------
                                                             Stratified by strata
```

The corresponding `stpm2` model is

```
. stpm2 group size number st2 st3 st4, df(4) scale(hazard) vce(cluster id)
> nolog tvc(st2 st3 st4) dftvc(2)

Log pseudolikelihood = -259.93122                  Number of obs   =        340

                                   (Std. Err. adjusted for 85 clusters in id)

------------------------------------------------------------------------------
             |               Robust
             |      Coef.   Std. Err.      z    P>|z|     [95% Conf. Interval]
-------------+----------------------------------------------------------------
xb           |
       group |  -.6061474   .3165317    -1.91   0.055    -1.226538    .0142434
        size |  -.0546432   .0969296    -0.56   0.573    -.2446218    .1353353
      number |   .2172699   .0679552     3.20   0.001     .0840803    .3504596
         st2 |  -1.644815   .3865122    -4.26   0.000    -2.402365    -.887265
         st3 |  -2.207566   .4910754    -4.50   0.000    -3.170056   -1.245076
         st4 |   -2.92798   .5450176    -5.37   0.000    -3.996195   -1.859766
       _rcs1 |   .8939912    .099383     9.00   0.000      .699204    1.088778
       _rcs2 |   .2631384   .0705043     3.73   0.000     .1249526    .4013242
       _rcs3 |  -.0808856   .0392069    -2.06   0.039    -.1577298   -.0040415
       _rcs4 |   .0746145   .0328121     2.27   0.023      .010304    .1389249
   _rcs_st21 |   1.919486   .7639084     2.51   0.012     .4222525    3.416719
   _rcs_st22 |   .8323456   .3945323     2.11   0.035     .0590764    1.605615
   _rcs_st31 |   2.079441   .9466471     2.20   0.028     .2240471    3.934836
   _rcs_st32 |    .572695   .4716519     1.21   0.225    -.3517257    1.497116
   _rcs_st41 |   2.119003   .9044294     2.34   0.019     .3463537    3.891652
   _rcs_st42 |   .2559404   .4304303     0.59   0.552    -.5876875    1.099568
       _cons |  -.0687489   .5398494    -0.13   0.899    -1.126834    .9893365
------------------------------------------------------------------------------
```

Three dummy covariates (`st2`–`st4`) for strata 2–4 have been created and included as time-dependent effects. Thus the shape of the baseline hazard is allowed to vary between the different repeated events. The coefficients of the covariate effects of interest are similar between the two modeling approaches. We have used 4 d.f. for the baseline and only 2 d.f. for the time-dependent effects. The model failed to converge when using 4 d.f. for the time-dependent effects of the repeated events. This failure is likely to be due to there being a small number of subjects with 4 events. We could have used different d.f. for each of the 4 strata by specifying them separately in the `dftvc()` option.

The PWP model uses the same data structure as the AG model and is `stset` in the same way. The PWP Cox model can be fit as follows:

```
. stcox group size number, nohr efron vce(cluster id) strata(strata) nolog
> noshow

Stratified Cox regr. -- Efron method for ties

No. of subjects      =           85              Number of obs    =        178
No. of failures      =          112
Time at risk         =         2480
                                                 Wald chi2(3)     =       7.17
Log pseudolikelihood =   -315.99082              Prob > chi2      =     0.0665

                                  (Std. Err. adjusted for 85 clusters in id)

                          Robust
          _t       Coef.   Std. Err.      z    P>|z|     [95% Conf. Interval]

       group   -.3334887   .2060021    -1.62   0.105    -.7372455     .070268
        size   -.0084947    .062001    -0.14   0.891    -.1300144    .1130251
      number    .1196172   .0516917     2.31   0.021     .0183033    .2209311

                                                          Stratified by strata
```

The difference from the code for the AG model is that we are now stratifying by event number. Thus the shape of the baseline hazard is different for each event number.

The corresponding stpm2 model is as follows:

```
. stpm2 group size number st2 st3 st4, df(4) scale(hazard) vce(cluster id)
> nolog tvc(st2 st3 st4) dftvc(2) difficult
note: delayed entry models are being fitted
Log pseudolikelihood = -149.77721                 Number of obs   =        178
                                 (Std. Err. adjusted for 85 clusters in id)

------------------------------------------------------------------------------
             |               Robust
             |      Coef.   Std. Err.      z    P>|z|     [95% Conf. Interval]
-------------+----------------------------------------------------------------
xb           |
       group |  -.3010988    .219141    -1.37   0.169    -.7306072    .1284097
        size |   .0020299   .0631778     0.03   0.974    -.1217963     .125856
      number |   .1458147   .0511189     2.85   0.004     .0456236    .2460058
         st2 |  -.8109816   .6202041    -1.31   0.191    -2.026559    .4045961
         st3 |   1.025842   .4011637     2.56   0.011      .239576    1.812109
         st4 |   .4610835   .6223859     0.74   0.459    -.7587706    1.680938
       _rcs1 |   .8333333   .0966027     8.63   0.000     .6439955    1.022671
       _rcs2 |   .2502149    .064926     3.85   0.000     .1229624    .3774675
       _rcs3 |  -.1008551   .0378385    -2.67   0.008    -.1750172   -.0266931
       _rcs4 |   .0431929   .0302382     1.43   0.153    -.0160728    .1024587
    _rcs_st21|   2.105856   1.031137     2.04   0.041     .0848649    4.126847
    _rcs_st22|   .8359231    .486194     1.72   0.086    -.1169996    1.788846
    _rcs_st31|   .4473373   .3088636     1.45   0.148    -.1580242    1.052699
    _rcs_st32|   .0839824    .161018     0.52   0.602    -.2316071    .3995719
    _rcs_st41|   .7837847      .3225     2.43   0.015     .1516964    1.415873
    _rcs_st42|   .0712918   .1945614     0.37   0.714    -.3100415    .4526251
       _cons |  -.5315121   .3867048    -1.37   0.169     -1.28944    .2264154
------------------------------------------------------------------------------
```

Again the coefficients of the covariate effects are similar between the two modeling approaches.

9.5.6 Summary

In this section, we have demonstrated that the approaches used within the Cox PH framework to model repeated events are easily extended to RP models.

9.6 Bayesian RP models

9.6.1 Introduction

There has been growing use of Bayesian methods in medical statistics and in many other areas of application. One of the key reasons for this is the freely available WinBUGS software (Lunn et al. 2009). There are those who, for philosophical reasons, advocate the use of Bayesian methodology. However, many users of WinBUGS do not consider themselves to be true Bayesian, but nevertheless are attracted to the flexibility to fit complex and nonstandard models that WinBUGS provides. For example, it is relatively simple to fit models in WinBUGS that account for measurement error (Mwalili, Lesaffre, and Declerck 2005), incorporate complex random effects for family data (Burton et al. 2005; Gauderman and Conti 2005), and combine data from numerous different sources while taking full parameter uncertainty into account (Spiegelhalter and Best 2003).

Here we will demonstrate how to fit an RP model in WinBUGS. We call WinBUGS from within Stata so that the data setup and any postestimation analysis can also be performed within Stata. To do this, we use the `winbugsfromstata` set of commands (Thompson, Palmer, and Moreno 2006).

This section is brief because we do not describe the Markov chain Monte Carlo (MCMC) estimation procedures used by WinBUGS and we have a rather superficial approach to the choice of prior distributions. However, we hope that you can see the potential to fit more complex models in this framework than is currently available when using Stata alone.

9.6.2 The "zeros trick" in WinBUGS

To fit an RP model in WinBUGS, we need to make use of what is known as the "zeros trick" (Spiegelhalter et al. 2003b) because there is no appropriate built-in distribution in WinBUGS with which to fit RP models. The trick enables us to specify a general likelihood. The probability density function of the Poisson distribution is

$$f(y|\lambda) = \frac{\lambda^y \exp(-\lambda)}{y!}$$

When $y = 0$, the density reduces to $\exp(-\lambda)$. Let L_i be the contribution to the likelihood for subject i and $\lambda = -\ln(L_i)$. If we can write down the likelihood function, then using the Poisson distribution with response $y = 0$ for all individuals enables us to fit a model. We may have to add a constant to λ to ensure that it is positive. There is also a "one trick" in WinBUGS that makes use of the binomial distribution.

9.6.3 Fitting a RP model

We start by fitting an RP model in the usual way using `stpm2`. We return to the Rotterdam breast cancer data and fit a PH model that includes two covariates, `age` and `hormon`. We have centered these covariates because doing so leads to better mixing (we need to take fewer samples in the MCMC estimation process). The `stpm2` model is shown below:

```
. stpm2 age hormon, scale(hazard) df(3) nolog
Log likelihood = -3666.2291                          Number of obs   =      2982

------------------------------------------------------------------------------
             |      Coef.   Std. Err.      z    P>|z|     [95% Conf. Interval]
-------------+----------------------------------------------------------------
xb           |
         age |  -.0048678   .0021431    -2.27   0.023    -.0090682   -.0006675
      hormon |   .2912813   .0813002     3.58   0.000     .1319358    .4506268
       _rcs1 |   .9808285   .0249242    39.35   0.000     .9319779    1.029679
       _rcs2 |    .269841   .0216561    12.46   0.000     .2273959    .3122861
       _rcs3 |  -.0087944    .010452    -0.84   0.400     -.02928     .0116911
       _cons |  -1.002159   .0284538   -35.22   0.000    -1.057927   -.9463901
------------------------------------------------------------------------------
```

We now fit the same model using WinBUGS. We need to write a WinBUGS program. It is listed below:

```
# Royston - Parmar Model
model  {
        C <- 10
        for(i in 1:N) {
                zeros[i] <- 0
                eta[i] <- gamma[1] + gamma[2]*rcs1[i] + gamma[3]*rcs2[i]
                            + gamma[4]*rcs3[i] + beta[1]*age[i]
                            + beta[2]*hormon[i]
                d.sp[i] <- gamma[2]*drcs1[i] + gamma[3]*drcs2[i]
                            + gamma[4]*drcs3[i]
                lnL[i] <- -(d[i] * log(max(d.sp[i] * exp(eta[i]),0.00001))
                            - exp(eta[i])) + C
                zeros[i] ~ dpois(lnL[i])
        }
# Prior Distributions
        for(j in 1:2) {
                beta[j] ~ dnorm(0,0.0001)
        }
        for(j in 1:4) {
                gamma[j] ~ dnorm(0,0.0001)
        }
# Hazard Ratios
        hr.age <- exp(beta[1])
        hr.hormon <- exp(beta[2])
}
```

Even if you have not used WinBUGS before, some of the code should be understandable. There is the linear predictor, `eta[i]`, which includes the intercept (`gamma[1]`), and three further `gamma[]` parameters for the three spline variables `rcs1`, `rcs2`, and `rcs3`. There is also the linear predictor for the derivative of the spline variables, `d.sp[i]`. This has the same parameters as in the linear predictor but uses the derivative variables `drcs1`, `drcs2`, and `drcs3`, as explained in section 5.2.1. These variables are then fed into the log likelihood, and the "zeros trick" is used. Because this is a Bayesian analysis, we need to give prior distributions for all unknown parameters. We use vague prior distributions because we want the "data to dominate" and to be able to compare the results with those obtained from stpm2. We do not want to go into details here, but there should be some caution and also appropriate sensitivity analysis when choosing prior distributions, particularly when the data are sparse (Lambert et al. 2005).

The winbugsfromstata set of commands enables us to write out the data file required by WinBUGS, set up a WinBUGS script file, call WinBUGS from within Stata, read in the WinBUGS output, and summarize and explore the WinBUGS output (Thompson, Palmer, and Moreno 2006).

First, we need to write the data to file in a format that is understandable by WinBUGS. We can use the wbdata command for this, as shown below:

```
. generate rcs1 = _rcs1
. generate rcs2 = _rcs2
. generate rcs3 = _rcs3
. generate drcs1 = _d_rcs1
. generate drcs2 = _d_rcs2
. generate drcs3 = _d_rcs3
. generate t = _t
. generate d = _d
. /* Save variables to WinBUGS data */
. scalar N = _N
. wbdata, contents(wbvector d rcs1 rcs2 rcs3 drcs1 drcs2 drcs3 age hormon,
> format(%3.0f %12.0g %12.0g %12.0g %12.0g %12.0g %12.0g %12.0g
> %12.0g %3.0f) + wbscalar, scalar(N) format(%2.0f))
> saving("WinBUGS/RP_rott_data.txt",replace) noprint
```

WinBUGS does not accept the underscore character in variable names, and so we have generated some new variables without the underscore character. We use the wbvector() option to store the required variables and the wbscalar() option to store the constant for the total number of observations. The text file, RP_rott_data.txt, containing the required data is then saved.

It is possible to run WinBUGS interactively, but we prefer to run it from Stata. To do so, we need to create a WinBUGS script file that gives the appropriate commands to WinBUGS to read in the data and initial values, fit the model, and store the results. We use the wbscript command to create the script file, but we first show the script file that wbscript creates:

```
display('log')
check('Z:/survbook/further_topics/do/WinBUGS/RP_rott_model.txt')
data('Z:/survbook/further_topics/do/WinBUGS/RP_rott_data.txt')
compile(1)
inits(1,'Z:/survbook/further_topics/do/WinBUGS/RP_rott_inits.txt')
gen.inits()
update(4000)
set('gamma')
set('beta')
set('ehr.age')
set('ehr.hormon')
thin.samples(10)
update(10000)
coda(*,'Z:/survbook/further_topics/do/WinBUGS/RP_rott_coda')
save('Z:/survbook/further_topics/do/WinBUGS/RP_rott_log.txt')
quit()
```

The first line opens a WinBUGS log window so that we can monitor the progress of our script and possibly see any error messages. The `check()` command asks WinBUGS to perform a syntax check of the model code that is stored in the file `RP_rott_model.txt`. We need to give the full path name. The `data()` command loads the data file created using the `wbdata` command above. The model and data are then compiled, with the 1 in the `compile(1)` command telling WinBUGS to run only one chain (running more than one chain is a good way of checking for convergence). The `inits()` command tells WinBUGS where a file containing initial values is stored, with the `gen.inits()` command generating any remaining initial values. We then run an MCMC "burn-in" chain of length 4,000 using `update()`, which is intended to allow the chain to stabilize. The various `set()` commands tell WinBUGS which of the parameters (and transformations of parameters) we wish to store from any further simulations. A further 10,000 values are then sampled and stored from the posterior distributions of our parameters of interest. The sampled values are then saved using the `coda()` command. Coda is a program written for S-plus and R, and it is designed to examine MCMC output. The Stata command `wbcoda` will be used later to read in the coda files. The log file is then saved (useful for debugging), and finally the `quit()` command closes WinBUGS.

The WinBUGS script file can be created using the `wbscript` command as follows:

```
. wbscript, sav("WinBUGS/RP_rott_script.txt", replace)
> model("`c(pwd)´/WinBUGS/RP_rott_model.txt")
> data("`c(pwd)´/WinBUGS/RP_rott_data.txt")
> inits("`c(pwd)´/WinBUGS/RP_rott_inits.txt")
> burn(5000) update(5000) set(gamma beta hr.age hr.hormon)
> log("`c(pwd)´/WinBUGS/RP_rott_log.txt")
> codafile("`c(pwd)´/WinBUGS/RP_rott_coda") noprint quit
```

WinBUGS requires us to give the full path name of the relevant files, and so we use the `` `c(pwd)' `` to denote the current working folder. It is useful and sometimes essential to specify initial values in WinBUGS. The `RP_rott_inits.txt` file contains them and is as follows:

```
list(beta=c(0,0), gamma=c(1,0,0,0))
```

Finally, we can call WinBUGS from within Stata using the `wbrun` command:

```
. wbrun, script("`c(pwd)'/WinBUGS/RP_rott_script.txt")
> win("C:\localapp\winbugs14\winbugs14.exe")
```

We need to tell the `wbrun` command where the script file is stored, as well as the location of the WinBUGS executable file. Running models in WinBUGS can take a long time, especially if there is a large amount of data. This rather simple model and a small dataset took almost three minutes to fit on a fairly standard laptop computer purchased in 2009.

When WinBUGS has finished running, we can load the results using the `wbcoda` command:

```
. wbcoda, root("WinBUGS/RP_rott_coda") clear
```

A description of the data gives

```
. describe
Contains data
  obs:         5,000
 vars:             9
 size:       200,000 (99.8% of memory free)
-------------------------------------------------------------------------------
              storage  display     value
variable name   type   format      label      variable label
-------------------------------------------------------------------------------
order           float  %9.0g
beta_1          float  %9.0g                  beta_1
beta_2          float  %9.0g                  beta_2
gamma_1         float  %9.0g                  gamma_1
gamma_2         float  %9.0g                  gamma_2
gamma_3         float  %9.0g                  gamma_3
gamma_4         float  %9.0g                  gamma_4
hr_age          float  %9.0g                  hr_age
hr_hormon       float  %9.0g                  hr_hormon
-------------------------------------------------------------------------------
Sorted by:  order
     Note:  dataset has changed since last saved
```

The `order` variable gives the iteration number of the MCMC chain. The remaining variables are those that we asked WinBUGS to monitor in the script file. These contain the 5,000 sampled values from the posterior distributions for our monitored parameters.

To obtain a summary of the distribution of each of the monitored variables we can use the `wbstats` command, as follows:

```
. wbstats gamma* beta* hr*
Parameter          n     mean        sd        se   median          95% CrI
gamma_1         5000   -1.003     0.030   0.0011   -1.003 (  -1.062,   -0.945 )
gamma_2         5000    0.981     0.026   0.0013    0.980 (   0.934,    1.031 )
gamma_3         5000    0.269     0.022   0.0011    0.269 (   0.228,    0.314 )
gamma_4         5000   -0.008     0.011   0.0004   -0.008 (  -0.030,    0.012 )
beta_1          5000   -0.005     0.002   0.0001   -0.005 (  -0.009,   -0.001 )
beta_2          5000    0.290     0.080   0.0025    0.292 (   0.129,    0.441 )
hr_age          5000    0.995     0.002   0.0001    0.995 (   0.991,    0.999 )
hr_hormon       5000    1.341     0.107   0.0034    1.340 (   1.138,    1.555 )
```

The estimates are very similar to those obtained from `stpm2`. For example, the HR and 95% CI for `hormon` is 1.34 [1.14, 1.57] when using `stpm2` and 1.34 [1.14, 1.56] for the WinBUGS model. Similarly, the HR for `age` is 0.9951 [0.9910, 0.9993] when using `stpm2` and 0.9951 [0.9908, 0.9995] for the WinBUGS model. This should not be too surprising because we are fitting the same model but using two different ways of estimating the parameters. Because we have used vague prior distributions for the model parameters in the WinBUGS model, we expect the results to be similar.

9.6.4 Summary

This has been a rather short introduction to fitting RP models in WinBUGS. For example, we have not covered how to check for convergence of the MCMC chains, how long a burn-in is necessary, and so on. We refer the interested reader to the WinBUGS manuals (Spiegelhalter et al. 2003b) and some useful books (Congdon 2006; Spiegelhalter, Abrams, and Myles 2003a). However, we hope we have showed the feasibility of fitting RP models in a Bayesian framework. An obvious and easy extension is to incorporate random effects into the model. One issue is that fitting these models takes much longer in WinBUGS than in Stata. There may be ways of speeding this up—for example, using the WinBUGS Development Interface (WBDev) (http://www.winbugs-development.org.uk/). We leave this aspect for others to explore.

9.7 Competing risks

Competing risks occur when an individual is at risk of more than one type of event, but can actually experience only one of them. The most common case is when the different events are death from different diseases, such as cancer, heart disease, or an infection. Competing risks are a special case of multistate models in which each of the different events are absorbing states (Andersen, Abildstrom, and Rosthøj 2002). In competing risks, a subject is at risk of dying from one of K different causes, but can only actually die of one cause.

The two most important measures in competing risks are the cause-specific hazard rate and the cumulative incidence function (CIF). The cause-specific hazard for cause

k, $h_k(t)$, gives the hazard rate at time t conditional on not having died of cause k or of any of the other $K-1$ causes of death. The cause-specific hazard, $h_k(t)$, can be estimated by treating events due to competing causes as censored observations. The K cause-specific hazard rates are usually estimated by fitting K separate models or by stacking the events (having K rows of data per individual) and fitting a model stratified by cause (Lunn and McNeil 1995).

The second important measure is the CIF, $C_k(t)$, for the kth competing risk. This gives the probability, as a function of time, that a subject dies of cause k in the presence of competing risks. It acknowledges that a subject cannot die of cause k if that subject has already died of one of the competing causes. The CIF is also known as the crude probability of death (Tsiatis 2005). It can be contrasted with the net probability of death (estimated from relative survival in chapter 8), which gives the probability of dying in a hypothetical world where it is impossible to die of other causes. CIFs give probabilities of death in the real world where individuals are always at risk of death from several different causes. We calculate cumulative incidences from a relative survival model in section 9.9. The CIF is defined as

$$C_k(t) = P(T \leq t \mid \text{cause} = k) = \int_0^t h_k(u) \exp\left\{-\int_0^u \sum_{k=1}^{k} h_k(v)\, dv\right\} du$$

$$= \int_0^t h_k(u) \prod_{k=1}^{K} S_k(u)\, du \qquad (9.1)$$

There are two distinct approaches to modeling competing-risks data:

1. **Model CIFs directly or more accurately on some transformation of the CIF.** This is what is done in the Fine and Gray model (Fine and Gray 1999), implemented in Stata as the `stcrreg` command (see [ST] **stcrreg**). These models are fit on the subhazard scale, where the subhazard is the CIF transformed to the hazard scale. When including covariates, `stcrreg` gives subhazard ratios.
2. **Model cause-specific hazards.** The hazard rate at time t for cause k gives the mortality rate of event k at time t for those subjects who are still at risk at time t—that is, those who have not died of cause k or any of the other causes or have not been censored. The corresponding CIF is found by estimating the hazard function for each cause and applying (9.1) to estimate the CIF for a specific cause k.

Here we show how RP models can be used in the cause-specific approach. Given that the survival probabilities and the hazard functions are needed to estimate the CIF, we feel that the use of RP models is particularly appealing compared with methods that use the Cox model, in which the hazard function is not directly estimated.

To illustrate the cause-specific approach, we use data for 506 men diagnosed with advanced prostate cancer who are randomly allocated to different levels of treatment of the drug diethylstilbestrol. The data have been used previously to illustrate Stata's `stcompet` command to nonparametrically estimate the CIF (Coviello and Boggess 2004). There are three different causes of death: cancer, `status=1`, cardiovascular disease (CVD), `status=2`, and other causes, `status=3`. The CIFs are estimated using the `stcompet` command, as follows:

```
. use prostatecancer
. stset time, failure(status==1)

     failure event:  status == 1
obs. time interval:  (0, time]
 exit on or before:  failure

------------------------------------------------------------------------------
      506  total obs.
        0  exclusions
------------------------------------------------------------------------------
      506  obs. remaining, representing
      155  failures in single record/single failure data
  18299.6  total analysis time at risk, at risk from t =         0
                             earliest observed entry t =         0
                                  last observed exit t =        76

. stcompet CI = ci, compet1(2) compet2(3) by(treatment)
```

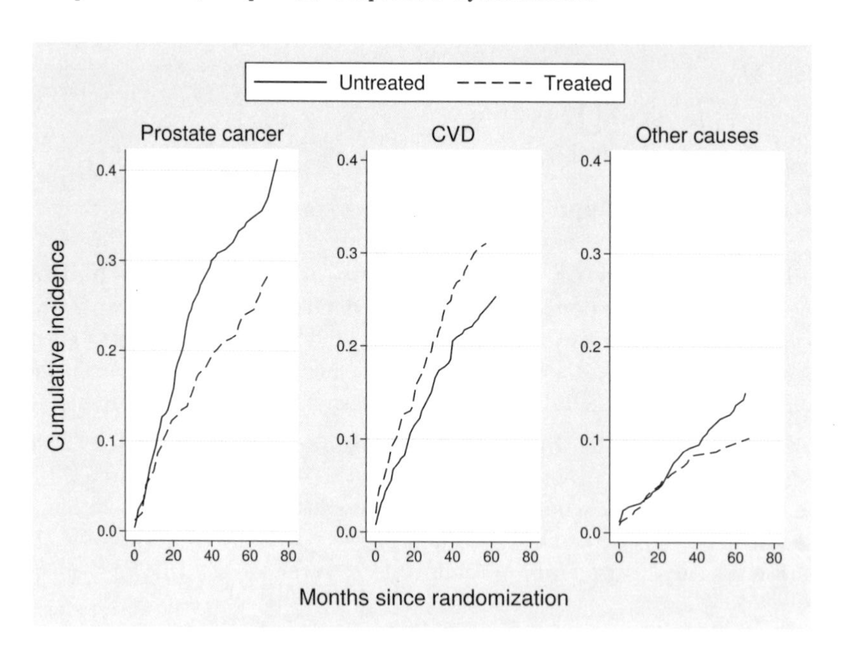

Figure 9.13. Estimated CIF for cancer, CVD, and other causes for men diagnosed with prostate cancer.

`stcompet` creates a new variable, `CI`, which contains the CIF for each of the three different causes of death. The resulting estimated CIFs are shown in figure 9.13. The treatment reduces the probability of dying due to cancer, but it somewhat increases the chance of death due to CVD. The reasons for this reduction are unclear just from the graphs. One possibility is that the risk of CVD death could be due to side effects of the drug, but it is more likely that if a man's risk of death due to prostate cancer is reduced, he has a greater opportunity to die of other causes such as CVD. This is an illustration of why consideration of both the cumulative incidence and cause-specific hazard functions are useful.

We now show how to use `stpm2` to obtain model-based estimates of the CIFs by estimating the cause-specific hazards. To do this in one model, we need to stack the data so that each individual has three rows of data, one for each of the competing events. To do this, we make use of the `expand` command:

```
. expand 3
(1012 observations created)
. bysort id: gen byte cause = _n
. generate byte cancer = cause == 1
. generate byte cvd = cause == 2
. generate byte other = cause == 3
. generate byte tx_cancer = treatment*cancer
. generate byte tx_cvd = treatment*cvd
. generate byte tx_other = treatment*other
. generate byte event = cause == status
```

We have also created indicator variables for each of the three competing causes and for interactions between `treatment` and the different causes. Because each individual has three rows of data—one for each of the three competing events—we need to create an indicator variable, `event`, to define which one of the events (if any) was the actual cause of death. We can now `stset` the data and use `stpm2` to fit the model, but we also use `stcox` so we can compare the estimates from the RP model with that from the Cox model.

```
. stset time, failure(event)
     failure event:  event != 0 & event < .
obs. time interval:  (0, time]
 exit on or before:  failure

------------------------------------------------------------------------------
     1518  total obs.
        0  exclusions
------------------------------------------------------------------------------
     1518  obs. remaining, representing
      356  failures in single record/single failure data
  54898.8  total analysis time at risk, at risk from t =         0
                             earliest observed entry t =         0
                                  last observed exit t =        76
```

```
. stcox tx_cancer tx_cvd tx_other, strata(cause) nolog noshow
Stratified Cox regr. -- Breslow method for ties
No. of subjects =         1518                Number of obs   =       1518
No. of failures =          356
Time at risk    =      54898.8
                                              LR chi2(3)      =      10.02
Log likelihood  =   -2023.7114                Prob > chi2     =     0.0184

------------------------------------------------------------------------------
          _t | Haz. Ratio   Std. Err.      z    P>|z|     [95% Conf. Interval]
-------------+----------------------------------------------------------------
   tx_cancer |   .6729649   .1098493    -2.43   0.015     .4887078    .9266924
      tx_cvd |    1.18494   .2008253     1.00   0.317     .8500285    1.651806
    tx_other |   .6352488   .1674886    -1.72   0.085     .3788938     1.06505
------------------------------------------------------------------------------
                                                             Stratified by cause
. stpm2 cancer cvd other tx_cancer tx_cvd tx_other, scale(hazard)
> rcsbaseoff nocons tvc(cancer cvd other) dftvc(3) eform nolog
Log likelihood = -1150.4866                     Number of obs   =       1518

------------------------------------------------------------------------------
             |     exp(b)   Std. Err.      z    P>|z|     [95% Conf. Interval]
-------------+----------------------------------------------------------------
xb           |
      cancer |   .2363179   .0275697   -12.37   0.000      .188015    .2970303
         cvd |   .1801868   .0238668   -12.94   0.000     .1389876    .2335983
       other |   .1008464    .018132   -12.76   0.000      .070895    .1434515
   tx_cancer |   .6722196   .1096964    -2.43   0.015     .4882109    .9255819
      tx_cvd |   1.188189   .2013301     1.02   0.309     .8524237     1.65621
    tx_other |   .6345498   .1672676    -1.73   0.084     .3785199    1.063758
_rcs_cancer1 |   3.501847     .44435     9.88   0.000     2.730788     4.49062
_rcs_cancer2 |   .8842712   .0742915    -1.46   0.143     .7500191    1.042554
_rcs_cancer3 |   1.046436   .0371625     1.28   0.201     .9760756    1.121868
   _rcs_cvd1 |   2.841936   .2619063    11.33   0.000     2.372299    3.404545
   _rcs_cvd2 |   .8772848   .0498866    -2.30   0.021     .7847607    .9807176
   _rcs_cvd3 |   1.008804   .0352009     0.25   0.802     .9421175     1.08021
 _rcs_other1 |   2.751505   .3563037     7.82   0.000     2.134738    3.546467
 _rcs_other2 |   .7962094   .0558593    -3.25   0.001     .6939208     .913576
 _rcs_other3 |   .9614597   .0512891    -0.74   0.461     .8660117    1.067428
------------------------------------------------------------------------------
```

The data have been `stset` in the usual way, but we have not used the `id()` option because we have overlapping time intervals. When using `stpm2`, we have used the `rcsbaseoff` option, which means that the baseline hazard has not been included, because we have fit a stratified model. This is done by including the three cause indicators (`cancer`, `cvd`, and `other`) as main effects and also as time-dependent effects using the `tvc()` option. There are now three separate baselines, one for each of the causes. The three interaction terms for treatment have also been included, and we can estimate the effect of treatment on the three different causes of death. The HRs for the treatment effect are 0.67 (95% CI; [0.49, 0.93]) for cancer, 1.19 [0.85, 1.66] for CVD, and 0.63 [0.38, 1.06] for other causes. Not surprisingly, the cause-specific HRs for the three treatment effects are very similar when comparing the RP estimates with those from the Cox model.

To estimate the CIFs, we need to obtain predictions of the survival and hazard function for each of the three causes for the two treatments. This is done in the following loop:

```
. range timevar 0.1 70 1000
(518 missing values generated)
. foreach cause in cancer cvd other {
  2.         predict s_`cause´_tx0, survival at(`cause´ 1)
>                zeros timevar(timevar)
  3.         predict s_`cause´_tx1, survival at(`cause´ 1 tx_`cause´ 1)
>                timevar(timevar) zeros
  4.         predict h_`cause´_tx0, hazard at(`cause´ 1)
>                timevar(timevar) zeros
  5.         predict h_`cause´_tx1, hazard at(`cause´ 1 tx_`cause´ 1)
>                timevar(timevar) zeros
  6. }
```

Overall survival can be estimated as the product of survival for the three different causes, as follows:

```
. generate s_all_tx0 = s_cancer_tx0 * s_cvd_tx0 * s_other_tx0
(518 missing values generated)
. generate s_all_tx1 = s_cancer_tx1 * s_cvd_tx1 * s_other_tx1
(518 missing values generated)
```

To estimate the CIF, we need to perform the integration in (9.1). It is not possible to obtain the answer analytically. Instead, we perform the integration numerically using the `integ` command.

```
. foreach cause in cancer cvd other {
  2.         gen f_`cause´_tx0 = s_all_tx0 * h_`cause´_tx0
  3.         gen f_`cause´_tx1 = s_all_tx1 * h_`cause´_tx1
  4.         integ f_`cause´_tx0 timevar, gen(CIF_`cause´_tx0)
  5.         integ f_`cause´_tx1 timevar, gen(CIF_`cause´_tx1)
  6. }
(518 missing values generated)
(518 missing values generated)
number of points = 1000
integral         = .3650361
number of points = 1000
integral         = .26941723
(518 missing values generated)
(518 missing values generated)
number of points = 1000
integral         = .25005096
number of points = 1000
integral         = .32487085
(518 missing values generated)
(518 missing values generated)
number of points = 1000
integral         = .14423041
number of points = 1000
integral         = .10145638
```

The resulting CIFs are plotted in figure 9.14, together with nonparametric estimates obtained from `stcompet`. The model-based curves and nonparametric estimates are broadly similar, despite the model-based estimates potentially being restricted by the assumption of PH. One of the advantages of using `stpm2` is the ease at which time-dependent effects could be incorporated for any or all of the three different causes of death.

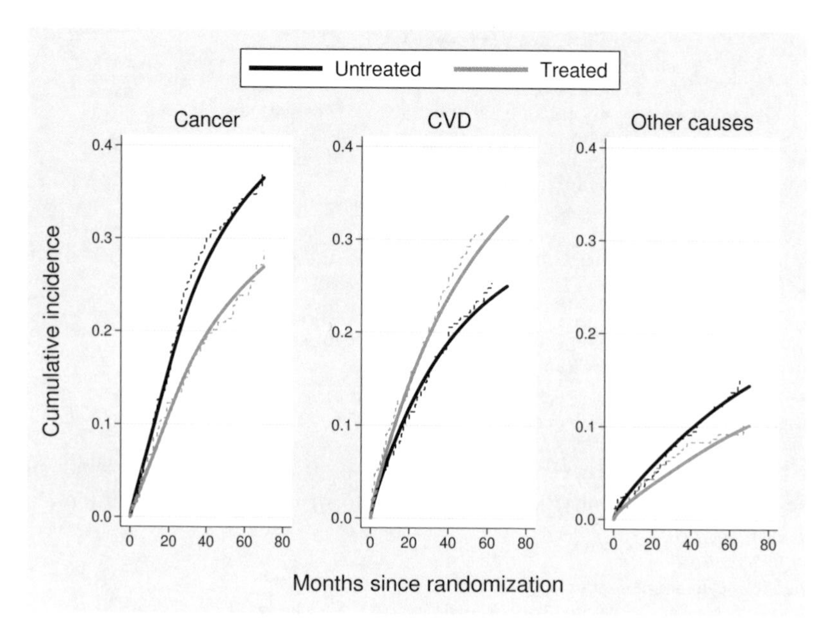

Figure 9.14. Advanced prostate cancer data. Estimated CIF for cancer, CVD, and other causes of death for men diagnosed with prostate cancer. Estimates were obtained from a cause-specific RP model. The dashed lines are the corresponding nonparametric estimates obtained from `stcompet`.

9.7.1 Summary

We have shown how CIFs can be estimated using RP models. The model is based on fitting cause-specific hazards models. In the code we have shown, we have not calculated CIs, although this would be relatively easy to do using either the bootstrap or the delta method, as in section 4.8.6. There are some advantages to modeling on the cumulative incidence scale (or some transformation of it). This is not currently possible with RP models, and is likely to be an area of further research.

9.8 Period analysis

9.8.1 Introduction

One important use of data from cancer registries is to monitor survival after a diagnosis of cancer for a range of cancer sites. Survival estimates are often compared over time and between regions or countries. As discussed in chapter 8, relative survival is often the method used to report population-based cancer survival because information on cause of death is not required. It is common to report mid- to long-term cancer survival at 5 or 10 years postdiagnosis. This raises an important issue when calculating these measures because the estimates include data for individuals diagnosed at least 5 or 10 years prior to the analysis date. In practice, even older data are included because of the lag time from data acquisition and cleaning to analysis.

When cancer survival is improving over time, the use of older data underestimates the survival proportion. One potential solution to this is to use *period analysis* to obtain more up-to-date estimates of patients' survival (Brenner and Gefeller 1997). This approach has become widely accepted in the analysis of population-based cancer survival. For example, it has been used in a number of recent international comparisons of cancer survival (Coleman et al. 2011; Møller et al. 2010). Period estimates of patient survival are usually calculated separately in subgroups of interest using life table methodology. In this section we first describe the motivation behind period analysis and then show that it is very simple to obtain model-based period estimates of cancer survival.

9.8.2 What is period analysis?

Up-to-date estimates of patient survival using period analysis are based on artificially truncating individuals' survival times prior to a recent cutoff in calendar time. This has the effect of using individuals diagnosed in a recent time period for short-term survival and individuals diagnosed further back in time for longer term survival. This is illustrated in figure 9.15, which shows the survival for four hypothetical individuals with survival experience between the start of 1996 and the end of 2005. For simplicity, all individuals are diagnosed with cancer on the first day of the year and die on the last day of the year. In a standard survival analysis, all individuals would become at risk on the date of diagnosis. This can be seen by their corresponding start and stop times in figure 9.15. These would correspond to the values of `_t0` and `_t` in Stata. The vertical reference lines show the start and end of the time window of interest for the period analysis; thus we are only interested in the survival experience from 2002–2005, inclusive. The survival times are potentially left-truncated, with the time of the left-truncation defined by the calendar time at the start of the window for the recent time period. In the figure, all of subject 1's survival experience is after the start of 2002 (the start of the time window) and thus their start and stop times are exactly the same as in a standard analysis. All of subject 4's survival experience is before the start of the time window, and thus that subject is excluded from the period analysis. Both subject 2 and 3 have survival experience that spans the start of the time window, and hence the time they start being at risk is changed for the period analysis. This change can be seen by the start times given in the figure—two years for subject 2 and five years for subject 6. Thus we ignore the short term survival for these two individuals, but they are not ignored completely in the analysis because they do contribute to longer term survival. Only individuals diagnosed recently (subject 1, in this case) contribute to short term survival.

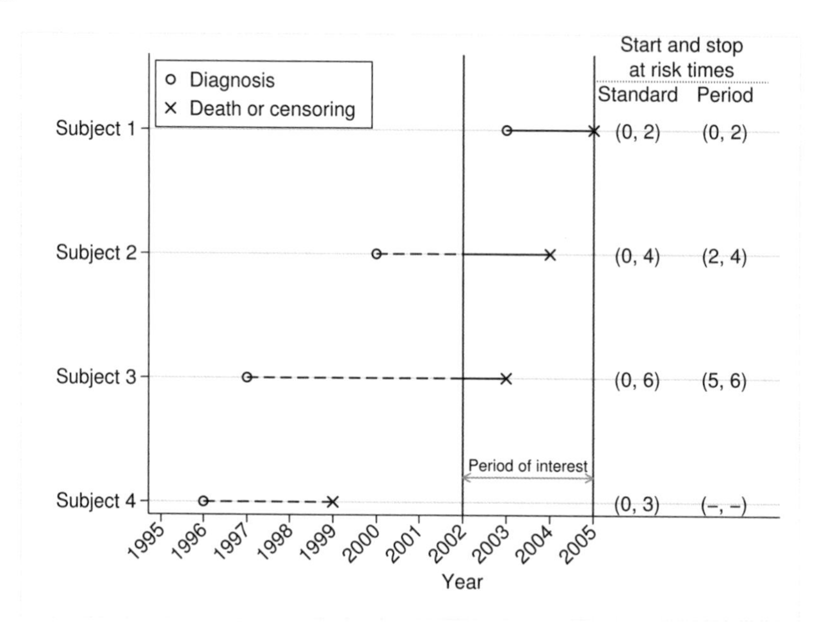

Figure 9.15. Schematic figure showing concept of delayed entry in period analysis.

Although artificial truncation of patient survival may initially seem like a strange thing to do, it is actually similar to methods used in demography to calculate life expectancy. For example, when calculating life expectancy, age-specific mortality rates (that is, hazards) of a recent population are used, not those from a cohort born 100 years ago.

One of the key assumptions of period analysis is that improvements in patient survival are generally seen in short-term survival and less so in longer-term survival. Although period analysis was at first criticized as a method, there have been a number of studies investigating its use on retrospective data that show that it actually works very well in practice (Brenner and Hakulinen 2002; Brenner, Gefeller, and Hakulinen 2004).

9.8.3 Application to England and Wales breast cancer data

Period analysis is incredibly simple in Stata through `stset`. To convert a standard analysis to a period analysis, all we have to do is adapt the `stset` command to define the start of the time window. The estimation commands remain the same. This is illustrated with the breast cancer data used in chapter 8 for relative survival models. We are interested in the five-year relative survival estimates by age group. In chapter 8, we used a previously created survival time, `survtime`, with `stset`. We can actually make use of the date of diagnosis, `datediag`, and the date of death or censoring, `dateexit`, with `stset` as follows:

```
. stset dateexit, failure(dead==1) id(ident) scale(365.24) origin(date diag)
> exit(time datediag + 5*365.24)

                id:  ident
     failure event:  dead == 1
obs. time interval:  (dateexit[_n-1], dateexit]
 exit on or before:  time datediag + 5*365.24
    t for analysis:  (time-origin)/365.24
            origin:  time datediag
------------------------------------------------------------------------------

   115331  total obs.
        0  exclusions
------------------------------------------------------------------------------

   115331  obs. remaining, representing
   115331  subjects
    47692  failures in single failure-per-subject data
   432461  total analysis time at risk, at risk from t =         0
                             earliest observed entry t =         0
                                  last observed exit t =         5
```

There is a small discrepancy in the total of 0.2 person-years compared with the total in section 8.4. The discrepancy is due to some rounding when the `survtime` variable was calculated. Otherwise, using `stset` incorporating the `datediag` and `dateexit` variables is the same as when using `survtime`. Now that we are using dates to `stset` the data, extension to period analysis is straightforward because we can use the `enter()` option to give the calendar time when individuals become at risk. The breast cancer data included women diagnosed between 1986 and 1990, inclusive. In this dataset, there is actually follow-up until 1995, but we will restrict follow-up to the end of 1990 to mimic the type of data that is usually obtained from cancer registries. We will use a one-year time window—that is, from the 1st of January 1990 until the 1st of January 1991. The updated `stset` command is as follows:

```
. stset dateexit, failure(dead==1) id(ident) scale(365.24)
> origin(datediag) exit(time mdy(1,1,1991)) enter(time mdy(1,1,1990))

                id:  ident
     failure event:  dead == 1
obs. time interval:  (dateexit[_n-1], dateexit]
 enter on or after:  time mdy(1,1,1990)
 exit on or before:  time mdy(1,1,1991)
    t for analysis:  (time-origin)/365.24
            origin:  time datediag

------------------------------------------------------------------------------
    115331  total obs.
     19640  obs. end on or before enter()
------------------------------------------------------------------------------
     95691  obs. remaining, representing
     95691  subjects
      8718  failures in single failure-per-subject data
  79415.43  total analysis time at risk, at risk from t =         0
                             earliest observed entry t =         0
                                  last observed exit t =  4.999452
```

We have used the mdy() function in the enter() option to give the date of the start of the time window. The output tells us that 19,640 observations are excluded because their survival time finishes on or before the 1st of January 1990. Having done this, all Stata st commands (for example, stcox, strate, and streg) take account of the delayed entry and hence perform a period analysis (Smith et al. 2004). User-written survival analysis commands, such as stpm2, also work if delayed entry has been incorporated, but it may be worth checking that it has actually been implemented. The life-table based period-analysis estimates of relative survival described by Brenner and Gefeller (1997) can be implemented using the strs command. However, we will fit RP models with delayed entry to obtain period-analysis estimates of relative survival. Before fitting a relative survival model, we need to merge in the expected mortality, as we did in chapter 8.

```
. generate age = int(min(agediag + _t,99))
. generate year = int(year(datediag) + _t)
(19640 missing values generated)
. merge m:1 sex region dep year age using popmort_uk, keepusing(rate)
> keep(match)
    Result                           # of obs.
    -----------------------------------------
    not matched                             0
    matched                            95,691  (_merge==3)
    -----------------------------------------
```

The modeling command is exactly the same as in chapter 8 because the delayed entry defined in our stset command is taken into account by stpm2.

```
. stpm2 agegrp2-agegrp5, scale(hazard) df(7) bhazard(rate) nolog
> tvc(agegrp2-agegrp5) dftvc(3)
note: delayed entry models are being fitted
Log likelihood = -24233.539                       Number of obs   =      95691

------------------------------------------------------------------------------
             |      Coef.   Std. Err.      z    P>|z|     [95% Conf. Interval]
-------------+----------------------------------------------------------------
xb           |
     agegrp2 |   .2116084    .055947     3.78   0.000     .1019542    .3212626
     agegrp3 |   .3893414   .0525807     7.40   0.000      .286285    .4923978
     agegrp4 |   .8334908    .052763    15.80   0.000     .7300773    .9369044
     agegrp5 |   1.359571    .055194    24.63   0.000     1.251393    1.467749
       _rcs1 |   1.196167   .0447309    26.74   0.000     1.108496    1.283838
       _rcs2 |  -.1040573   .0310448    -3.35   0.001    -.1649041   -.0432105
       _rcs3 |   .0115074   .0103255     1.11   0.265    -.0087302     .031745
       _rcs4 |   .0735219   .0084617     8.69   0.000     .0569373    .0901066
       _rcs5 |   .0230572   .0035651     6.47   0.000     .0160697    .0300448
       _rcs6 |   .0027781   .0020977     1.32   0.185    -.0013333    .0068895
       _rcs7 |  -.0035721   .0015318    -2.33   0.020    -.0065744   -.0005698
_rcs_ageg~21 |  -.2206054   .0544849    -4.05   0.000    -.3273938    -.113817
_rcs_ageg~22 |   .0037501   .0363832     0.10   0.918    -.0675596    .0750598
_rcs_ageg~23 |   -.054056   .0176451    -3.06   0.002    -.0886398   -.0194722
_rcs_ageg~31 |  -.4292558   .0494359    -8.68   0.000    -.5261484   -.3323633
_rcs_ageg~32 |   .0237341   .0331912     0.72   0.475    -.0413195    .0887877
_rcs_ageg~33 |   -.093292    .016314    -5.72   0.000    -.1252668   -.0613171
_rcs_ageg~41 |  -.5806478   .0480046   -12.10   0.000    -.6747351   -.4865606
_rcs_ageg~42 |   .1113016   .0328638     3.39   0.001     .0468898    .1757134
_rcs_ageg~43 |  -.0947236   .0158956    -5.96   0.000    -.1258785   -.0635688
_rcs_ageg~51 |  -.6513244   .0481047   -13.54   0.000    -.7456079    -.557041
_rcs_ageg~52 |    .108751    .033157     3.28   0.001     .0437644    .1737375
_rcs_ageg~53 |   -.131883   .0174319    -7.57   0.000    -.1660488   -.0977171
       _cons |  -2.394757   .0414345   -57.80   0.000    -2.475967   -2.313546
------------------------------------------------------------------------------
```

stpm2 has given a note to tell us that there is delayed entry. As in chapter 8, individual parameters are difficult to interpret, and so we predict the five-year relative survival by age group.

```
. range temptime 0.003 5 200
(95491 missing values generated)
. predict s1_period, survival zeros timevar(temptime)
. forvalues i = 2/5 {
  2.         predict s`i´_period, survival at(agegrp`i´ 1) zeros
> timevar(temptime)
  3. }
. list s1_period-s5_period if temptime == 5, noobs

  +-------------------------------------------------------------+
  | s1_period   s2_period   s3_period   s4_period   s5_period |
  |-------------------------------------------------------------|
  | .71587798   .70034626   .70134475   .65492001   .49031619 |
  +-------------------------------------------------------------+
```

If the data are stset again for the same five-year period but without the one-year window—that is, a standard (relative) survival analysis and the model refit—the following estimates are obtained:

```
. list s1_standard-s5_standard if temptime == 5, noobs
```

s1_stan~d	s2_stan~d	s3_stan~d	s4_stan~d	s5_stan~d
.70086966	.67277961	.68021521	.64559112	.50382664

For all age groups except the oldest, the period estimates are higher than the standard estimates. This indicates that there is probably some trend over the 5-year period in terms of improved survival and that by use of period analysis we have obtained more up-to-date estimates. A trend over this period could of course be examined in a model. The existence of such a trend can also be incorporated into a period analysis (Brenner, Gondos, and Arndt 2007; Brenner and Hakulinen 2007, 2008) to obtain more precise and up-to-date period-analysis estimates of patient survival.

9.9 Crude probability of death from relative survival models

9.9.1 Introduction

In chapter 8, we showed how relative survival models can be fit by incorporating each individual's expected mortality or survival into both RP and Poisson models. In this section, we show how, after fitting a relative survival model, we can borrow some ideas from competing-risks theory to obtain an analogue of the CIF described in section 9.7. Recall that in relative survival, we assume that overall survival is the product of the expected survival and the relative survival—that is,

$$S(t) = S^*(t) R(t)$$

and that the overall hazard rate is the sum of the background hazard and the excess hazard rates—that is,

$$h(t) = h^*(t) + \lambda(t)$$

If we assume independence between mortality due to cancer and mortality due to other causes, then we interpret relative survival as net survival—that is, survival in a hypothetical world where it is impossible to die of any cause other than the disease of interest. This is sensible when we want to compare survival over time and between countries or regions, because mortality due to other causes varies over time and between places. However, to a patient and their doctor, it is more relevant to know the patient's "real-world" probability of dying of cancer and of other causes. In competing risks, this is known as the CIF, but in population-based cancer studies it is usually referred to as the crude probability of death (Cronin and Feuer 2000). The excess hazard rate, $\lambda(t)$, is an estimate of the cause-specific hazard rate due to the disease of interest, and $h^*(t)$ is an estimate of the cause-specific hazard rate for other causes. Thus we can adapt the standard cumulative incidence (9.1) for competing risks for our relative survival model to obtain the crude probability of death due to cancer,

$$Cr_c(t) = \int_0^t S^*(u) R(u) \lambda(u) \, du \tag{9.2}$$

and the crude probability of death due to other causes,

$$Cr_o(t) = \int_0^t S^*(u) R(u) h^*(u) du \tag{9.3}$$

Thus $Cr_c(t)$ gives the probability of dying from the cancer of interest at time t in the presence of the competing risk of death due to other causes, and $Cr_o(t)$ gives the probability of dying from other causes at time t in the presence of the competing risks of death due to cancer. For more details of the general approach, see Lambert et al. (2010).

9.9.2 Application to England and Wales breast cancer data

We return to the England and Wales breast cancer data used in chapter 8. When estimating crude probabilities, we are usually interested in using them for individual patients. The effect of age on the probability of both death due to cancer and death due other causes is important, and we want to make predictions for individual patients rather than have broad age categories. In section 8.9, we used FPs to model the effect of continuous age in a relative survival model. Here we use splines. We first need to load and `stset` the data and merge in the expected mortality in the same way as we did in chapter 8.

```
. use EW_breast, clear
(England & Wales breast cancer survival)
. stset survtime, failure(dead==1) exit(time 5) id(ident)
                id:  ident
     failure event:  dead == 1
obs. time interval:  (survtime[_n-1], survtime]
 exit on or before:  time 5
------------------------------------------------------------------------------
   115331  total obs.
        0  exclusions
------------------------------------------------------------------------------
   115331  obs. remaining, representing
   115331  subjects
    47692  failures in single failure-per-subject data
 432458.2  total analysis time at risk, at risk from t =         0
                             earliest observed entry t =         0
                                  last observed exit t =         5
. generate age = int(min(agediag + _t,99))
. gen year = int(year(datediag) + _t)
. merge m:1 sex region dep year age using popmort_uk, keepusing(rate)
> keep(match)
    Result                           # of obs.
    -----------------------------------------
    not matched                             0
    matched                           115,331  (_merge==3)
    -----------------------------------------
```

We now generate the spline variables for age at diagnosis, `agediag`.

```
. rcsgen agediag, gen(agercs) df(4) orthog
Variables agercs1 to agercs4 were created
. global knotsage `r(knots)´
. matrix Rage = r(R)
```

We have used 4 d.f. (5 knots) for the effect of age at diagnosis. We have stored the knot locations and the R matrix because we need to generate some of the spline variables again later. We now fit the RP model using `stpm2`, using 7 d.f. for the baseline and allowing the effect of the age at diagnosis to be time dependent by including it in the `tvc()` option. We use 4 d.f. for the time-dependent effect of each spline term.

```
. stpm2 agercs*, scale(hazard) df(7) tvc(agercs*) dftvc(3) nolog
  (output omitted)
Log likelihood = -137819.18                     Number of obs   =     115331
```

	Coef.	Std. Err.	z	P>|z|	[95% Conf.	Interval]
xb						
agercs1	.4703492	.0051977	90.49	0.000	.4601619	.4805365
agercs2	-.223165	.0051568	-43.28	0.000	-.2332722	-.2130579
agercs3	-.01518	.0052148	-2.91	0.004	-.0254009	-.0049591
agercs4	-.0235297	.0043852	-5.37	0.000	-.0321244	-.0149349
_rcs1	.9893405	.0066387	149.03	0.000	.9763289	1.002352
_rcs2	-.0421117	.0046434	-9.07	0.000	-.0512126	-.0330108
_rcs3	-.0272257	.0019123	-14.24	0.000	-.0309737	-.0234777
_rcs4	.0238995	.001179	20.27	0.000	.0215888	.0262103
_rcs5	.0036782	.0006998	5.26	0.000	.0023066	.0050498
_rcs6	.0013535	.000468	2.89	0.004	.0004362	.0022707
_rcs7	-.000058	.0003147	-0.18	0.854	-.0006749	.0005588
_rcs_ager~11	-.1527932	.0075542	-20.23	0.000	-.1675993	-.1379872
_rcs_ager~12	.0137041	.0051444	2.66	0.008	.0036211	.023787
_rcs_ager~13	-.0375437	.0017548	-21.39	0.000	-.0409831	-.0341043
_rcs_ager~21	-.0304847	.0071458	-4.27	0.000	-.0444902	-.0164792
_rcs_ager~22	.003856	.0048435	0.80	0.426	-.0056372	.0133491
_rcs_ager~23	-.0002861	.0016856	-0.17	0.865	-.0035898	.0030175
_rcs_ager~31	-.0373475	.006755	-5.53	0.000	-.0505871	-.0241079
_rcs_ager~32	.0065441	.0045576	1.44	0.151	-.0023885	.0154768
_rcs_ager~33	-.0045959	.0017155	-2.68	0.007	-.0079582	-.0012336
_rcs_ager~41	.0054249	.0041502	1.31	0.191	-.0027093	.0135592
_rcs_ager~42	-.0011411	.0028567	-0.40	0.690	-.0067402	.004458
_rcs_ager~43	-.0022261	.0013407	-1.66	0.097	-.0048537	.0004016
_cons	-1.188481	.0052986	-224.30	0.000	-1.198866	-1.178096

We do not even try to interpret the parameters, but we want to predict first the net probability of death—that is, $1 - R(t)$—and then the crude probability of death for both cancer and other causes using (9.2) and (9.3). The England and Wales breast cancer dataset is fairly large at 115,331 observations, so the predictions and plotting of graphs can take a long time. One way of speeding things up is to use out-of-sample prediction. We do it by dropping all variables from the dataset and then creating a new dataset of 1,000 observations and making predictions for that dataset, but making sure we use the covariate values that are of interest. We have modeled age continuously using spline functions, and so we need to choose some relevant ages to make predictions for; here we choose ages 35, 45, 55, 65, 75, and 85.

```
. drop _all
. set obs 1000
obs was 0, now 1000
. range temptime 0.003 5
. gen _t = .
(1000 missing values generated)
. foreach agediag in 35 45 55 65 75 85 {
  2.         capture drop agercs*
  3.         tempvar a
  4.         gen `a´ = `agediag´
  5.         quietly rcsgen `a´, knots($knotsage) gen(agercs) rmatrix(Rage)
  6.         drop `a´
  7.         predict s`agediag´, survival timevar(temptime)
  8.         gen netprob`agediag´ = 1 - s`agediag´
  9. }
```

We first drop all observations in our dataset using `drop _all`. We use the `range` command to produce our new time variable. The `_t` variable needs to exist when using the `predict` command after `stpm2`, and so we create it (even though it is missing for all values). We then loop over the ages of interest to obtain the predicted relative survival functions. Because we use splines for the effect of age, we need to know the values of the spline variables at each age. That is why we save the knot locations and R matrix above. We used a similar trick in section 7.7. The net probability of death due to cancer for our selected ages is shown in figure 9.16. The net probability of death due to cancer is worse with increasing age, with the exception that the 35-year-old women do slightly worse than those aged 45 and 55. It is important to remember that these are estimates of the probabilities of death in the hypothetical world where you cannot die of other causes. As we discussed above, it can be more relevant to estimate probabilities of death in the real world where patients are at risk of death due to the other causes; that is, we want to estimate the crude probability of death.

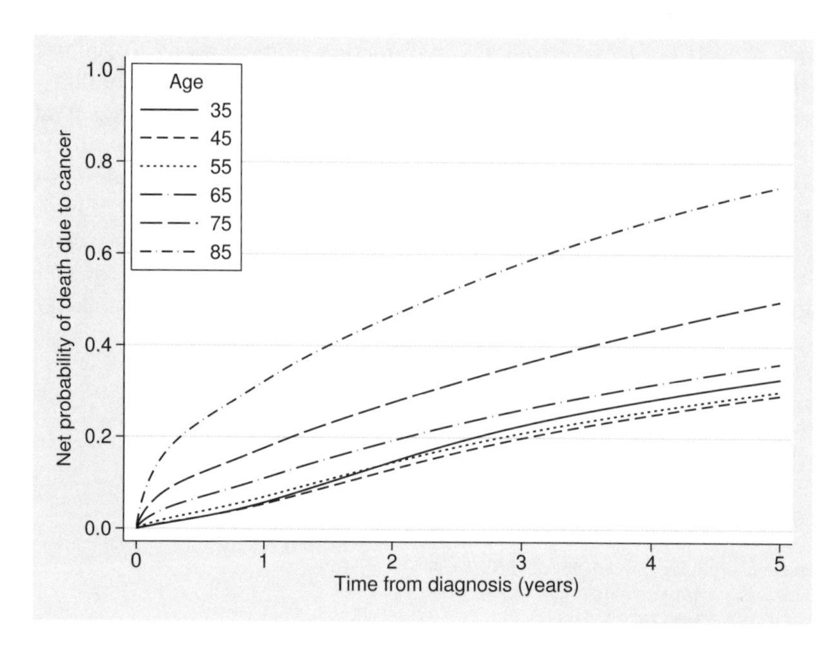

Figure 9.16. England and Wales breast cancer data. Estimated net probability of death due to cancer for selected ages.

To perform the integration in (9.2) and (9.3), we split the time scale into many (usually 1,000) intervals. We then calculate the integrand for each time point in both equations and simply sum the estimates, taking account of the width of the time intervals. One advantage of performing the numerical integration in this way is that it allows us to obtain CIs of the crude probability of death; see Lambert et al. (2010) for details of the necessary calculations. We have written a postestimation command, `stpm2cm`, that performs these calculations. Again we loop over our selected ages to obtain the predictions.

```
. foreach agediag in 35 45 55 65 75 85 {
  2.          capture drop agercs*
  3.          tempvar a
  4.          gen `a´ = `agediag´
  5.          quietly rcsgen `a´, knots($knotsage) gen(agercs) rmatrix(Rage)
  6.          drop `a´
  7.          local atlist agercs1 `=agercs1[1]´ agercs2 `=agercs2[1]´
>                  agercs3 `=agercs3[1]´ agercs4 `=agercs4[1]´
  8.          stpm2cm using popmort_uk, mergeby(sex region dep year age) maxt(5)
>                  at(`atlist´) diagage(`agediag´) diagyear(1990) sex(2)
>                  attyear(year) attage(age) stub(crudeprob`agediag´)
>                  tgen(t`agediag´) mergegen(region 1 dep 3)
>                  nobs(1000) survprob(survprob)
  9. }
```

There are a lot of options for `stpm2cm`. The main reason for this is that the expected survival needs to be calculated, and that is done by calling `strs` (described in section 8.5), which merges in the expected survival from the population mortality file (`popmort_uk.dta`); thus `stpm2cm` requires many options of `strs`. Among other variables, `stpm2cm` generates the crude probability of death due to the disease of interest in *stubname* `_d` and the crude probability of death due to other causes in *stubname*`_o` through use of the `stub(`*stubname*`)` option. The estimated crude probability of death due to cancer for the selected ages can be seen in figure 9.17. As age increases, there is a greater difference between the estimated net (shown in figure 9.16) and crude probability of death due to cancer, with the crude probability of death always being lower. The reason for this is that mortality due to other causes plays a greater role as age increases.

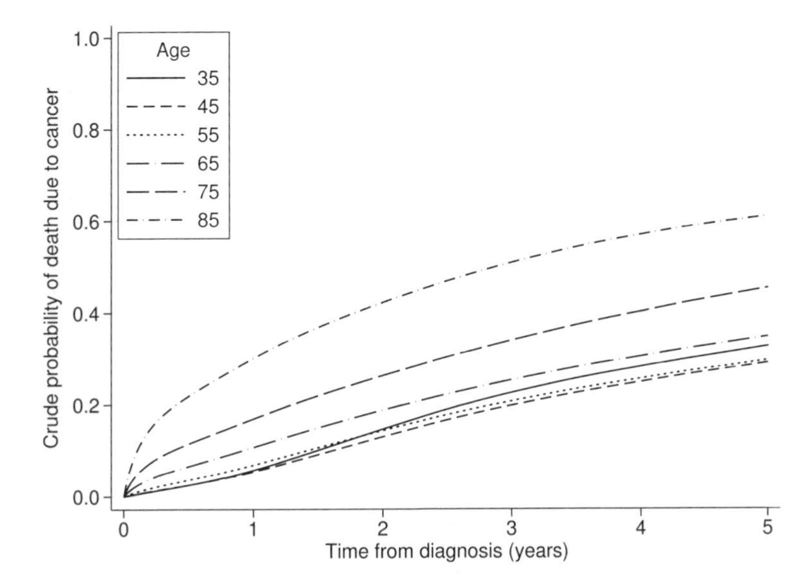

Figure 9.17. England and Wales breast cancer data. Estimated crude probability of death due to cancer for selected ages.

It is useful to show the crude probability of death due to cancer and due to other causes on the same graph. We usually stack the probabilities so that at each time point the cumulative probability of death due to cancer, probability of death due to other causes, and probability of being alive can be seen. The following code produces a stacked graph for each of the selected ages and then combines them into a single graph:

```
. foreach age in 35 45 55 65 75 85  {
  2.    generate crudeprob`age´_do = crudeprob`age´_o + crudeprob`age´_d
  3.    twoway (area crudeprob`age´_d t`age´, color(gs1))
> (rarea crudeprob`age´_d crudeprob`age´_do t`age´, color(gs5))
> (area crudeprob`age´_do t`age´, base(1) color(gs12)),
> scheme(lean2)
> legend(order(1 "Dead (breast cancer)" 2 "Dead (other causes)" 3 "Alive")
> cols(3) span size(*0.8) symxsize(*0.8))
> xtitle("", size(*1.5)) ytitle("", size(*1.5))
> ylabel(0(0.2)1, angle(horizontal) format(%3.1f) labsize(*1.5) grid)
> xlabel(,labsize(*1.5)) title("Age `age´", ring(0)) plotr(m(zero)) nodraw
> name(stack`age´,replace)
  4. }
. grc1leg stack35 stack45 stack55 stack65 stack75 stack85, nocopies
> scheme(lean2) name(stackprob, replace) b1title("Years from diagnosis")
> l1title("Probability of death") plotregion(style(none))
> graphregion(margin(0 0 0 0))
```

The graph can be seen in figure 9.18. The increase with age for both the crude probability of death due to the cancer and due to other causes can immediately be seen. Unsurprisingly, the crude probability of death due to other causes for a woman aged 35, 45, or 55 is very small because expected mortality is very low.

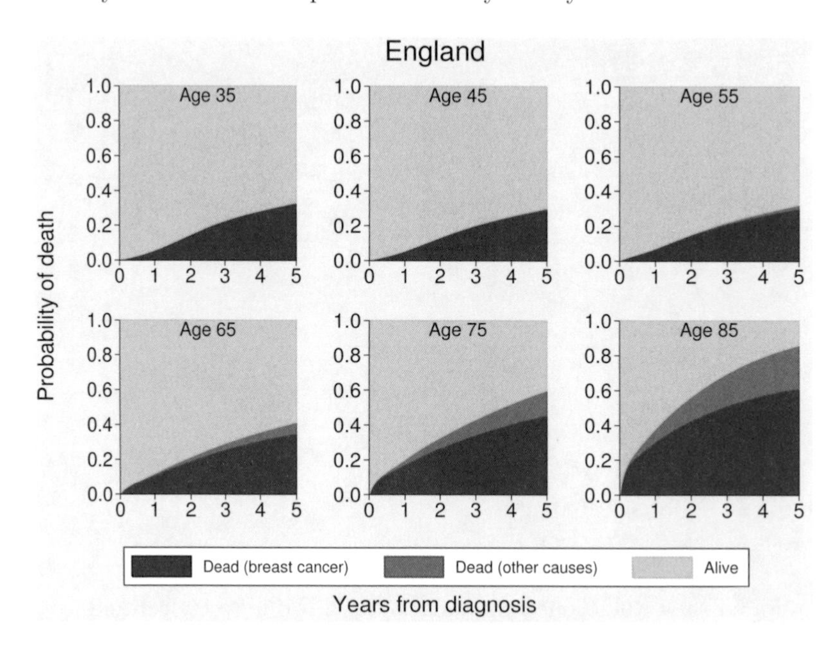

Figure 9.18. England and Wales breast cancer data. Estimated crude probability of death due to breast cancer and due to other causes for selected ages.

9.9.3 Conclusion

The estimation of the crude probabilities of death after fitting a relative survival model is essentially the same as the estimation of the CIF in a competing-risks setting. The difference is that we assume that we know the cause-specific hazard rate for other causes, rather than estimating it. Within relative survival, crude probabilities had previously only been estimated using life table methods (Cronin and Feuer 2000). In a model-based approach, it is possible to obtain predictions for any covariate pattern. Prediction of crude probabilities of death is important when making treatment decisions—particularly in the elderly, for whom mortality due to other causes is higher. However, for predictions to be clinically useful, it is important to record and model as many relevant covariates as possible. Within cancer, stage of disease and other measures of disease severity are of particular importance.

9.10 Final remarks

As time has gone on, we have found that flexible parametric survival modeling, particularly the RP approach, offers opportunities to simplify and extend standard methods of survival analysis in ways that we had not predicted a priori. We expect the process to continue. An application we and collaborators are already working on is so-called cure models, in which a proportion of patients is presumed to be cured of a condition of interest (for example, cancer) after a certain lapse of time.

In a way, we see parametric survival analysis as belonging more to the mainstream of statistical thought and practice than the "semiparametric" body of techniques that originated with the Cox PH model and has been continued and extended by applying the counting-process approach to many statistical modeling contexts. Two significant advantages flow from the anchoring of flexible parametric models in traditional methodology: "prediction" (for example, of hazard and survival functions) is easier; and because estimation is within the likelihood framework, we can more easily compare models and perform other aspects of inference.

In conclusion, we hope that the tools, analyses, and examples described in our book will help applied statisticians to investigate and analyze their survival data in Stata in a more inquisitive and detailed way than they would have done hitherto.

References

Akaike, H. 1973. Information theory and an extension of the maximum likelihood principle. In *Second International Symposium on Information Theory*, ed. B. N. Petrov and F. Csaki, 267–281. Budapest: Akademiai Kiado.

Altman, D. G. 1998. Confidence intervals for the number needed to treat. *British Medical Journal* 317: 1309–1312.

Altman, D. G., and P. K. Andersen. 1999. Calculating the number needed to treat for trials where the outcome is time to an event. *British Medical Journal* 319: 1492–1495.

Altman, D. G., and P. Royston. 2000. What do we mean by validating a prognostic model? *Statistics in Medicine* 19: 453–473.

Andersen, P. K., S. Z. Abildstrom, and S. Rosthøj. 2002. Competing risks as a multi-state model. *Statistical Methods in Medical Research* 11: 203–215.

Andersen, P. K., Ø. Borgan, R. D. Gill, and N. Keiding. 1997. *Statistical Models Based on Counting Processes*. Corrected ed. New York: Springer. http://www.worldcat.org/isbn/0387945199.

Andersen, P. K., and R. D. Gill. 1982. Cox's regression model for counting processes: A large sample study. *Annals of Statistics* 10: 1100–1120.

Aranda-Ordaz, F. J. 1981. On two families of transformations to additivity for binary response data. *Biometrika* 68: 357–363.

Begg, C. B., and D. Schrag. 2002. Attribution of deaths following cancer treatment. *Journal of the National Cancer Institute* 94: 1044–1045.

Bennett, S. 1983. Analysis of survival data by the proportional odds model. *Statistics in Medicine* 2: 273–277.

Bhaskaran, K., O. Hamouda, M. Sannes, F. Boufassa, A. M. Johnson, P. C. Lambert, K. Porter, and CASCADE Collaboration. 2008. Changes in the risk of death after HIV seroconversion compared with mortality in the general population. *Journal of the American Medical Association* 300: 51–59. http://dx.doi.org/10.1001/jama.300.1.51.

Brenner, H., and O. Gefeller. 1997. Deriving more up-to-date estimates of long-term patient survival. *Journal of Clinical Epidemiology* 50: 211–216.

Brenner, H., O. Gefeller, and T. Hakulinen. 2004. Period analysis for 'up-to-date' cancer survival data: Theory, empirical evaluation, computational realisation and applications. *European Journal of Cancer* 40: 326–335.

Brenner, H., A. Gondos, and V. Arndt. 2007. Recent major progress in long-term cancer patient survival disclosed by modeled period analysis. *Journal of Clinical Oncology* 25: 3274–3280. http://dx.doi.org/10.1200/JCO.2007.11.3431.

Brenner, H., and T. Hakulinen. 2002. Advanced detection of time trends in long-term cancer patient survival: Experience from 50 years of cancer registration in Finland. *American Journal of Epidemiology* 156: 566–577.

———. 2007. Maximizing the benefits of model-based period analysis of cancer patient survival. *Cancer Epidemiology, Biomarkers & Prevention* 16: 1675–1681. http://dx.doi.org/10.1158/1055-9965.EPI-06-1046.

———. 2008. Period versus cohort modeling of up-to-date cancer survival. *International Journal of Cancer* 122: 898–904. http://dx.doi.org/10.1002/ijc.23087.

Breslow, N. E., and N. E. Day. 1987. *Statistical Methods in Cancer Research: Vol. 2—The Design and Analysis of Cohort Studies.* Lyon: IARC.

Burnham, K. P., and D. R. Anderson. 2004. Multimodel inference: Understanding AIC and BIC in model selection. *Sociological Methods & Research* 33: 261–304.

Burton, P. R., K. J. Scurrah, M. D. Tobin, and L. J. Palmer. 2005. Covariance components models for longitudinal family data. *International Journal of Epidemiology* 34: 1063–1077. http://dx.doi.org/10.1093/ije/dyi069.

Carstensen, B. 2006. Demography and epidemiology: Practical use of the Lexis diagram in the computer age or: Who needs the Cox model anyway? Reprt presented at the Annual Meeting of the Finnish Statistical Society, Oulu, Finland.

———. 2007. Age–period–cohort models for the Lexis diagram. *Statistics in Medicine* 26: 3018–3045. http://dx.doi.org/10.1002/sim.2764.

Cheung, Y. B., F. Gao, and K. S. Khoo. 2003. Age at diagnosis and the choice of survival analysis methods in cancer epidemiology. *Journal of Clinical Epidemiology* 56: 38–43.

Clark, T. G., M. E. Stewart, D. G. Altman, H. Gabra, and J. F. Smyth. 2001. A prognostic model for ovarian cancer. *British Journal of Cancer* 85: 944–952.

Clayton, D., and E. Schifflers. 1987. Models for temporal variation in cancer rates. II: Age–period–cohort models. *Statistics in Medicine* 6: 469–481.

Cleves, M., R. G. Gutierrez, W. W. Gould, and Y. V. Marchenko. 2010. *An Introduction to Survival Analysis Using Stata.* 3rd ed. College Station, TX: Stata Press.

Coleman, M. P., P. Babb, P. Damiecki, P. Grosclaude, S. Honjo, J. Jones, G. Knerer, A. Pitard, M. J. Quinn, A. Sloggett, and B. De Stavola. 1999. *Cancer Survival Trends in England and Wales, 1971–1995: Deprivation and NHS Region*. London: Office for National Statistics.

Coleman, M. P., D. Forman, H. Bryant, J. Butler, B. Rachet, C. Maringe, U. Nur, E. Tracey, M. Coory, J. Hatcher, C. E. McGahan, D. Turner, L. Marrett, M. L. Gjerstorff, T. B. Johannesen, J. Adolfsson, M. Lambe, G. Lawrence, D. Meechan, E. J. Morris, R. Middleton, J. Steward, M. A. Richards, and the ICBP Module 1 Working Group. 2011. Cancer survival in Australia, Canada, Denmark, Norway, Sweden, and the UK, 1995–2007 (the International Cancer Benchmarking Partnership): An analysis of population-based cancer registry data. *Lancet* 377: 127–138.

Coleman, M. P., M. Quaresma, F. Berrino, J.-M. Lutz, R. De Angelis, R. Capocaccia, P. Baili, B. Rachet, G. Gatta, T. Hakulinen, A. Micheli, M. Sant, H. K. Weir, J. M. Elwood, H. Tsukuma, S. Koifman, G. A. E. Silva, S. Francisci, M. Santaquilani, A. Verdecchia, H. H. Storm, J. L. Young, and the CONCORD Working Group. 2008. Cancer survival in five continents: A worldwide population-based study (CONCORD). *Lancet Oncology* 9: 730–756.

Collett, D. 2003. *Modelling Survival Data in Medical Research*. 2nd ed. London: Chapman & Hall/CRC.

Congdon, P. 2006. *Bayesian Statistical Modelling*. London: Wiley.

Cook, R. J., and D. L. Sackett. 1995. The number needed to treat: A clinically useful measure of treatment effect. *British Medical Journal* 310: 452–454.

Coviello, V., and M. Boggess. 2004. Cumulative incidence estimation in the presence of competing risks. *Stata Journal* 4: 103–112.

Cox, D. R. 1957. Note on grouping. *Journal of the American Statistical Association* 52: 543–547.

———. 1972. Regression models and life-tables (with discussion). *Journal of the Royal Statistical Society, Series B* 34: 187–220.

Cronin, K. A., and E. J. Feuer. 2000. Cumulative cause-specific mortality for cancer patients in the presence of other causes: A crude analogue of relative survival. *Statistics in Medicine* 19: 1729–1740.

Cupples, L. A., D. R. Gagnon, R. Ramaswamy, and R. B. D'Agostino. 1995. Age-adjusted survival curves with application in the Framingham Study. *Statistics in Medicine* 14: 1731–1744.

de Boor, C. 2001. *A Practical Guide to Splines*. Revised ed. New York: Springer.

Dickman, P. W., J. Adolfsson, K. Åström, and G. Steineck. 2004a. Hip fractures in men with prostate cancer treated with orchiectomy. *Journal of Urology* 172: 2208–2212.

Dickman, P. W., A. Sloggett, M. Hills, and T. Hakulinen. 2004b. Regression models for relative survival. *Statistics in Medicine* 23: 51–64. http://dx.doi.org/10.1002/sim.1597.

DiMatteo, I., C. R. Genovese, and R. E. Kass. 2001. Bayesian curve-fitting with free-knot splines. *Biometrika* 88: 1055–1071.

Durrleman, S., and R. Simon. 1989. Flexible regression models with cubic splines. *Statistics in Medicine* 8: 551–561.

Ederer, F., L. M. Axtell, and S. J. Cutler. 1961. The relative survival rate: A statistical methodology. *National Cancer Institute Monograph* 6: 101–121.

Ederer, F., and H. Heise. 1959. Instructions to IBM 650 programmers in processing survival computations. Methodological note No. 10, End results evaluation section. National Cancer Institute, Bethesda, MD.

Estève, J., E. Benhamou, M. Croasdale, and L. Raymond. 1990. Relative survival and the estimation of net survival: Elements for further discussion. *Statistics in Medicine* 9: 529–538.

European Collaborative Study. 1991. Children born to women with HIV-1 infection: Natural history and risk of transmission. *Lancet* 337: 253–260.

Faes, C., M. Aerts, H. Geys, and G. Molenberghs. 2007. Model averaging using fractional polynomials to estimate a safe level of exposure. *Risk Analysis* 27: 111–123. http://dx.doi.org/10.1111/j.1539-6924.2006.00863.x.

Fine, J. P., and R. J. Gray. 1999. A proportional hazards model for the subdistribution of a competing risk. *Journal of the American Statistical Association* 94: 496–509.

Gamel, J. W., and R. L. Vogel. 2001. Non-parametric comparison of relative versus cause-specific survival in Surveillance, Epidemiology and End Results (SEER) programme breast cancer patients. *Statistical Methods in Medical Research* 10: 339–352.

Gauderman, W. J., and D. V. Conti. 2005. Commentary: Models for longitudinal family data. *International Journal of Epidemiology* 34: 1077–1079.

Gönen, M., and G. Heller. 2005. Concordance probability and discriminatory power in proportional hazards regression. *Biometrika* 92: 965–970.

Grambsch, P. M., and T. M. Therneau. 1994. Proportional hazards tests and diagnostics based on weighted residuals. *Biometrika* 81: 515–526.

Gutierrez, R. G. 2002. Parametric frailty and shared frailty survival models. *Stata Journal* 2: 22–44.

Hakulinen, T. 1982. Cancer survival corrected for heterogeneity in patient withdrawal. *Biometrics* 38: 933–942.

Hakulinen, T., and L. Tenkanen. 1987. Regression analyses of relative survival rates. *Applied Statistics* 36: 309–317.

Harrell Jr., F. E. 2001. *Regression Modeling Strategies: With Applications to Linear Models, Logistic Regression, and Survival Analysis.* New York: Springer.

Hastie, T., and R. Tibshirani. 1993. Varying-coefficient models (with discussion). *Journal of the Royal Statistical Society, Series B* 55: 757–796.

Hosmer Jr., D. W., S. Lemeshow, and S. May. 2008. *Applied Survival Analysis: Regression Modeling of Time to Event Data.* 2nd ed. New York: Wiley.

Kelly, P. J., and L. L. Y. Lim. 2000. Survival analysis for recurrent event data: An application to childhood infectious diseases. *Statistics in Medicine* 19: 13–33.

Korn, E. L., B. I. Graubard, and D. Midthune. 1997. Time-to-event analysis of longitudinal follow-up of a survey: Choice of the time-scale. *American Journal of Epidemiology* 145: 72–80.

Laird, N. M., and D. Olivier. 1981. Covariance analysis of censored survival data using log-linear analysis techniques. *Journal of the American Statistical Association* 76: 231–240.

Lambert, P. C., P. W. Dickman, C. P. Nelson, and P. Royston. 2010. Estimating the crude probability of death due to cancer and other causes using relative survival models. *Statistics in Medicine* 29: 885–895.

Lambert, P. C., and P. Royston. 2009. Further development of flexible parametric models for survival analysis. *Stata Journal* 9: 265–290.

Lambert, P. C., A. J. Sutton, P. R. Burton, K. R. Abrams, and D. R. Jones. 2005. How vague is vague? A simulation study of the impact of the use of vague prior distributions in MCMC using WinBUGS. *Statistics in Medicine* 24: 2401–2428. http://dx.doi.org/10.1002/sim.2112.

Lambert, P. C., J. R. Thompson, C. L. Weston, and P. W. Dickman. 2007. Estimating and modeling the cure fraction in population-based cancer survival analysis. *Biostatistics* 8: 576–594. http://dx.doi.org/10.1093/biostatistics/kxl030.

Lunn, D., D. Spiegelhalter, A. Thomas, and N. Best. 2009. The BUGS project: Evolution, critique and future directions. *Statistics in Medicine* 28: 3049–3067. http://dx.doi.org/10.1002/sim.3680.

Lunn, M., and D. McNeil. 1995. Applying Cox regression to competing risks. *Biometrics* 51: 524–532.

Makuch, R. W. 1982. Adjusted survival curve estimation using covariates. *Journal of Chronic Diseases* 35: 437–443.

Mallows, C. 1998. The zeroth problem. *American Statistician* 52: 1–9.

Medical Research Council Renal Cancer Collaborators. 1999. Interferon-α and survival in metastatic renal carcinoma: Early results of a randomised controlled trial. *Lancet* 353: 14–17.

Mok, T. S., Y.-L. Wu, S. Thongprasert, C.-H. Yang, D.-T. Chu, N. Saijo, P. Sunpaweravong, B. Han, B. Margono, Y. Ichinose, Y. Nishiwaki, Y. Ohe, J.-J. Yang, B. Chewaskulyong, H. Jiang, E. L. Duffield, C. L. Watkins, A. A. Armour, and M. Fukuoka. 2009. Gefitinib or carboplatin-paclitaxel in pulmonary adenocarcinoma. *New England Journal of Medicine* 361: 947–957. http://dx.doi.org/10.1056/NEJMoa0810699.

Møller, H., F. Sandin, F. Bray, A. Klint, K. M. Linklater, A. Purushotham, D. Robinson, and L. Holmberg. 2010. Breast cancer survival in England, Norway and Sweden: A population-based comparison. *International Journal of Cancer* 127: 2630–2638.

Moons, K. G. M., D. G. Altman, Y. Vergouwe, and P. Royston. 2009. Prognosis and prognostic research: Application and impact of prognostic models in clinical practice. *British Medical Journal* 338: 1487–1490.

Mwalili, S. M., E. Lesaffre, and D. Declerck. 2005. A Bayesian ordinal logistic regression model to correct for interobserver measurement error in a geographical oral health study. *Applied Statistics* 54: 77–93.

Nelson, C. P., P. C. Lambert, I. B. Squire, and D. R. Jones. 2007. Flexible parametric models for relative survival, with application in coronary heart disease. *Statistics in Medicine* 26: 5486–5498. http://dx.doi.org/10.1002/sim.3064.

———. 2008. Relative survival: What can cardiovascular disease learn from cancer? *European Heart Journal* 29: 941–947. http://dx.doi.org/10.1093/eurheartj/ehn079.

Nieto, F. J., and J. Coresh. 1996. Adjusting survival curves for confounders: A review and a new method. *American Journal of Epidemiology* 143: 1059–1068.

Norman, P. E., J. B. Semmens, M. M. D. Lawrence-Brown, and C. D. J. Holman. 1998. Long term relative survival after surgery for abdominal aortic aneurysm in Western Australia: Population based study. *British Medical Journal* 317: 852–856.

Patel, K., R. Kay, and L. Rowell. 2006. Comparing proportional hazards and accelerated failure time models: An application in influenza. *Pharmaceutical Statistics* 5: 213–224.

Prentice, R. L., B. J. Williams, and A. V. Peterson. 1981. On the regression analysis of multivariate failure time data. *Biometrika* 68: 373–379.

Reid, N. 1994. A conversation with Sir David Cox. *Statistical Science* 9: 439–455.

Royston, P. 2000. Choice of scale for cubic smoothing spline models in medical applications. *Statistics in Medicine* 19: 1191–1205.

———. 2001. Flexible parametric alternatives to the Cox model, and more. *Stata Journal* 1: 1–28.

———. 2006. Explained variation for survival models. *Stata Journal* 6: 83–96.

Royston, P., and D. G. Altman. 1994. Regression using fractional polynomials of continuous covariates: Parsimonious parametric modelling (with discussion). *Applied Statistics* 43: 429–467.

Royston, P., D. G. Altman, and W. Sauerbrei. 2006. Dichotomizing continuous predictors in multiple regression: A bad idea. *Statistics in Medicine* 25: 127–141. http://dx.doi.org/10.1002/sim.2331.

Royston, P., and M. K. B. Parmar. 2002. Flexible parametric proportional-hazards and proportional-odds models for censored survival data, with application to prognostic modelling and estimation of treatment effects. *Statistics in Medicine* 21: 2175–2197. http://dx.doi.org/10.1002/sim.1203.

Royston, P., M. K. B. Parmar, and D. G. Altman. 2008. Visualizing length of survival in time-to-event studies: A complement to Kaplan–Meier plots. *Journal of the National Cancer Institute* 100: 92–97.

———. 2010. External validation and updating of a prognostic survival model. Department of Statistical Science, University College London: London.

Royston, P., and W. Sauerbrei. 2004. A new measure of prognostic separation in survival data. *Statistics in Medicine* 23: 723–748.

———. 2008. *Multivariate Model-Building: A Pragmatic Approach to Regression Analysis Based on Fractional Polynomials for Modelling Continuous Variables.* Chichester, UK: Wiley.

Royston, P., and E. M. Wright. 1998. A method for estimating age-specific reference intervals ("normal ranges") based on fractional polynomials and exponential transformation. *Journal of the Royal Statistical Society, Series A* 161: 79–101.

Sauerbrei, W., and P. Royston. 1999. Building multivariable prognostic and diagnostic models: Transformation of the predictors by using fractional polynomials. *Journal of the Royal Statistical Society, Series A* 162: 71–94.

Sauerbrei, W., P. Royston, and H. Binder. 2007a. Selection of important variables and determination of functional form for continuous predictors in multivariable model building. *Statistics in Medicine* 26: 5512–5528.

Sauerbrei, W., P. Royston, and M. Look. 2007b. A new proposal for multivariable modelling of time-varying effects in survival data based on fractional polynomial time-transformation. *Biometrical Journal* 49: 453–473.

Schemper, M., S. Wakounig, and G. Heinze. 2009. The estimation of average hazard ratios by weighted Cox regression. *Statistics in Medicine* 28: 2473–2489. http://dx.doi.org/10.1002/sim.3623.

Schwarz, G. 1978. Estimating the dimension of a model. *Annals of Statistics* 6: 461–464.

Silverman, B. W. 1985. Some aspects of the spline smoothing approach to non-parametric regression curve fitting. *Journal of the Royal Statistical Society, Series B* 47: 1–52.

Smith, L. K., P. C. Lambert, J. L. Botha, and D. R. Jones. 2004. Providing more up-to-date estimates of patient survival: A comparison of standard survival analysis with period analysis using life-table methods and proportional hazards models. *Journal of Clinical Epidemiology* 57: 14–20. http://dx.doi.org/10.1016/S0895-4356(03)00253-1.

Spiegelhalter, D. J., K. R. Abrams, and J. P. Myles. 2003a. *Bayesian Approaches to Clinical Trials and Health-Care Evaluation.* Chichester, UK: Wiley.

Spiegelhalter, D. J., and N. G. Best. 2003. Bayesian approaches to multiple sources of evidence and uncertainty in complex cost-effectiveness modelling. *Statistics in Medicine* 22: 3687–3709. http://dx.doi.org/10.1002/sim.1586.

Spiegelhalter, D. J., A. Thomas, N. Best, and D. Lunn. 2003b. *WinBUGS User Manual, version 1.4.* Cambridge, UK: MRC Biostatistics Unit.

Stamey, T. A., J. N. Kabalin, J. E. McNeal, I. M. Johnstone, F. Freiha, E. A. Redwine, and N. Yang. 1989. Prostate specific antigen in the diagnosis and treatment of adenocarcinoma of the prostate. II. Radical prostatectomy treated patients. *Journal of Urology* 141: 1076–1083.

Therneau, T. M., and P. M. Grambsch. 2000. *Modelling Survival Data: Extending the Cox Model.* New York: Springer.

Thiébaut, A. C. M., and J. Bénichou. 2004. Choice of time-scale in Cox's model analysis of epidemiologic cohort data: A simulation study. *Statistics in Medicine* 23: 3803–3820. http://dx.doi.org/10.1002/sim.2098.

Thompson, J., T. Palmer, and S. Moreno. 2006. Bayesian analysis in Stata with WinBUGS. *Stata Journal* 6: 530–549.

Tsiatis, A. A. 2005. Competing Risks. In *Encyclopedia of Biostatistics*, 2nd edition, ed. P. Armitage and T. Colton, 1025–1035. Hoboken, NJ: Wiley.

Tukey, J. W. 1957. On the comparative anatomy of transformations. *Annals of Mathematical Statistics* 28: 602–632.

van Houwelingen, H. C. 2000. Validation, calibration, revision and combination of prognostic survival models. *Statistics in Medicine* 19: 3401–3415.

Wei, L. J., D. Y. Lin, and L. Weissfeld. 1989. Regression Analysis of multivariate incomplete failure time data by modeling marginal distributions. *Journal of the American Statistical Association* 84: 1065–1073.

Whitehead, J. 1980. Fitting Cox's regression model to survival data using GLIM. *Journal of the Royal Statistical Society, Series C* 29: 268–275.

Author index

T

V

W

Y

Subject index